Senior Living Communities

Senior Living Communities

Operations Management and Marketing for Assisted Living, Memory Care, Independent Living, and Continuing Care Retirement Communities

Third Edition

Benjamin W. Pearce

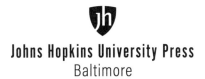

Johns Hopkins University Press

Baltimore

© 1998, 2007, 2024 Johns Hopkins University Press
All rights reserved. Published 2024
Printed in the United States of America on acid-free paper
9 8 7 6 5 4 3 2 1

Johns Hopkins University Press
2715 North Charles Street
Baltimore, Maryland 21218
www.press.jhu.edu

Library of Congress Cataloging-in-Publication Data is available.

ISBN 978-1-4214-4806-0 (paperback)
ISBN 978-1-4214-4807-7 (ebook)

A catalog record for this book is available from the British Library.

Special discounts are available for bulk purchases of this book.
For more information, please contact Special Sales at
specialsales@jh.edu.

To my parents, Robert and Dixie Pearce,
who taught me to respect elderly people, and to my grandmother
Ellen Pearce, with whom I spent summers during wheat harvest
in my youth, who taught me how to love them

Contents

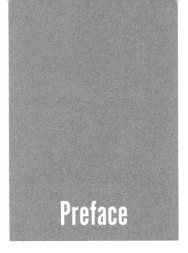

Senior living communities include a diverse range of properties that provide housing and care for many different types of residents. Operations and marketing of these communities effectively require a detailed understanding of the considerable complexity of this business model. With the advent of infectious diseases worldwide, that complexity has increased dramatically.

Prior to COVID-19, valuation capitalization rates were at an all-time low, and the values of senior living properties being purchased by sophisticated institutional investors were at record highs. With the onset of the COVID-19 pandemic, most operators were fundamentally impacted in ways for which they found themselves unprepared. Operators faced significant headwinds as expenses increased while at the same time occupancy and revenue softened.

COVID-19 mortality rates across senior housing increased as the health and caregiving complexity of residents increased, with the highest percentages occurring in memory care settings and skilled nursing facilities. Concurrently as caregiving staff became exposed and infected during the pandemic, many faced unproductive quarantine periods at home. Some left the business entirely to seek other, safer opportunities where they could have less exposure for themselves and their families. Meanwhile, employers in other sectors with staff shortages saw the pandemic as an opportunity to recruit hardworking health care employees to their businesses.

Operators ultimately recognized the pandemic as an opportunity to reset expenses and cost creep from staffing and operations to regain efficiency. In response to unforeseen COVID-related expenses, operators offset these costs with reductions in controllable expenses and lower staffing levels, while at the same time increasing service fees to the families. The combined effect has already allowed companies to emerge from the pandemic leaner and with improved expense margins.

Demographics, however, will continue to be strong for senior living communities. According to the most recent data available, there are more than 810,000 people who reside in approximately 30,000 assisted living facilities. The US population of adults older than 85 will double by 2036 and triple by 2049. Seven out of 10 of these people will require assisted living care in their lifetime, and the United States will need nearly a million new senior living units to accommodate this burgeoning cohort of the population by 2040.[1] Senior housing is not income dependent and is generally funded through the sale of accumulated assets and personal wealth. Approximately 80 percent of seniors over the age of 75 are homeowners.[2] A home purchased in 1987 is worth four times more today, and a modest $10,000 investment made in 1981 is now worth $1 million.[3] Investors therefore remain encouraged by the outlook of long-term demand and prospects for rate growth, which is expected to mitigate expense pressures.

According to the Seniors Housing Quarterly Unit Absorption report, record levels of senior housing absorption are now being achieved.[4] The temporary mandatory and voluntary admission restrictions during pandemic outbreaks, combined with the reduction in the construction of new units in the marketplace, has fueled record absorption during the recovery period with pent-up demand. Senior housing has been a very popular alternative to institutionalization and will continue to be the preferred choice as seniors look for supportive services throughout their aging process. Demographics will continue to drive demand, and government programs will be overrun by those seeking to utilize their benefits. The combined effect will drive higher acuity residents into senior housing where they can access care more efficiently and at a lower cost than skilled nursing. This higher acuity resident will require more monitoring and complex care solutions than ever before in assisted living and will change the face of the industry. Operators will need to think more strategically and monitor the care needs of their residents while navigating the maze of post-acute options and payor sources. Assisted living that was once the "residential" option may ultimately become part of accountable care organizations that form a complete care continuum linked electronically to physicians and hospitals. The addition of medically oriented assisted living beds and on-site clinics will bring aging-in-place options that are very desirable to residents, enabling them to use their Medicare benefits, but will also add considerably to the complexity of the business model.

This third edition has been updated with the latest in strategic planning and operational practices designed to pragmatically address this new operational complexity. The book offers unique and much-needed benchmarking and best practices specific to the senior living industry that focus on prevention and carefully managing residents with chronic diseases.

Managing care needs within a resident population starts with gathering information about their functional status, then monitoring trends in those functionalities and implementing interventions at the right time to fully support the resident's changing needs.

Once these changes are identified, if caught early and treated, the interventions can help to avoid further deterioration and resident risk. This book provides detailed steps that can help providers create their own system for monitoring, identify functional trends, provide menus of interventions for residents at risk (nutritional, falls, behavioral, depression, and cognitive), and offer communication strategies with interested parties to coordinate their mutual awareness and support. There are also details on how to calculate staffing needs for low, medium, and high levels of acuity. Itemized are the most common survey deficiencies that are found and cited by state regulators, as well as typical standard of care violations that are targeted in senior living litigation that I have seen as an expert witness in reviewing cases for both plaintiff and defense attorneys. In addition, the benefits of using electronic health records and their necessity to meet meaningful-use requirements are offered as Medicare and Medicaid programs expand into assisted living.

This book also provides insights into new relevant details in the successful design, operation, marketing, and management of both existing and future senior living communities. This edition expands, updates, and sharpens the vision of the critical tactical details that impact the successful operation of senior living communities. The reader will learn how to operate competitively by developing new state-of-the-art communities and optimizing the performance of existing properties.

The appendixes contain information to help operators clarify goals and direction for their communities beyond the day-to-day challenges. "Sample SWOT Analysis and Strategic Plan" (appendix A), "Senior Living Metrics Glossary" (appendix B), "Operations Audit" (appendix C), "Executive Director Responsibilities" (appendix D), and "Critical-Path Tasks for Preopening" (appendix E) all provide clarity to a vision of excellence. In appendix D, I have added a detailed checklist for executive directors to organize what they should be doing daily, weekly, monthly, quarterly, and annually to cover all the management expectations of their leadership position.

I have presented what I have learned over the past 40 years managing hundreds of senior living communities across the country in a pragmatic, clear, concise, no-nonsense presentation. These lessons from field experience, combined with the comprehensive operational strategies detailed in this book, can serve as a road map that the reader can overlay onto their own operations. The goal herein is to shorten the learning curve for operators, marketers, and developers to understand current and future industry fundamentals while benefiting the seniors living in these communities, the staff who serve them, and the families who have entrusted their loved ones to their care.

NOTES

1. E. Rubin, "Assisted Living Statistics: Current Data and Trends, Consumer Affairs, updated March 17, 2023, https://www.consumeraffairs.com/assisted-living /statistics.html.

2. S&P / Case-Shiller U.S. National Home Price Index, FRED Economic Data, https://fred.stlouisfed.org/se ries/CSUSHPISA.

3. "Here's What a $10,000 Investment in an S&P 500 Index Fund in 1980 Would Be Worth Today," Nasdaq News & Insights: Personal Finance, February 8, 2018, https://www.nasdaq.com/articles/heres-what-10000 -investment-sp-500-index-fund-1980-would-be-worth -today-2018-02-08.

4. Caroline Clapp, "NIC MAP Vision 4Q22 Key Take-aways: Record Senior Housing Demand Drove Higher Occupancy," January 26, 2023, https://blog.nic.org/nic -map-vision-4q22-key-takeaways-senior-housing-de mand-increased-2.8.

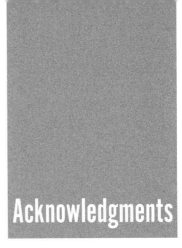

Acknowledgments

I am pleased at how well this book has been received in the industry and am excited to offer this third edition. My goal is to establish a standard against which excellence in the delivery of senior housing can reasonably be measured, to reach out to operators beyond my sphere of influence, and to help improve the lives of the elderly people they serve. I have drawn on many sources of information, including technical books, operations manuals, my own operational experience, and discussions and private communications with colleagues.

I thank the many colleagues whose comments on various drafts of parts of this book have improved its accuracy and added significantly to its innovation. Although I have endeavored to make this book as complete and as pragmatic as possible, even after working in this business all my adult life, I am continually learning new ways to serve the needs of elderly people better and more efficiently.

I am indebted to the following colleagues, whose advice, input, and criticisms of various parts of this book have added to its practicality, balance, and fairness: Angela G. Sullivan, MS, RD, CNSD; Steven C. Samuels, MD; Ralph Bellande; Megan Buffington; Bridget Gibbons; Jennie Wu, Raymond Goodman, Kittye S. Harman, REH; Darla Lambertson, RN; Cheryl Lucas, CDM; and Karen Pearce, RN, MSN, ANP-BC.

I also wish to recognize the talented executive directors and administrators whom I have been so fortunate to lead. They have provided me with success, encouragement, and friendship. Together we have learned what this book has to offer, and I extend to them my respect, admiration, and gratitude: they have brought a sparkle to the eyes of many elderly people.

Finally, I thank my wife, Karen, and my children, Benjamin, Rachel, and Micaela, for their patience and support, without which I could not have completed this book.

I

Administration

Introduction

The dramatic growth and development of the senior housing business have attracted numerous new participants. Many of these operators have learned, primarily by trial and error, how to deliver consistent, high-quality services to elderly people. For others, the attempt to capitalize on the growing demand for senior housing has been an expensive and frequently disastrous venture, to say nothing of the toll it has taken on seniors who bought into the dream of attractive housing and services and were later entangled in a developer's financial nightmare.

This book describes operational and marketing strategies widely practiced by the most successful operators in the United States today, as well as the regulatory and financial climate in which senior living communities exist. I identify the best practices employed to operate and market efficiently five types of facilities: independent living facilities, assisted living facilities, congregate seniors housing facilities, continuing care retirement communities, and skilled nursing facilities.

Independent Living Facilities

An independent living facility (ILF) is a multifamily complex catering to seniors. It generally consists of homes, condominiums, apartments, or mobile or motor homes in which residents maintain an independent lifestyle. It offers minimal or no services beyond the maintenance of the building and grounds. Some independent living communities also include housing units subsidized by the federal government.

Assisted Living Facilities

An assisted living facility (ALF) is a type of living arrangement that combines shelter with various personal support services, such as meals, housekeeping, laundry, and property maintenance. Assisted living is designed for seniors who do not need nursing home care but do need regular help with activities of daily living (ADLs), such as ambulation, bathing, dressing, grooming, preparing and eating meals, and toileting. Units may or may not have full kitchens, although most provide at least a kitchenette. Assisted living facilities may include those termed board-and-care homes, personal care homes, and supervised care facilities. Usually, service is provided on a month-to-month basis or through home health agency billings and Medicare.

Congregate Seniors Housing

Congregate seniors housing (CSH) refers to multifamily complexes catering to seniors, with centralized dining services, shared living spaces, and access to social and recreational activities. Many congregate-care facilities offer transportation services, personal care services, rehabilitative services, spiritual programs, housekeeping, and other support services. Apartments may be rented on a monthly or annual basis or may have a condominium or fee-simple structure.

Continuing Care Retirement Communities

Continuing care retirement communities (CCRCs), also referred to as life-care communities, provide a continuum of care, including housing, health care, and various support services. These communities provide services specified by contract, usually for the rest of the resident's life. The services provided range from support of independent living to skilled nursing care. Health care services may be provided directly or through access to affiliated health care facilities. Most communities offer a wide variety of contract options. Fees may be structured as a refundable entry fee plus a monthly service fee, as a condominium, as a rental, or as an endowment; long-term care insurance may be mandatory. Residency agreements usually are offered in three versions: extensive (providing for unlimited long-term care), modified (providing a specified amount of long-term care per year), or fee-for-service (providing guaranteed health care as needed at market rates).

Skilled Nursing Facilities

Skilled nursing facilities (SNFs) provide skilled nursing care and/or rehabilitation services to injured, sick, or disabled persons. These facilities are often referred to as nursing homes, but technically, nursing homes lack skilled services where patients are under the care of trained registered nurses in a medical setting under a doctor's supervision. A nursing home is a permanent residence for people who need care 24 hours per day, 7 days per week, while a skilled nursing facility is a temporary residence for patients undergoing medically necessary rehabilitation treatments. Skilled nursing facilities provide more complex medical care and rehabilitation, while long-term care facilities offer more permanent support and custodial care. There are several types of financial arrangements in skilled nursing, including private pay, where the patient is responsible personally for all costs and services during their stay; Medicaid, which will provide nursing home care for persons who require that level of care and meet the program's financial requirements; and Medicare, where the patient has benefits and is admitted to skilled nursing after a mandatory 3-day qualifying hospital stay.

Medicare patients who must be admitted to a nursing home are required to be fully hospitalized (3-day qualifying stay) prior to nursing home admission if they expect Medicare to pay for their nursing home stay. If a patient had been put on observation status instead of fully admitted, then there will be no Part A nursing home reimbursement—which can amount to thousands of dollars or more and can quickly deplete the patient's financial resources. If Medicare is to cover any nursing home costs, the patient *must be formally admitted* to the hospital for at least 3 midnights. Medicare will cover up to 20 days at 100 percent providing the patient has a physician-ordered medical need. After that, and if the patient is deemed medically stable, Medicare pays 80 percent, and the patient or patient's supplemental insurance pays the remaining 20 percent. If a patient was coded as "inpatient" for observation only and goes for rehabilitation after their hospital stay, Medicare will not cover their room and board as they were never admitted to the hospital as an inpatient; they may still be able to receive Part B therapy.

The Medicare program does not pay for long-term custodial care. The Medicaid program (Title 19 of the Social Security Act) is a state-administered health insurance program that is jointly funded by the federal and state governments. The states operate individual Medicaid programs under broad federal guidelines. Medicaid serves many people who have extreme medical costs that can completely deplete income and assets. Eligibility is calculated by deducting medical care cost from their income and assets. This allows individuals to spend down their assets to become Medicaid eligible. Unlike Medicare, Medicaid is an entitlement program based upon income and assets. Qualifying for Medicaid not only involves financial criteria but also has physical requirements. Applicants must demonstrate through a physical exam that he or she is unable to perform their activities of daily living, including feeding, dressing, bathing, toileting, and continence. If it cannot be shown to Medicaid that their care is medically necessary, the Medicaid application will be denied.

The Patient-Driven Payment Model (PDPM) is the proposed new Medicare payment rule for skilled nursing facilities. It is intended to replace the current RUG-IV system with a completely new way of calculating reimbursement. Under PDPM, therapy minutes are removed as the basis for payment in favor of resident classifications and anticipated resource needs during the course of a patient's stay.

PDPM assigns every resident a case-mix classification that drives the daily reimbursement rate for that individual. This system is based upon outcomes and successes in treatment for Medicare providers. Providers who overdeliver care won't get paid for services beyond the reimbursement level for each classification, but underdelivering care will lead to poor outcomes and potential Medicare audits and take-backs.

Other than the provision of differing levels of health care, the operational management of different types of senior living communities has only subtle differences. Where these differences are material to my discussion, they are noted.

THE OUTLOOK FOR THE INDUSTRY

Now more than ever, businesses are seeking new and more efficient ways to operate. Changes in the senior living industry over the last several years have forced out marginal operators and resulted in the recapitalization of millions of dollars in real estate. The dramatic growth of the industry during the late 1970s was spurred in part by multifamily developers who were unable to thrive when faced with interest rates of 20 percent plus prime and needed to add services to make their projects viable. Multifamily developments were made more attractive through the introduction of services that allowed a marginal increase in the average net income per unit (capitalizing on an economy of scale in overhead) to meet the lenders' cash-flow requirements.

Original assumptions about the size of the market and fill-up rate were grossly overstated, and this error has made lending institutions more cautious. After many projects failed, lenders became reluctant to underwrite new projects until their portfolios of existing projects met certain performance thresholds. Some opted out of the business entirely. Lenders remain uncertain about whether to underwrite the industry as real estate or as a business. It seems that new development is viewed more as real estate, whereas acquisitions are valued on the basis of operating cash flow and revenue multipliers. Even now, as providers are demonstrating a more positive track record, lenders are still choosy about the projects they underwrite. They are more attracted to projects that provide a continuum of care than to rental housing. Seniors are themselves becoming more informed about housing and care options and tend to prefer projects that allow them the greatest flexibility and choice throughout their lives.

Even though the congregate projects of the 1980s are mostly full, rising interest rates remain a concern, complicated by the recent tendencies of the Federal Reserve to control inflation in the expanding economy. Current operators of congregate communities will attempt to offset the effects of rising interest rates during the next upward cycle by adding yet another level of service to their communities. This time, it will probably take the form of home health care or other support services for residents, designed to increase the average net revenue per unit. Such options will be popular among the residents, who will view them as cost-effective alternatives to admission to a nursing home. In addition, many residents may qualify for intermittent home health care benefits through Medicare Parts A and B.

DEMOGRAPHICS THAT WILL DICTATE CHANGE

The 2016 American Community Survey estimated the number of people in the United States aged 65 and over as 49.2 million. Of them, more than half (28.7 million, or 58%) were aged 65 to 74. The 75 to 84 age group was around 14.3 million, or 29 percent—more than double the number and proportion (6.3 million, or 13%) for those 85 and older.[1]

The projected future growth of the 85 and older population has taken demographers and social scientists by surprise. By 2050, there will be an estimated 19 million people in the United States aged 85 and older. In the past, statisticians have tended to underestimate improvements in mortality. If one were to examine these same projected numbers 20 years ago, the numbers would be a lot lower than they are today. But with improvements in mortality that have taken place over the past 40 or so years, by all accounts it appears that in fact this "oldest old" population (i.e., people aged 85 and older) will grow tremendously over the next few decades.[2]

In less than two decades, the graying of America will be inescapable: older adults are projected to outnumber kids for the first time in US history. Already, the middle-aged outnumber children, but the country will reach a new milestone in 2034 (previously 2035). That year, the US Census Bureau projects, older

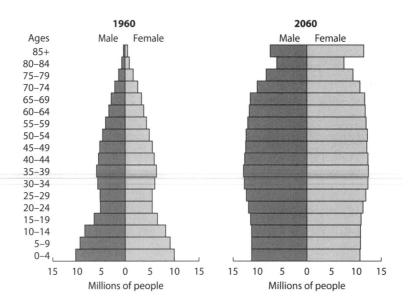

Figure 1.1   From Pyramid to Pillar: A Century of Change, Population of the United States

Source: U.S. Census Bureau, March 2018, https://www.census.gov/library/visualizations/2018/comm/century-of-change.html.

adults will edge out children in population size. People aged 65 and over are expected to number 77 million, while children under age 18 will number 76.5 million. Americans are having fewer children, and the baby boom of the 1950s and 1960s has yet to be repeated. Fewer babies coupled with longer life expectancy equals a country that ages faster. With this swelling number of older adults, the country could see greater demands for health care, in-home caregiving, and assisted living facilities (figure 1.1).[3]

Health deteriorates significantly with aging, with very old people becoming increasingly vulnerable to a barrage of chronic, debilitating conditions and diseases. For a long time, nursing homes were the only senior care option available. In the 1980s, a more person-centered care model was born—enter assisted living.[4] A rapidly growing senior population implies the need for additional assisted living communities, but so does the current generation of middle-aged adults who will require senior housing over the next several decades. Baby boomers are retiring with unprecedented financial assets and strong opinions about the future of senior living. Many want high-quality accommodations and care, in addition to the ability to explore personal passions and interests after retirement.

With 7 out of 10 people requiring assisted living care in their lifetime, demand is expected to grow by an additional 1 million beds by 2040. More than 810,000 Americans currently reside in assisted living communities, accounting for 88 percent of all senior residential care community residents.

From now until 2030, 10,000 baby boomers will reach retirement age each day, and many will seek assisted living options once they're no longer able to care for themselves independently. By 2040, over 80 million people in the United States will be over 65 years old, with that number growing to nearly 95 million by 2060, according to the US Census Bureau. With the over-65 population projected to double by 2060, the number of seniors requiring care will increase dramatically. This almost doubling of the senior population over the next four decades is projected to necessitate almost 1 million additional assisted living beds.[5]

As the population ages and dementia becomes more prevalent, the percentage of assisted living residents experiencing cognitive decline increases. In 2019, 42 percent of seniors in assisted living had Alzheimer's disease or another type of dementia, according to the Alzheimer's Association 2020 Alzheimer's Disease Facts and Figures report.[6] To cater to this population, many assisted living communities have added memory care wings or sections. Over 23 percent of assisted living communities cater either exclusively to residents with dementia or offer secure separate environments for memory care.

Many families are surprised to learn that Medicare and Medicaid don't typically pay for assisted living and that other types of insurance often only cover a small percentage of monthly rent. Most families use private funds to pay for assisted living. This means they use a combination of personal savings, pension payments, and/or retirement or investment income. Other options they use include home equity and bridge loans, pension payouts, or even funds donated by younger family members.

As of the first quarter of 2020, about 27 percent of senior housing communities in the United States were primarily nursing care, while 26 percent were primarily assisted living. The Genworth Cost of Care Survey 2021 reported that the national median cost for a private one-bedroom room in assisted living per month was $4,500, which breaks down to around $148 per day (and adds up to $54,000 per year).[7] To put that into some context, the same survey said a private room in a nursing home will cost around $9,034 a month, which is $297 per day ($108,405 per year). Home health aide services average $154 per day ($56,210 per year), based on an 8-hour day, 5 days a week (more time-intensive care will likely be more expensive). This cost varies widely in different states, with the median monthly cost at $6,500 in Massachusetts and at $3,350 in South Dakota.

Few people have insurance coverage that protects them against the high costs of long-term care. Traditional Medicare, the public health insurance program for people over 65, does not cover long-term care beyond some skilled care right after hospitalization for an injury or illness. Some Medicare Advantage plans from private insurers offer supplemental coverage for services like meal delivery and rides to medical appointments, but it is limited.

After impoverishing themselves, most people must depend on Medicaid, a means-tested welfare program, to pay for long-term care. Medicaid, the joint federal and state program that covers low-income Americans, is the largest single funding source of long-term care. Medicaid accounted for $1 of every $6 spent on health care in this country in 2019, the most recent data available.[8] Although income limits vary by state, you typically can't get Medicaid unless you exhaust most of your savings and other assets beyond your primary home and vehicle.

TRENDS IN TAX POLICY

It is only a matter of time before legislators seek to finance the costs of health care by using the largest and most readily available private resource in the country—the approximately $700 billion in home equity owned by Americans over the age of 65. The American Seniors Housing Association (ASHA), in its address to the US House of Representatives Ways and Means Subcommittee on Health, suggested that several tax policies be amended to include incentives for the use of home equity to finance health care for seniors. Among the alternatives are the following:

1. Revise section 1034 of the Internal Revenue Code to defer the recognition of income from the prior sale of a principal residence, to the extent that such proceeds are used as an entrance fee for or to gain admission to a "qualified retirement community." Currently one's principal residence, regardless of value, is an asset exempt from Medicaid calculations.

2. Increase the limit for the exclusion of gain from the sale of a principal residence if the proceeds are used for senior housing or long-term care. Internal Revenue Code section 121 was amended to change the limit for the exclusion of gain from the sale of a principal residence from $125,000 to $250,000 ($500,000 for a couple). Additional exclusions in the future may be (a) placed in trust for the sole purpose of providing long-term care; (b) used to gain entrance to an ongoing residence in a qualified CCRC, assisted-living facility, or licensed congregate community; or (c) used to purchase long-term care insurance.

3. Provide for tax-free withdrawals from IRAs, 401(k) savings plans, and other qualified pension plans; allow accelerated death benefits to be paid from life-insurance policies on people who are terminally ill or permanently residing in a nursing home; and provide tax deductions for long-term care premiums: the older the insured, the greater the deduction. "Rollover privileges should be extended to those who reinvest in regulated IRA

type funds, the proceeds of which are used to fund congregate or assisted living residences structured with rental rather than entry fee or endowment programs."[9]

4. Provide tax credits for expenses incurred in providing custodial care for a parent or grandparent in the taxpayer's home. This provision of the Family Reinforcement Act would require a physician to certify that the care receiver cannot perform at least two ADLs without substantial assistance or exhibits a similar level of disability as a result of a cognitive impairment.

5. Waive the 7.5 percent adjusted gross income threshold for amounts paid for medical care, including amounts paid for long-term care insurance premiums for the taxpayer, his or her spouse, or a dependent. Also clarify that the costs of assisted living services are included in the definition of deductible medical expenses under the Internal Revenue Code.[10] The Internal Revenue Code section 7702B(c), "chronically ill individual," allows the deduction of the cost of maintenance or personal care services required by an individual who is unable to perform at least two ADLs or who has severe cognitive impairment, and who requires supervision to protect him- or herself and others from threats to health and safety, if such services are provided pursuant to a plan of care prescribed by a licensed health care practitioner. A letter from the resident's physician should suffice to meet this condition. Meals are eligible for only a 50 percent deduction. If an individual does not meet the requirements of this law, only that portion of the monthly expense that is attributable to medical care is tax-deductible. These costs generally include extended-care costs and medications.

Whether, or to what extent, health care services provided in a senior community are currently tax-deductible is not easy to determine. Section 213 of *Selected Federal Taxation Statutes and Regulations* states, "There shall be allowed as a deduction the expenses paid during the taxable year not compensated for by insurance or otherwise for medical care of the taxpayer, his spouse or a dependent to the extent where that expense exceed 7.5 percent of adjusted gross income." The definition of medical care is further explained in section 1016: "If an individual is in a nursing

home or a home for the aged because of his physical condition and the availability of medical care is a principal reason for his presence there, the entire cost of maintenance, including meals and lodging, is deductible." The key distinction is the purpose of living in the facility. If it is for personal or family reasons, then only the portion of the cost attributable to medical or nursing costs is deductible. Service fees in assisted living facilities typically bundle medical care costs with room and board, making it difficult to determine or justify what portion of the rent covers medical care. Further, most assisted living facilities explicitly state that they are not medical care facilities. According to the Assisted Living Federation of America, assisted living facilities are "a type of living arrangement which combines shelter with various personal support services, such as meals, housekeeping, laundry, and maintenance. Assisted living is designed for seniors who need regular help with activities of daily living (ADLs), but do not need nursing home care." Under this definition, it may be hard to argue that costs associated with these facilities are tax-deductible.

Publication 502 of the Internal Revenue Service, titled *Medical and Dental Expenses*, helps clarify the question. "You can include in medical expenses the cost of medical care in a nursing home or home for the aged for yourself, your spouse, or your dependents. This includes the cost of meals and lodging in the home if the main reason for being there is to get medical care. Do not include the cost of meals and lodging if the reason for being in the home is personal. You can, however, include in medical expenses the part of the cost that is for medical or nursing care." This means that in an assisted living facility, unless the purpose of the stay is to receive medical care, the cost of lodging and meals may not be deductible.

If an individual is chronically ill, however, as defined under the section titled "Qualified Long-Term Care Services," all costs associated with the care and supervision of the individual may be tax-deductible, subject to the 7.5 percent limit. *Chronically ill* is defined in Publication 502: "A chronically ill individual is one who has been certified by a licensed health care practitioner within the previous 12 months as: 1) Being unable, for at least 90 days, to perform at least two activities of daily living without substantial assistance from another individual, due to the loss of functional capacity. Activities of daily living are eating, toileting, transferring, bathing, dressing, and continence or 2) Requiring substantial supervision to be protected from threats to health and safety due to severe cognitive impairment." With the enactment of the Kennedy-Kassebaum bill, the law is now clear. Congress stated that the tax code should provide equal consideration for people with Alzheimer's disease or other irreversible dementia. The only cloudy area remaining is the fee structure of the facility in which they reside.

Another important tax consideration is the entrance fee, life-care fee, or "founder's fee." "You can include in medical expenses a part of the life care fee or 'founder's fee' you pay either monthly or as a lump sum under an agreement with a retirement home. The part of the payment you include is the amount properly allocable to medical care." Many of today's assisted living communities charge an entrance or maintenance fee. This fee is intended to cover administrative processing and the maintenance of the property, rendering it a nondeductible expense according to the Internal Revenue Service. If this fee is charged and used for the initial assessment and the development of the plan of care, it may be considered a medical expense and qualify as a deductible medical expense. Communities that are dedicated to caring for people with Alzheimer's disease and related dementia, and render substantial supervision to protect residents from threats to health and safety due to their severe cognitive impairment, appear to meet the test.

Further legislation and changes in the tax code may be inevitable if the government is to meet the growing health care needs of elderly US residents. Such amendments would significantly affect the delivery of senior housing in the coming decade and could offset the incentive for residents to stay in their own homes, supported by home health care, and encourage them instead to move into continuing care communities with their life savings and home equity intact. Although the tax advantages of such legislation could have a significant negative effect on rental communities, there will always be people who prefer the flexibility and freedoms rental housing affords.

THE EFFECTS OF NATIONAL HEALTH CARE POLICY

Changes in regulations and interpretations of government programs for coverage of long-term disability and illness have varying implications for provid-

ers of services to seniors. Since Medicare began to determine coverage for levels of care based on diagnosis, nursing homes have evolved to provide subacute and special care. When the Omnibus Budget Reconciliation Act of 1987 introduced guidelines to redefine long-term care standards, intermediate care effectively became assisted living as we know it today. The costs of compliance with federal and state regulations governing long-term care have become prohibitive.[11]

As state budgets are stretched to the breaking point by growth in Medicaid spending, states will tighten their control on the certificate-of-need approval process to limit their financial liability. This trend will enable existing nursing homes to increase their margins slowly in response to the decreasing supply. In addition, nursing home operators are moving in the direction of specialized care, subacute care, and managed care to improve their financial performance.

Washington lawmakers are calling for enhanced matching rates for home- and community-based services and propose to raise the current matching rate by 30 percent. State and federal policy makers have estimated that 20 to 25 percent of nursing home residents who need assistance with ADLs do not require round-the-clock nursing care. Only those who require acute and chronic care will need to be displaced to skilled nursing environments. Nursing homes will therefore be forced to deal with residents requiring higher levels of care within the same or even lower reimbursement structures (rates are calculated based on prior years' operations) and to compete for staff with flexible, government-funded home health care agencies and assisted living communities. The private-pay market, typically consisting of residents requiring lower levels of care (83 percent of nursing home residents deplete their assets within one year), will ultimately recognize the inherent benefits, freedom, and economy of less institutional settings in which they can receive virtually the same care.

The Health Security Act of 1993 provides assessment and care to those requiring help with three or more ADLs or who have severe cognitive impairment. The act specifies that the funds be used in home- or community-based settings such as retirement and assisted living projects. Clearly, the assisted living and home health care business has prospered at the expense of the long-term care industry. This growth opportunity will continue to bring new players into the industry who lack the marketing or operational experience necessary to succeed. The inevitable failures in this growing health care segment will lead to increased regulation and the associated higher costs of compliance. Assisted living appears to be serving the intermediate care market and even competing for the private nursing home market through innovative, lightly regulated nursing care arrangements. In fact, skilled nursing visits are now being provided to assisted living residents through home health agencies.

Moderate-income residents who do not qualify for Medicaid but cannot afford to pay privately will have access to personal care assistance, interpreted as the type of assistance that is provided in assisted living in a senior nursing facility setting. For operators of senior communities, however, this approach may prove to be a double-edged sword. If residents have access to supportive services and home health care in independent living apartments, perhaps federal assistance will enable operators to increase the average revenue per unit, and residents' financial resources will last longer. On the other hand, the average need for care in these communities will increase, the average length of stay will decrease, and the units vacated will need to be marketed to a less active clientele. This could be a dangerous strategy in the long run. As buildings age, a new developer may come to town with an attractive project with which existing operators cannot compete for independent, active, and affluent prospects. Many retirement communities have been run into the ground by marketing defensively to manage their turnover rather than proactively to build a waiting list as a means of managing their revenue and level of care.

■ **STRATEGIC PARTNERSHIPS**

Medicare reform seeks to better link hospitals and doctors to the supervision of their patients' post-acute care. In response, some larger senior living providers are developing care continuums that are linked to these physician and hospital payers and referral sources through IT connections and on-site medical clinics, drawing patients from both ends of the continuum.

By adding more medically oriented assisted living beds and on-site clinics to their housing campuses, operators will provide residents a rental aging-in-

place alternative to the CCRC. The marketing pitch is that you can forego a CCRC entrance fee payment but still gain access to a full shelter care continuum, all under the close supervision of your medical care provider and all without paying an entrance fee.

Linking these post-acute destinations is important to hospitals, because they need to worry about Medicare readmission penalties.

- The Hospital Readmissions Reduction program, mandated by the Affordable Care Act, cuts reimbursement rates for facilities with readmission rates above the national average.
- Hospitals are penalized for readmissions within 30 days back into their institution (since 2012).
- Penalties for each readmission can be substantial.
- The hospital isn't just penalized for those readmissions that exceed a predetermined percentage. The hospital's entire Medicare reimbursement for that year is reduced.
- Prior to the change above, there are times when a hospital may not be able to admit someone to the hospital on an inpatient status (because there's not sufficient medical necessity), but it may not be safe to send the person home either. Instead, the hospital will keep that person in the hospital and code them as being "under observation" (historically for 48 hours, 2 days, or 2 midnights) with an outpatient status.
- To avoid these penalties, hospitals are putting many more people on "observation," which is outpatient status, for long periods of time, and patients are not being coded with inpatient status. This distances the hospitals from the 30-day readmit financial penalty—as they never coded the patient to inpatient status.
- It shifts the risk and the financial burden to the Medicare patient.

Emerging IT systems allow physicians and discharge planners to communicate with post-acute providers in real time so as to ensure they are receiving the appropriate level of post-acute transitional follow-up and not returning to the hospital due to provider neglect. By courting newly emerging accountable care organizations (ACOs) and hospital discharge planners to refer acute care discharges to their new SNFs, ALFs, and linked home health agencies, these senior housing providers can now offer medical and insurance referral sources a full post-acute care continuum for their patients that is coordinated and has ongoing communication with these payer/provider entities. An ACO is a network of doctors and hospitals that shares responsibility for providing care to patients. In the new law, an ACO would agree to manage all of the health care needs of a minimum of 5,000 Medicare beneficiaries for at least three years.

ACOs would make providers jointly accountable for the health of their patients, giving them strong incentives to cooperate and save money by avoiding unnecessary tests and procedures. For ACOs to work they'd have to seamlessly share information. Those that save money while also meeting quality targets would keep a portion of the savings. But some providers could also be at risk of losing money. The US Department of Health and Human Services (HHS) estimates that ACOs could save Medicare up to $960 million in the first three years. That's far less than 1 percent of Medicare spending during that period. If the program is successful, it can be expanded by the Secretary of Health and Human Services. In Medicare's traditional fee-for-service payment system, doctors and hospitals generally are paid more when they give patients more tests and do more procedures. That drives up costs, experts say. ACOs wouldn't do away with fee-for-service but would create savings incentives by offering bonuses when providers keep costs down and meet specific quality benchmarks, focusing on prevention and carefully managing patients with chronic diseases. In other words, providers would get paid more for keeping their patients healthy and out of the hospital.

Strategic partnerships with hospital systems will play a critical role in the expansion of assisted living facilities. The number of Medicare beneficiaries enrolled in managed care plans continues to grow at a rate of more than 30 percent per year. Medicare payments currently make up 40 percent or more of a typical hospital system's revenue base, and, with this increasing penetration of Medicare risk plans, hospitals will increasingly serve as managers for low-cost health care services.

Assisted living provides a level of services between home care and acute care. As managed care providers seek high-quality, lower-cost alternatives to home care and nursing home care, the inclusion of assisted living in a hospital system's range of services will enhance its attractiveness to managed care payers. In addition, as assisted living residents age in place, they require more ancillary services—such as therapies, pharmacy services, and home care—which the hospital system can also undertake to provide. In this way, the system can maximize revenue by controlling market share across the continuum and retain its customer base.

For the hospital system, joint ventures or other strategic alliances with existing private and public assisted living providers can provide management services while generating significant ancillary referral. Such a partnership can make effective use of excess capital and property and enable the system to provide a fuller range of health care services. For the assisted living provider, an affiliation with a local hospital system can significantly increase market acceptance within the community and provide access to attractive financing options available to the hospital.

FINANCIAL RESOURCES

The availability of financing has traditionally been the primary determinant of the growth and direction of senior housing projects. Developers are now becoming more creative, as some of the nation's largest pension funds have begun to invest in the demographically driven senior living industry. Although traditional financing resources remain basically intact, new financing vehicles have surfaced now that the majority of the projects constructed in the early to mid-1990s have been occupied. This new availability may spur another growth phase for the industry as established operators demonstrate a positive track record. The following financial resources are among the most popular.

- **Tax-exempt bonds for 501(c)(3) organizations.** Debt that is normally issued through a government conduit is usually tax-exempt. Typical final maturity is thirty years, with a level, self-amortizing debt-service schedule. These bonds can sometimes be issued to for-profit providers.
- **State financing initiatives.** These are especially common in connection with high-priority senior service-delivery systems like assisted living. Industrial revenue bonds (IRBs) have also been available at the local level. These instruments can either be written in the form of level, self-amortizing bonds

or have requirements for balloon principal reductions at regular intervals. Some IRB issues may have minimum low-income requirements and rent caps.

- **Investment pools such as real estate investment trusts (REITs) and pension funds.** These take an equity position through which they own the real estate and lease it back to an operating company, either in the form of a sale-leaseback arrangement, with some rent escalation tied to an increase in revenue, or through participating mortgages. REITs are a more expensive vehicle, but because they can accept higher risks, returns can be higher. A bank may finance a project at 250 basis points over the yield curve, whereas an REIT will do so at 500 basis points over the curve.

- **Tax-exempt and taxable bonds.** The Tax Reform Act of 1986 prohibits for-profit developers from financing new congregate projects using industrial revenue bonds. The law does permit the issuance of residential rental-project bonds to for-profit owners. Rates are slightly higher than those for 501(c)(3) bonds and are subject to the alternative minimum tax; there are limits on volume, and an allocation must be obtained from the home state. There is strong demand for unrated tax-exempt bonds issued on behalf of nonprofit institutions such as the Massachusetts Industrial Finance Agency (MIFA) or other state finance agencies. To access this financing market, project operators may wish to affiliate with health care and religious institutions that can serve as the owners, with operators providing management and development services on a fee basis. Tax-exempt mutual funds are currently aggressive in providing project financing for as much as 90 percent of total project costs, with limited guarantee requirements. Interest rates for unrated tax-exempt bonds may vary, depending on the credit resources and sponsorship of the project.

- **Conventional loans by commercial banks and insurance companies.** Commercial banks are slowly returning to the market to finance real estate and health care projects. Commercial lenders are credit-oriented and will focus on the capital resources, quality, and experience of the project team. Typical projects require 25 to 30 percent in equity and additional creditworthy recourse and lease-up guarantees. The significant advantages of working with a commercial bank are the reduced loan processing time (typically four to six months) and freedom from imposed regulatory or construction cost (i.e., prevailing-wage) requirements. Commercial banks usually have a regional focus. They generally allocate less than 5 percent of their total loan portfolio to health care properties that are currently dominated by skilled nursing facility (SNF) loans. Finally, as the industry becomes more vertically integrated, providing an on-site continuum of care, conventional lenders are becoming more likely to finance independent communities, where there is less risk.

- **Participating mortgages.** These are loans that share in cash flow or appreciation.

- **Debt securitization financing for single borrowers with multiple assets that can be cross-collateralized.** Securitization is the process by which mortgage loans are combined into pools of $100 million or more to produce rated securities for sale to institutional investors. Many lenders are interested in bundling loans, either to diversify their in-house portfolio or to pool the loans for the ultimate sale of interests in the pool to institutional investors. Ratings range from AAA for the most creditworthy to B for deeply subordinated classes. As the underwriting criterion most closely scrutinized by the rating agencies is cash flow, Wall Street finances only operating communities and does not provide construction financing. In some joint ventures between commercial banks and other lenders, such as investment banking firms, one party supplies the construction financing and the other provides the take-out financing or securitization. Loan-to-value ratios of 65 to 70 percent and debt-service coverage ratios of 1.25 to 1.45 are typical. Loan coupons are set based on a spread over US Treasury securities (typically with a spread of 3.0 to 3.85 percent) with a maturity comparable to the term of the mortgage loan.[12]

- **The Department of Housing and Urban Development (HUD) 232 mortgage insurance program.** This program was created by the National Housing Act in 1959 and was originally designed for nursing homes and intermediate care facilities. In 1985, HUD 232 was expanded to include board-and-care homes that HUD defines as "residential facilities that provide room, board, and continuous protective oversight for individuals who cannot live independently, but who do not require the more extensive care offered by intermediate care facilities or nursing homes."

The HUD 232 program provides mortgage insurance to help sponsors finance their projects more easily and cheaply by providing credit enhancement. The insurance guarantees that the federal government will repay the loans if the borrower fails to meet the mortgage payments. It is available for mortgages for new construction, purchase of facilities, rehabilitation of existing structures, and mortgage refinancing.

The major drawback of the HUD program is the time needed to process applications (currently estimated at twelve months) and to secure project approvals. Most HUD regional offices are significantly understaffed and cautious about underwriting assisted living projects. In addition, construction contracts must be written at prevailing wages rather than as less costly open-bid jobs.

Moreover, facilities providing direct medical care are not eligible for this insurance. Most assisted living facilities do not provide such care and are therefore eligible for HUD 232 mortgage insurance.

Despite its drawbacks, the HUD 232 financing program offers significant benefits. It can be particularly useful to providers of assisted living because it has no low-income criteria and so can be used by facilities that plan to charge market rents.

Financing under HUD 232 is nonrecourse. Funds must be borrowed for a 30- to 40-year period at fixed interest rates. Regulation of operations is minimal. Equity requirements are 10 percent for new construction plus additional support for working capital and startup. HUD recognizes the appraised value of the land owned by the sponsor as counting toward the 10 percent equity contribution.

- **Private funding sources.** The US assisted living facility market size was valued at USD 91.8 billion in 2022, and it is expected to expand at a compound annual growth rate (CRGR) of 5.53 percent from 2023 to 2030.[13] The industry showed phenomenal growth from mid-1990 until 2020, with many top operators more than doubling their residential capacity. But the industry was hit hard in 2020 by the COVID-19 pandemic. According to the CDC, around 2.1 million people, representing 0.6 percent of the US population, lived in residential care or assisted living facilities during the pandemic. A number of these facilities became hotspots for the transmission of the novel coronavirus, and 42 percent of the total COVID-19 deaths in the US were of assisted living residents. So during COVID, actual results fell behind projections, driving some smaller operators to liquidate resulting in industry consolidation.

- **The Department of Housing and Urban Development (HUD) 213 mortgage insurance program for cooperative housing**. Section 213 insures mortgage loans to facilitate the construction, substantial rehabilitation, and purchase of cooperative housing projects. Each member shares in the ownership of the whole project with the exclusive right to occupy a specific unit and to participate in project operations through the purchase of stock. Insured mortgages may be used to finance construction, acquisition of existing or rehabilitated detached, semidetached, row, walk-up, or elevator type housing projects consisting of five or more units. The program has statutory per unit mortgage limits which may vary according to the size of the unit, the type of structure, and the location of the project. There are also loan-to-replacement cost limitations. Contractors for new construction and substantial rehabilitation housing projects must comply with prevailing wage requirements under the Davis-Bacon Act. Section 213 loans have very attractive features such as 98 percent loan-to-value and 40-year amortization and are nonrecourse. Applicants must meet the 90 percent presale requirements, but co-ops are attractive to independent seniors with moderate incomes who want the benefits of a senior community and control over how the community is managed. Members in the co-op are guaranteed the right to a particular unit and receive the same tax benefits as homeowners. Members also accumulate equity on their shares. Co-op members still pay a fixed basic fee that covers operating expenses, property taxes, maintenance, insurance, and utilities. The co-op does not provide care, which the members can contract for through home health agencies and private caregivers.

■ LENDERS' AND INVESTORS' CONCERNS

As they analyze prospective investments, lenders and investors are primarily concerned with managing risk. Because of the recent preponderance of failed projects, lenders have grown wary of the industry, requiring high equity contributions, while buyers have begun to demand high internal rates of return to support expected market yields. The market has run the course from aggressive and speculative to conservative and risk-averse.[14] Operators who have established a reputation for consistently meeting investment expectations and absorption projections in the past have a better chance of securing acceptable rates and loan ratios from lenders. The following points outline the most significant concerns of lenders and investors:

1. The developer's or sponsor's experience, track record, and depth of management.
2. The viability of the project concept and long-run exit strategy.
3. Aggressive market-area definition and assumptions.
4. Implied market-penetration rates.
5. Aggressive or optimistic forecasts of fill-up and absorption rates, with appropriate financial reserves (typically, capital and operational reserves of 30 to 35 percent).
6. The competitiveness of the project with other existing and future projects.
7. Cost containment or value engineering, minimizing operating expenses and maximizing returns on capital expenditures.
8. The affordability and perceived value of the project in the eyes of consumers.
9. Long-run actuarial integrity.
10. The level and validity of presales.
11. Capitalization rates. These can go up because of the perception of increased risks associated with financing senior housing. Generally, as the health care component of the project increases, so does the capitalization rate (see table 1.1), because of the higher intensity of management as well as the increased costs and risks associated with regulatory compliance. Capitalization rates are most often defined as the expected annual yield of a property if it were purchased for cash. For example, if the net cash flow of a property were $1,000,000 in the first 12 months after purchase on a purchase price of $10,000,000, the capitalization ("cap") rate would be 10 percent. (See chapter 2 for a detailed discussion of capitalization rates.)
12. Debt service coverage ratios (DSCRs). These have increased for senior housing from 1.2 to 1.3 and even 1.35. The DSCR is calculated by dividing the net project cash flow by the debt service. A DSCR of 1.25 means that for every $1.00 in debt service, the project produces $1.25 in cash flow.

Table 1.1	Capitalization Rates by Type	
Level of care	Average rate (%)	Range (%)
Independent living facility	6.0	5.3–6.5
Assisted living facility	6.4	6.1–7.5
Memory care facility	7.8	7.1–8.1
Skilled nursing facility	11.7	19.9–12.3

Source: JLL Research Report Seniors Housing and Care Investor Survey and Trends COVID-19 Update 2020.

■ CAPITAL AVAILABILITY AND UNDERWRITING

Even though many of the industry's troubled facilities (owned and managed by inexperienced or undercapitalized firms) have been transferred to industry professionals and firms with demonstrated expertise in developing and managing senior housing, lenders will remain cautious until the failure rate of their underwriting falls into line with the risk assumed. After 15 to 20 years of successful operation in this industry, developers still face several underwriting issues:[15]

Industry track record. Many defaults were due to erroneous assumptions about marketing. Developers aggressively predicted that people 65 years of age or older would move to communities from as far away as fifteen miles. But operators found their communities being filled by people 80 years of age or older who, for the most part, moved from only five to seven miles away. Underfunding of marketing and operating-deficit reserves was based on unrealistic expectations of fill-up. Further consolidation, favoring operators with successful portfolios, will lead to more refined criteria for underwriting.

Is it real estate or is it a business? Investors are more comfortable with office, retail, industrial, and apartment investments than with assisted living. The degree of management intensity has often deterred investors. They now realize, however, that the greatest opportunity for profit in senior housing acquisitions will come from adding services and improving operational and marketing efficiencies.

Lack of expertise in senior housing. Investors' in-house investment staff or advisers and consultants have not been knowledgeable enough to analyze developers' projections properly. Their experience has been gained through reactive evaluation of failing or nonperforming projects. Lenders are now turning to competent industry consultants, in addition to their own staff, to perform due-diligence analysis before making loan commitments. The industry is very susceptible to staffing shortages and communicable disease outbreaks, where traditional multifamily investments have been more predictable and better understood. Lending opportunities will continue to improve as lenders develop more sophisticated underwriting and creditworthiness criteria.

Disappointing historical results of senior housing investments. Poor past performance—attributable to flawed assumptions about the market, underfunding of marketing, poor sales ability, unrealistic lease-up projections, and inadequate operating reserves—has resulted in unsatisfactory cash yields and write-downs in investment value. Successful projects are motivated by market forces rather than by site availability.

Success of alternative classes of asset. The poor performance of real estate portfolios has diverted capital to better-performing classes of asset, including stocks, fixed-income instruments, venture capital, and private placements.

◼◼◼◼ LEGAL AND LEGISLATIVE ISSUES

In response to the growth of the senior housing industry, many states have enacted or are now enacting legislation to regulate senior housing developments and subsequent operations. Although life-care or continuing care retirement communities are typically the most heavily regulated, most states have adopted regulations for assisted living communities that are increasingly complex. Regulatory changes have tended to address the care of frailer and sicker residents and concerns about inappropriate retention, adequacy of care, and the shortage of trained staff. Newer provisions govern resident assessments, medication management, staffing numbers, staff training, criminal background checks, admission and retention criteria, disclosure requirements, and resident agreements.

Many state regulatory agencies have imposed definitions of assisted living or continuing care retirement communities. Although regulations governing these facilities vary widely among states, they are primarily concerned with ensuring that prospective residents have adequate, accurate information with which to make decisions about joining and remaining in a community. Some states have established precise regulations governing the development and operation of such communities. Still others have imposed civil or criminal penalties for failure to comply with legislation. States also continue to address the need for specialized care for residents with Alzheimer's disease and other dementias: 44 states now have specific requirements for residential care facilities serving people with dementia. These requirements address disclosure, services available, admission and discharge criteria, staffing, staff training, activities, environment, and security. Scenarios for state regulations governing the development of senior housing fall into four major categories:

1. **Preopening request.** The community may be required to obtain state certification and to disclose financial information to prospective residents. Some states also impose a minimum presale occupancy requirement before granting a permit to begin construction.

2. **Contracts between the residents and the community.** Regulations may address the form and content of the resident contract, promotional materials, residents' rights, resident councils, liens, and terms of withdrawal from the community.

3. **Health care request.** The community may be required to obtain a certificate of need (CON). This involves an extensive and expensive approval process in which the developer is required to demonstrate that a need exists for the project in the chosen location. Many states have enacted CON legislation to control the supply of nursing home beds so that excessive supply will not result in competitive practices that could compromise the quality of care. Because Medicaid is the single fastest-growing component of many state budgets, the CON process has also been used by legislators to limit states' potential financial liability.

4. **Financial requirements.** Regulations may call for escrow deposits before and after occupancy, reserve

requirements, performance bonding, annual audits, and restrictions on fee adjustments and refunds.

The retirement community must also comply with regulations not specific to the industry, such as zoning and building codes. Depending on its source of permanent financing, the community may be subject to further requirements, such as low-income qualification for a percentage of its residents (as required under many IRB financing rules).

■ FINANCIAL CONCERNS FOR SENIORS

To succeed, businesses must understand the characteristics and concerns of the market they serve. Not only does this understanding enable the provider to market to and serve its existing clientele, it also provides the insight needed for planning. Operators of senior living communities should understand the major financial difficulties facing seniors, some of which they themselves may be unaware of or grossly underestimate. These include the following:

Inflation. Seniors typically underestimate their current cost of living by $400 to $500 per month. They may forget to account for real estate taxes and other costs that are not paid on a monthly basis. When they learn the cost of living in a retirement community, they may experience sticker shock, for their biggest fear is to outlive their savings.

Reluctance to sell a home. Seniors typically think that their homes are worth more than prevailing market conditions indicate, and they are therefore loath to sell. This is especially true of people who may be subconsciously looking for excuses to delay the move to a retirement community. In addition, Americans have traditionally used real estate as a vehicle to transfer inheritance to their children and thus protect their largest asset from estate taxes. If the parents retain ownership of a home, their children inherit the "stepped-up" basis or fair market value of the home and therefore avoid the capital gains tax on the original purchase price of the home.

Future health care costs. Although many seniors worry about health care and related costs, they may rationalize that they will be covered by Medicare or their complex supplemental insurance policies. Many of their children also share this belief. Nationally, however, Medicare covers only about 3 percent of nursing home costs.

Living with dramatically lower interest yields from conservative savings portfolios. In the early 1990s, interest earned on seniors' cash or cash equivalents plummeted by 50 percent or more compared to returns in the mid- to late 1980s. Returns dropped again after the stock market slide following the attacks of September 11, 2001. Recently COVID-19, world instability, and inflation at the gas pump and in grocery stores have significantly impacted the stock market and consequently seniors' investment values. After accounting for Social Security payments and other noncash investments, seniors in the $30,000 annual-income category derive up to 50 percent of their income from cash or near-cash investments. Many seniors have watched in horror as their monthly income has declined while their health care costs have increased.

■ RISKS

Satisfying the concerns of investors and lenders requires that most developers and subsequent operators incorporate pro forma safeguards and contingencies into their projections. These margins of safety may mean the difference between success and failure for a single project or an entire company. They include the following:

■ A well-conceived community should not rely on more than 5 percent of its age- and income-qualified prospects as a penetration rate to reach stabilized occupancy. The higher the penetration, the longer the expected time to stabilization. Communities with 10 percent or higher penetration may take more than 24 months to reach this threshold. (See chapter 14 for a detailed discussion on penetration rates.)

■ Bottom-fishing for troubled projects may not always be a successful strategy. Many troubled communities may have been overvalued and undercapitalized, based on unrealistic projections of fill-up. They may incorporate other fatal flaws, involving design, location, and mix of products or services. Even experienced operators may not be able to overcome these obstacles. Many acquisitions are currently being purchased for replacement value.

■ Developers must build first-class projects that are appropriate for the geographic location and provide the best possible value for the residents. They must strike a balance between conserving capital and investing where the returns are the greatest. All development must be built around what the primary market prospects can afford. The economics of community enhancements must also be closely scrutinized. For example, for every $10,000 per unit of capital savings (or expenditure), the effect on the residents' monthly service fee is approximately $95 (assuming a 9 percent cost of capital, a 1.2 DSCR, and 95 percent stabilized occupancy).[16]

■ The COVID-19 pandemic has had a major impact on senior living. After a 12-year growth cycle and the lowest capitalization rate valuations of all time, the disease (which has had disproportionately high mortality rates on the elderly) has brought unprecedented challenges. Short-term occupancy rates have plummeted due to losses of existing residents, while mandatory isolation strategies promulgated by state and federal health officials have restricted marketing efforts to replace them. Concurrently, employees who were already scarce looked to other professions entirely to avoid contact with the vulnerable elderly population so as not to bring a contagious disease home to their family. Supply chain shortages caused by the pandemic also triggered price increases across the board from vendors. These increases in operating expenses are a primary driver of valuations. Personal protective equipment, staff shortages, and vendor price increases have effectively driven down profitability and consequently returns for investors. While these expense premiums are expected to normalize postpandemic, some long-term impacts on staffing are likely to soften net operating income and consequent capitalization rate valuations.

Demographics show that the "silver tsunami" will continue to roll. With the over-85 population doubling by 2036 and tripling by 2049, the United States will need nearly 1 million new senior living units by 2040.[17] We will see an investor migration somewhat away from traditional assisted living and more toward unlicensed high margin independent living, where the residents will arrange for their own care by collectively negotiating with home health agencies. We will also see an increase temporarily in proprietary ownership rather than development fueled by institutional or publicly traded stockholders, as these investors are particularly sensitive to overall returns and their dollars will be attracted to higher margin investments.

■ OPPORTUNITIES

Even during this period of rapid expansion in the senior living industry, there are still opportunities for developers with insight into their local markets to grow and compete effectively. Successful operators employ the following strategies to strengthen their market position:

■ Adding assisted living to the continuum of living arrangements in an existing community, developing a freestanding assisted-living community, or developing a dementia care unit within the community

■ Bringing state-of-the-art independent living with a continuum of care to areas with residents who are aging in place and will require gradually increasing levels of care

■ Developing new start-up projects offering a full continuum of care (CCRCs) in underserved markets

■ Taking advantage of evolving private-public partnerships and affinity groups, especially with respect to managed care

■ Purchasing existing full or nearly full rental communities from banks or other institutions willing to write down or recapitalize the asset to meet the developer's investment criteria

■ Developing a relationship with a provider who has a record of successful development and who could capitalize on the company's reputation and management

■ Converting existing, functionally obsolete properties in strong market areas to full-service retirement centers offering affordable access for middle income seniors, or developing cooperatives using HUD 213 financing.

■ DEVELOPMENT OPPORTUNITIES FOR ASSISTED LIVING

ADVANTAGES

1. Market penetration rates required from age- and income-qualified seniors for a typical project are low, ranging from 1 to 4 percent. Demographic data should be adjusted to include only single-occupant households and exclude populations already institutionalized.

2. Market awareness of the concept has increased. Assisted living has been embraced by senior consumers and their families, as well as by professional referral sources and legislators, as a cost-effective alternative for the 15 to 20 percent of nursing home residents who are primarily private payers.

3. Assisted living is popular among adult children (ages 45 to 60) who are trying to deal with the needs of aging parents. These people, who influence their parents' decisions, prefer the idea of assisted living to that of skilled nursing settings.

4. When added to an existing community, assisted living draws on many resources already in place and further amortizes existing fixed overhead. It can add positive annual cash flow after debt service of $4,000 to $7,000 per unit. It is also an effective response to aging in place, because it allows the senior population to remain as independent as possible.

5. Assisted living can compete for traditional private-pay nursing home residents. The market is rapidly expanding as skilled nursing facilities move toward subacute care, rehabilitation, and other specialized care. The light care private-pay segment will expand, and well-positioned freestanding operators will take advantage of this growth. As a rule, the cost of providing assisted living services to light care residents is only about two-thirds the cost of providing similar services in a skilled nursing facility. Assisted living providers are delivering a needed product that can be adapted to the market. Nursing home operators are confined by government mandates that are based on a medical model and by the delivery and compliance costs associated with it.

6. The demand for care of residents with dementia is growing, and some providers may direct all of their resources to providing such care in a more cost-efficient setting, such as assisted living.

7. Current Medicaid funding is allocated 57 percent from the federal government and 43 percent from the states. This relationship could change, forcing the states to enact legislation to expand the delivery of services to lower levels of care. Several states have already established moratoriums on the CON process to halt the construction of additional skilled nursing beds.

8. As managed care becomes more widespread, physician groups will control more health care dollars. Medicare risk programs will encourage physicians to look to assisted living communities with respite or transitional care units, rather than the traditional acute care or skilled nursing environments, for the rehabilitation of certain classes of patients, such as those who have undergone knee or hip replacement or are in need of stabilization.

9. Some community hospitals are paid a daily rate when a health maintenance organization (HMO) controls the length of a patient's stay. After surgery, the HMO encourages the physician to discharge the patient to a lower-level setting for recovery and rehabilitation. Although lower-level settings provide a wide range of care, the common challenges of managing this care highlight the need for a seamless delivery system.

10. Most long-term care insurance policies are now written with coverage for assisted living and home health care. Insurers have learned that these less-expensive environments can provide satisfactory care at a fraction of the cost of nursing homes.

CHALLENGES AND RISKS

1. In most states, varying levels of assistance in daily living can be offered with limited levels of regulation. As this market cools as a result of increased supply (on which there are currently no CON restrictions), market saturation and increased regulation are inevitable. Projects that are likely to stand the test of time are those that (a) are well conceived and backed by experienced, reputable operators; (b) are tightly integrated into continuum-of-care companies; and (c) have a realistic exit strategy. Regulators understand that the business aims to contain costs, and states are moving toward spending Medicaid dollars for the delivery of these services in the assisted living arena. They therefore have a strong incentive not to overburden the industry with regulations.

2. Future regulation could entail significant costs to bring a project into compliance. To avoid such costs, projects should be conceived and operated according to high self-imposed standards that might become mandatory in the future. Developers are increasingly building independent living

communities that deliver higher returns without the licensing, regulatory, and staffing risks associated with assisted living. The level of care is becoming increasingly complex in assisted living, and this higher acuity translates to a higher capitalization rate and lower values.

3. The current demand for nursing home beds is not a reliable predictor of the projected demand for assisted living. As much as 70 percent of nursing care may involve Medicaid reimbursement, whereas assisted living is a private-pay market. Many seniors in the service area may not be able to pay privately for assisted living.

4. Marketing plans must take account of high turnover rates. New facilities always draw the most attention, even from residents of other nursing homes and retirement communities. Reverse effects can also transpire with older developments. Turnover rates can be as high as 50 percent annually; for a 90-unit project, this translates to 45 units per year.

5. The average price of assisted living is usually about 66 to 75 percent of prevailing nursing rates in the area. The maximum level of consumer affordability for privately paid assisted living is typically 80 to 85 percent of cash flow disposable income applied to the monthly fee.

Financial Qualifications: Private Payer

Independent $3,200 × 12 = $38,400
(@ 75 percent) $38,400 ÷ 0.75 = $51,200 per year or
                 $4,266 per month

Assisted living $4,500 × 12 = $54,000
(@ 85 percent) $54,000 ÷ 0.85 = $63,529 per year or
                 $5,294 per month

An independent resident leasing a unit for $3,200 per month would need to have an annual income of $51,200 to qualify. An assisted living resident would need $63,529 in annual income to qualify. The remainder will come from a depletion of their assets.

The long-term strategy must be to keep development costs and overhead to a minimum and strike a balance between spending capital dollars and building value as it is perceived by the residents.

6. Concerns about the availability of funding for home care may deter people from leaving their homes and moving into a group residential setting, where costs can be more easily controlled by economies of scale.

7. As competition increases, maintaining full occupancy will be difficult. Today's average profit margins of 40 percent will be harder to achieve; congregate operators are already experiencing downward trends. Steep price competition, the development of more-affordable models, and residents' needs and expectations of more-intensive services will drive down operating margins across the country.

8. Nursing homes may enter the market, expanding their licenses to include assisted living units within their skilled nursing facilities or to convert partial or entire wings from skilled care to custodial care, assisted living, transitional, and subacute care.

9. The COVID-19 pandemic has posed a real challenge to the senior housing sector. People living in senior housing facilities faced higher risk of severe and long-term complications from the virus because of age and underlying health conditions. Between the fourth quarter of 2019 and the second quarter of 2021, occupancy rates in senior housing dropped from 87.9 percent to 78.7 percent as many people opted for alternative living arrangements. The occupancy rate has increased since but as of the second quarter of 2022, it remained below the levels before the pandemic.[18] Historically, assisted living communities and other long-term care facilities have experienced more turnover and higher attrition rates than comparable industries. The COVID-19 pandemic has exacerbated this problem.

As of September 2021, only 4 percent of assisted living facilities reported they were fully staffed, while over 30 percent reported a high level of staffing shortages, according to a survey from the American Health Care Association and NCAL.[19] This translates to significantly higher employee turnover and lower staff retention than before the pandemic. Staff shortages also bring with them unplanned overtime and premium pay to ensure shift coverage. Further, assisted living communities are expecting to incur significant expenses in response to COVID-19, both in terms of sanitation supplies and supply chain shortages, especially in personal protective equipment (PPE), food, and cleaning supplies.

As the population ages, assisted living facilities will have to address these staffing concerns. Experts believe that increased wages may be able to counter shortages as the pandemic continues to wane.

The COVID-19 pandemic also affected many families' decisions to move their loved ones into assisted living communities. As of April 2020, about 18 percent of families who moved a relative into senior living said COVID-19 affected their choices of both when and where to move. According to A Place for Mom's January 2022 family survey, that number dropped to only 5 percent, implying increased post-vaccine comfort.

▰▰▰▰ DEVELOPMENT OPPORTUNITIES FOR CONTINUING CARE RETIREMENT COMMUNITIES

ADVANTAGES

1. CCRCs represent a major growth area that is compatible with and likely to benefit from health care reform.
2. They address the continuum of needs and the sensitivities of today's informed senior market. They are also well suited to a more affluent and sophisticated clientele.
3. CCRCs may provide significant tax advantages for individuals if Internal Revenue Code section 1034 (rollover) and section 121 (exclusion of gain) are amended to include these types of property. An additional segment of the homebound elderly market will then have a financial incentive to move out of their homes. Approximately 94 percent of America's elderly people have their health care needs provided for at home.
4. Lenders and investors recognize the inherent value of CCRCs as a business investment rather than as real estate.
5. State governments looking for ways to defray their expanding health care budgets may facilitate the development and financing of new construction.
6. CCRCs structured with a nonprofit operating entity will benefit from the aging in place of their residents and unit turnover. Residents' responsibility for operating expenses will minimize disruption and costs.
7. Few current regulations limit expansion in these market segments. CONs will be awarded more freely for CCRCs than for freestanding nursing homes.

CHALLENGES AND RISKS

1. The lengthy development process—up to three years—is complicated by the involvement of multiple regulatory agencies.
2. Sites with sufficient acreage and optimal location will be increasingly scarce and expensive.
3. Performance and value are more closely associated with the accuracy of actuarial predictions than with operational skill and efficiency.

In sum, legislators, investors, and lenders nationwide are headed in the most prudent and politically popular direction for health care for elderly people. The development of CCRCs, freestanding assisted living facilities, and home health care will expand dramatically over the next ten years. The entry of inexperienced or undercapitalized operators into these arenas will lead to future consolidation. Although well-established, competent operators will benefit from this trend, lending institutions and investors may be wary, having felt the sting of the consolidation in congregate developments during the 1980s and 1990s and again during the COVID-19 pandemic.

NOTES

1. A. W. Roberts, S. U. Ogunwole, L. Blakeslee, and M. A. Rabe, *The Population 65 Years and Older in the United States: 2016*, United States Census Bureau, October 2018, https://www.census.gov/content/dam/Census/library/publications/2018/acs/ACS-38.pdf.
2. National Library of Medicine, "Size and Demographics of Aging Populations," https://www.ncbi.nlm.nih.gov/books/NBK51841/.
3. J. Vespa, "The Graying of America: More Older Adults than Kids by 2035," United States Census Bureau, last revised October 8, 2019, https://www.census.gov/library/stories/2018/03/graying-america.html.
4. K. B. Wilson, "Historical Evolution of Assisted Living in the United States, 1979 to the Present," *Gerontologist* 47, no. suppl_1 (December 2007): 8–22, https://academic.oup.com/gerontologist/article/47/suppl_1/8/614189.
5. Roberts et al., *The Population 65 Years and Older.*
6. Alzheimer's Association, *2022 Alzheimer's Disease Facts and Figures*, https://www.alz.org/media/Documents/alzheimers-facts-and-figures.pdf.
7. Genworth, "Cost of Care Survey," https://www.genworth.com/aging-and-you/finances/cost-of-care.html.

8. K. Painter, "Understanding Long-Term Care Insurance," AARP, October 13, 2021, https://www.aarp.org/caregiving/financial-legal/info-2021/understanding-long-term-care-insurance/.

9. American Seniors Housing Association, *Seniors Housing: The Market-Driven Solution to Long-Term Care* (Washington, DC: ASHA, 1994), 12.

10. American Seniors Housing Association, *Seniors Housing Update* (Washington, DC: ASHA, 1994), 2.

11. There are currently federal and state regulations governing skilled nursing. While some federal laws and regulations apply to assisted living communities (e.g., the Department of Labor's administration of the Fair Labor Standards Act), state-level regulation of assisted living services and operations ensures an efficient, comprehensive licensure system because the states can effectively coordinate their full range of housing and service programs available to seniors and individuals with physical, intellectual, or developmental disabilities.

12. R. Anthony, "Capital Markets Financing for the Small Borrower," *Spectrum* 8, no. 5 (September 1994): 29–32.

13. "U.S. Assisted Living Facility Market Size, Share & Trends Analysis Report by Age (More than 85, 75–84, 65–74, Less than 65), Region (West, South, Midwest), and Segment Forecasts, 2023–2030," Grand View Research, https://www.grandviewresearch.com/industry-analysis/us-assisted-living-facility-market.

14. American Seniors Housing Association, *Selected Seniors Housing Transactions* (Washington, DC: ASHA, 1994), 5.

15. W. H. Elliot, J. L. Beck, and D. S. Schless, *Seniors Housing Finance: Trends and Prospects* (Washington, DC: American Seniors Housing Association, 1992), 21.

16. J. Moore, "Strategic Industry Focus Needed," *Contemporary Long-Term Care* 16 (March 1993): 24, 94.

17. E. Rubin, "2021 Assisted Living Statistics: Current Data and Trends," ConsumerAffairs, January 19, 2023, https://www.consumeraffairs.com/assisted-living/statistics.html.

18. Statista, "Senior Housing Occupancy Rate in the United States from the 4th Quarter of 2019 to 2nd Quarter of 2022," https://www.statista.com/statistics/1195721/us-senior-housing-occupancy/.

19. National Center for Assisted Living, "Survey: Assisted Living Incurring Significant Costs and Financial Hardship in Response to COVID-19," August 2020, https://www.ahcancal.org/News-and-Communications/Fact-Sheets/FactSheets/Survey-AL-COVID-Costs.pdf.

2

Financial Principles

The successful operation of a senior living community depends largely on balancing the owner's financial objectives with the interests of the residents and the employees. These interests often conflict, and the ability to reconcile them is the hallmark of a seasoned executive director. In this chapter, I discuss how to evaluate the performance of a senior living community under various models of ownership, and I offer some general guidelines for doing so.

This chapter also offers a very brief overview of accounting principles. The senior managers of a community must be comfortable with their budgets and understand the financial principles affecting community operations. The average executive director or middle-management supervisor, with little or no training in accounting, may find company financial statements confusing. But if one studies their form and function and learns the meaning of a few accounting terms, these statements are not hard to understand, and they reveal a great deal about the community's financial health and the effects of individual departments' performance.

TYPES OF OWNERSHIP

Three basic types of ownership are common to the senior living business: proprietary (with and without entry fees), nonprofit–tax exempt, and nonprofit taxable. Here I briefly define each type and review their respective advantages, disadvantages, and general financial considerations.

Proprietary

Projects with proprietary ownership are commonly referred to as for-profit communities. Generally they are sponsored by a privately owned corporation or a publicly traded entity. In publicly owned companies, equity is usually divided into common or preferred stock, held as retained earnings, or distributed to stockholders' equity accounts. Profits may be distributed as dividends. Private companies are generally capitalized by a group of investors or through private funds and are under no obligation to disclose financial results except to their investors.

The owner or partners each have an equity account to which profits are distributed. They expect a return on their invested dollars, much as one would expect interest to be earned on money in the bank, the fundamental difference being the rate of return and the corresponding risk on the investment. The primary operational advantage of proprietary ownership is the owners' degree of control of the real estate and operations.

Proprietary developers have historically concentrated on the construction and operation of independent or congregate and assisted living projects, leaving the continuing care communities largely to nonprofit sponsors. In recent years, however, proprietary interests have entered the CCRC arena in larger numbers, mainly because of the evolution of the market. Seniors have become more educated about their options. The communities that provide the widest choices of living units and services are becoming increasingly attractive. There will always be a market for independent or congregate projects, however. Many seniors see congregate living as an acceptable, flexible, and cost-effective alternative to nursing home placement and, most important, may not feel comfortable about investing hard-earned capital in a senior living project. Many senior living investors see less risk and better margins in facilities that provide basic services and leave the complex and unpredictable business of care delivery to be contracted directly by the residents. Much of the recent development has and will follow this trend as the increase in regulatory oversight combined with the lack of available staff drives up labor costs and drives down profitability and returns. Under this independent living model, the unlicensed facility will provide limited meals and maintenance, and the residents will contract for their care on an as-needed basis with home health agencies or private parties.

There are several financial benchmarks for privately owned communities. As a newly developed community fills, it will first reach a break-even point for operations. This is the point at which revenues collected from residents equal the cost of operating the community. The next break-even threshold is reached when revenues have increased to cover the cost of operations plus debt service. After this point, any surplus cash flow is first earmarked for capital improvements and to refinance construction or pay down working-capital loans. Because of the inherent risk, construction and working-capital loans usually bear a higher interest rate than the permanent loan that replaces them. The longer they remain outstanding, the greater the interest expense borne by the project. Permanent mortgage financing usually replaces construction financing after the operating net income of the project exceeds the debt service of the permanent loan by about 10 to 20 percent. Therefore, for each month that occupancy fails to reach this threshold and the construction loan remains in place, the project incurs a higher interest expense than was projected in the financial pro forma, and in essence experiences a construction cost overrun.[1]

At this point in the project, the investor still has generally not seen any return on investment. The investment flow is used to pay down short-term working capital, and it could easily be two years before the project produces any real return. This period, known as the *discounted payback period* (DPP), is the time required to recover the original investment plus working-capital contributions from the present value of the project's future cash flows. The cumulative shortfall balance is a year-end or month-end balance of the negative cash flow. Over time, as the community fills, this balance should reach zero. When operations cover debt service and capital improvements, the investment flow reverses and begins to offset the cumulative shortfall balance.

For comparison with other investment opportunities, all future investment flows must be converted to their present value. Return on investment for the project will be spread over the number of years that the investor maintains ownership. To determine the value of these future returns today, we must calculate the *present value* (PV) of the projected future cash flows of the project. This calculation converts future cash inflows and outflows to their present value using the project's cost of capital as the discount rate. The *net present value* (NPV) is the cost of the investment subtracted from the present value of the future cash flows. The NPV represents the amount that the project will return after factoring in the cost of capital. Simply put, the DPP is the number of years it takes for the cumulative present value of the investment to equal zero.

The investor's *return on equity* (ROE) is calculated by dividing the community's cash flow by the investor's equity contribution. Generally the investor compares this return (including the time value of money during the fill-up stage), on stabilization of the community's occupancy, to the opportunity cost or return in an alternative investment. Return on equity will generally increase with the occupancy of the community, as the fixed costs of the operation are absorbed by the initial tenants, and the variable costs of additional tenants once the property has exceeded 90 percent occupancy are marginal. As cash flow is calculated after debt service, any increase in the interest rate of adjustable-rate financing will reduce the investor's return. This can be particularly devastating if management is unable to pass the increased costs on to the residents, who are generally on fixed incomes. *Return on assets* (ROA) is calculated by dividing the project's cash flow by the total asset value (total project costs, including land, buildings, and furniture, fixtures, and equipment) less accumulated depreciation. ROA will always be less than ROE unless the project is not leveraged.

Another measure of financial return is *internal rate of return* (IRR). This measure is widely used by investors to evaluate the net return. The IRR is calculated by a process of iteration to find the discount rate that equates the present value of future cash flows (usually 5- or 10-year periods) with the cost of the investment. For the project to add value to the company, the IRR must be greater than the cost of capital (i.e., greater than the interest rate on the borrowed funds). Most investors calculate their pretax IRRs on a leveraged and an unleveraged basis—that is, before and after debt service. The leveraged IRR will of course always be greater.

If the flow of cash is negative or does not cover all current obligations, the owner may need to convert some other assets to cash, secure short-term or long-term financing, or bring in additional investment partners. The owner in a private company will increase her investment, but a public company may sell a new issue of stock. Most primary lenders consider this working capital as the owner's "risk money" and will expect her to raise it rather than ask the lending institution to supply it.

Nonprofit–Tax Exempt

A nonprofit organization exists by a charter issued by the secretary of state of the incorporating state and must function within the definition of the charter. Most nonprofit retirement communities have been designed after the model of a continuing care retirement community. The typical nonprofit CCRC is not owned by stockholders or a private corporation but rather by its members. Usually the organization is sponsored by a nonprofit affinity group, such as a religious order, and governed by a board of trustees. In most cases, at least one of the resident members of the community sits on the board as a voting or nonvoting participant. The board is usually responsible for setting overall policy and delegates the day-to-day operations to management. The system works best when the board provides management with the flexibility to run the property, and management in

turn demonstrates a willingness to tap into the expertise and business acumen of the various board members. CCRCs by definition operate under considerable external competitive and regulatory pressures as well as internal organizational ones.

Newly developed communities are generally required by state regulations to meet presale thresholds before receiving construction approval. The proportion of the advance fees collected that can be used to fund construction of the community varies by state. Most states require the escrowing of resident advance fees during the development period and occasionally even after start-up. Generally, presale levels above 75 percent indicate a reasonably rapid absorption of the community on opening. Presale levels below 50 percent suggest a weak market and are cause for serious concern. Entry fees are usually shielded from federal tax, and some states allow ad valorem tax exemption as well as favorable sales-tax and payroll-tax treatment. These projects may also have access to borrowing sources such as tax-exempt bonds, which can carry attractive rates.

The main disadvantage of the nonprofit community is that control is vested in a board of directors who are typically well intentioned but without financial resources, industry-specific operational experience, or personal investment. Currently, residents cannot pass through any rollover of capital gains or realize the benefits of any real estate–related deductions. In addition, as the cost of the operations is directly borne by the residents, any increases in debt service are passed directly to them. By the same token, however, residents themselves are motivated to control the expansion of services and resulting expenses.

Some life-care communities have been criticized because their fee calculations have not been based on sound actuarial data. Communities that have relied on the advance payment of entrance fees to partially offset operational losses have, on reaching stabilized occupancy, found themselves without adequate turnover to cover the operational shortfalls. This risk has been especially acute in communities that have introduced home health care to residents in their apartments in an effort to minimize obligations to provide care in the more expensive skilled-nursing facility.

Surplus cash from operations is usually used to fund capital improvements or resident reserve funds, or else it is invested. The accumulation of significant amounts in the reserve can jeopardize the community's 501(c)(3) nonprofit status and render the organization liable to taxes. Therefore, management must carefully balance the operation to maintain its nonprofit status while providing for the future cash requirements of debt service, capital improvements, and increased operating expenses. The last is especially important for newer communities with a substantial nursing home component that, when fully occupied, will significantly increase operational expenses.

Nonprofit Taxable

Nonprofit taxable operations typically are designed in the form of cooperatives or condominiums. These operations provide certain tax advantages to their members, such as rollover of capital gains and pass-through of real estate taxes and interest. Real estate taxes and surcharges are reduced, owing to investment in the membership fee that is not producing income. Residents can benefit from the appreciation of their units and retain control of their assets. To many seniors who are used to a lifetime of home ownership, these features are attractive.

The disadvantages include higher financial requirements for entry and substantially more complex residency agreements. In addition, condominiums and cooperatives usually fall under the auspices of the state real estate commission and exist at the complicated interface of tax laws, real estate laws, and CCRC regulations (where they exist), some of which may be in conflict.

A nonprofit operation is generally governed by a board of directors composed of members, the developer, and outside local interests. The board usually hires a management company to oversee operations. Usually the developer structures the program so that its own management company is awarded the management contract; however, most states limit the term of these contracts to a maximum of three years. Surplus cash flow is either used to fund capital improvements or invested.

OPERATIONAL BUDGETING

The annual budget process is one of the exercises almost universally dreaded by middle management. It does, however, provide management the opportunity to evaluate individual operations annually for efficiency, form, and function. Systematic financial planning not only makes financial targets more attainable but also facilitates accurate cash-flow planning and forecasts. Accurate financial forecasts may enable owners to acquire financing at lower rates or distribute greater returns to investors. The goal of the budget process is to forecast whether the expenses of running the business (cash outflows) will exceed revenues collected from the residents and to decide how to cover a projected deficit or, conversely, how to distribute a projected surplus. The budgeting process itself can also help reveal areas in the operation where the setting of measurable goals would be especially beneficial to all interested parties.

Budgeting Revenue

Budgeting revenue is usually based on the projected monthly average revenue per unit. Occupancy projections for the year are multiplied by the average revenue per unit to obtain the total expected unit revenue for each month of the budget period. Average revenue per unit is calculated based on prior-period actual results and then adjusted for expected increases in rent or monthly service fees. These figures are calculated for each different type of unit by isolating the revenue for each type of unit and dividing by the total number of units that were occupied for the previous full month. This approach assumes that all units are occupied and producing revenue for throughout the budget period: in other words, the budget will not account for prorations on units that are vacated or newly occupied part way through the budget month. (Some operators do not offer prorations and require prepayments on move-ins and advance notice for move-outs. This arrangement minimizes lost revenue, but it may not always be enforceable.)

Increases in rent or monthly service fee should be budgeted starting in the month in which they are expected to occur. Under local landlord-tenant legislation, it may be necessary to provide advance notice to residents. Some operators raise fees for all residents once per year at the same time rather than at the anniversary date of the residency agreement. This method can be used only if the fee increases are universally applied. Under this scenario, moreover, the management always runs the risk of an organized protest by residents, especially in for-profit operations. If the management has not adequately prepared residents to expect fee increases, it may find itself on the defensive. Conversely, if fees are increased on the anniversary date of the individual residency agreement, different increases can be applied to similar apartments with a much lower risk of any collective action. In addition, when only a few of the residents' renewals become due each month, it is easier to deal with individual concerns privately.

Interest rates strongly affect the residents' investment returns and the project's debt service. For a resident to qualify financially to live in a congregate community, most operators require that the monthly service fee be no more than 70 percent of the resident's monthly disposable income (85 percent for assisted living). Therefore, for a resident to afford a monthly service fee of $3,100 per month, or $37,200 per year, he will require $53,142 ($37,200 ÷ 0.70 = $53,142) in annual income from investments and Social Security. Assuming a 7 percent annual return on his investments, the resident will require approximately $759,171 ($53,142 ÷ 0.07 = $759,171) in assets to produce this income (not including Social Security payments). Every 1 percent increase in interest rates will increase the income produced from these assets by $7,591 annually or $632 per month (not including compounding). For a 250-unit community valued at $20 million, with a 75 percent loan to value and financed with $15 million on a floating-rate note, the same 1 percent increase in interest rates will cost the owner $150,000 more in interest expense per year. When this amount is divided among 250 residents, the $50 per month fee increase required to cover the increase in interest expense will amount to 1.6 percent, not including any increases in operating expenses. Clearly, in this example the residents' ability to absorb the community's increase in debt service and operational expenses in an expanding economy will be adequate. If interest rates fall, however, residents' earnings can fall dramatically, to the point where residents cannot absorb cost increases, and the community may need to consider refinancing as a vehicle for underwriting the ever-increasing cost of operations.

Budgeting Expenses

The development of an annual budget generally involves comparing each expense account of the general ledger to community historical results, industry standards, and assumptions as outlined in the original financial projections or pro forma. For new communities, in the absence of historical data, the first budget is generally built from projections in combination with industry standards. Each year thereafter, as the community matures, operating results help to refine the budget's accuracy.

For mature projects, historical data are generally collected and then annualized and compared to financial projections and ownership objectives. During the fill-up stage of the project, however, the budgeting process is referred to as "zero based"—that is, built without the use of historical data or from scratch. Some companies build their budgets every year using the zero-base method, arguing that basing projections on prior results compounds any intrinsic inefficiencies of the system. Reviewing each department budget line item from scratch each year can be an involved process, yet it may uncover areas where costs can be trimmed and therefore justify the extra work: after all, the costs of operating the community are ultimately borne by the residents, some of whom may not be able to afford continuous annual increases.

In constructing budgets, expenses that do not depend on changes in the community occupancy (fixed costs) should be separated from those that vary according to occupancy (variable costs). There are fixed and variable expenses in each department. For example, fixed expenses for food and beverages include the chef's salary, cooking utensils, kitchen equipment and operations, and utilities. Variable expenses that generally increase proportionally with occupancy include those for food, staffing, and supplies.

Tracking departmental monthly expenditures with a declining-balance ledger can simplify budgetary compliance. This is simply a ledger sheet or spreadsheet listing at the top each expense category, along with its corresponding monthly budgeted amount. As materials or supplies are received, the department head assigns each invoice or packing-slip item to the appropriate account and enters it into her ledger. The expense is subtracted from the monthly total budget to determine the remaining amount in each category. As the month progresses, the department manager will have an accurate picture of the amount of money remaining. As the budgeted amount in each category becomes exhausted, additional orders for supplies can be placed for receipt in the following month. In this way, the department head does not have to wait to see the financial statement to determine whether her department expenses are over or under budget. The declining-balance ledger is an excellent planning tool that is particularly helpful to new staff, and its use should be standard procedure for all department heads.

Nonprofit communities by definition have the objective of balancing revenues with expenses, plus perhaps a small surplus to cover a reserve fund and any unexpected contingencies. They can generally provide more services to their residents for the same or a lower monthly fee than their for-profit counterparts. This is partly because profit considerations are not taken into account during budgeting, but also because their tax-exempt status shelters them from real estate and sales taxes, and most communities are self-managed by a board of directors or by sponsors. In a large 350-unit CCRC with an annual operating budget of $9.4 million, costs for taxes and management could easily total $1.3 million. In a community of this size, then, the difference between a for-profit and a nonprofit operation represents a 14 percent savings to the residents of the nonprofit community for an equivalent service package, not including the premium for profit and risk.

Many owners are now including clauses in their management agreements to specify performance thresholds based on the community's EBITDAR, defined as earnings before interest expense (net of interest income), taxes (federal, state, local, and property), depreciation, amortization, and rent or lease expense (property and capital leases). This approach segregates noncontrollable expenses from operations costs and allows targeting a percentage of revenue or minimum dollar amount to cover debt. The EBITDAR calculation reflects true operational expenses and is not subject to fluctuations in interest expense (especially important for variable-rate financing). Using EBITDAR net income, owners can establish a predebt value for the revenue stream created by the property using capitalization rates. See the section on capitalization rates for a detailed discussion on project valuation.

Industry standards for budgeting expenses in various departments are detailed in the corresponding chapters in this book. The relationships are presented as ratios for variable expenses and itemized for fixed expenses, where appropriate, for a typical 200-unit congregate community. These figures can be adjusted upward or downward according to community size and occupancy. Clearly, the development of a community budget and allocation of financial resources will vary greatly according to state regulations, labor markets, community size, competition, service package, and, most important, owner philosophy. Alternative choices for various levels of service and quality are offered for management consideration throughout the text.

◼◼◼◼ FIXED-ASSET CAPITALIZATION

Fixed-asset capitalization, also known as capital improvement, is a process of assessing the current and projected physical state of a property, establishing the costs of maintaining or modernizing it, and planning for needed improvements.

Some financing vehicles require the maintenance of minimum replacement reserves. The adequacy of these reserves should be reevaluated regularly. They usually involve substantial amounts of capital that may not be required if needs are accurately assessed through the capital planning process.

Clearly, understanding current and future physical needs can help managers control their cash flow, take advantage of favorable credit opportunities, and avoid refinancing in unfavorable markets. Owners, managers, and maintenance staff should engage in this process together. Capital planning is a valuable diagnostic tool for projecting and managing the community's current and long-term physical, financial, and human requirements. See chapter 13 for a complete description of how to develop a comprehensive capital replacement plan.

◼◼◼◼ ACCOUNTING

The following brief accounting overview is designed to familiarize managers with some basic accounting principles and their application to operations management in senior living communities. Whether the community objective is to achieve a profit from the operations or merely to balance revenues with expenses, it is important to understand the accounting of the community's finances.

Several governing bodies in the accounting profession are dedicated to defining generally accepted accounting principles (GAAP).[2] These groups publish formal statements and pronouncements on how to handle all kinds of accounting issues, and their publications serve as the authoritative sources on GAAP-basis accounting. Here I generally follow the most current provided by the following texts: (1) The Financial Accounting Standards Board (FASB), *Statements of Financial Accounting Standards*; (2) *FASB Interpretations*; (3) the American Institute of Certified Public Accountants (AICPA), *Accounting Research Bulletins*; and (4) *The Opinions of the Accounting Principles Board* (APB).

Accounting Methods

There are two primary methods of recognizing revenues and expenses: the *accrual basis* and the *cash basis*. It is important to understand both of these methods and the differences between them.

The *accrual basis* of accounting recognizes revenues in the period in which they are earned—that is, when goods have been sold or a service rendered. It recognizes expenses in the period they are incurred—that is, when a legal liability exists. This means that earnings and expenses are recorded as they happen, regardless of whether any cash changes hands at the time.

The *cash basis* of accounting, in contrast, accounts only for cash receipts and cash expenditures, not revenues and expenses. Thus, transactions are recorded only when there is a flow of cash into or out of the business. For example, when a guest is served a $12 meal in the dining room, the business has earned the $12 for that meal. The resident who hosted the guest will pay for the meal next month. Under the *accrual* method of accounting, the business records, or accrues, the cost of the meal this month as a revenue and a balance due (account receivable) from the resident; in contrast, under the cash method of accounting, the business does not recognize the amount due for the meal until the following month, when the resident pays for it.

The senior housing industry lends itself well to the accrual basis of accounting, as residents usually are charged and pay for their services on a monthly basis. The expenses of delivering these services are also budgeted monthly and yield a clear picture of the financial balance of the operation.

General Ledger

A *general ledger* is the final accounting record of the financial condition and results of operations of a business. All financial business activity is categorized by account codes and recorded in the general ledger. The general ledger keeps track of all account balances as well as the transactions coded to each account. There are two major types of general ledger accounts: *balance sheet accounts*, which keep track of the company's financial condition in the categories of assets, liabilities, and equity; and *income statement accounts*, which keep track of the company's operating results in the categories of revenues and expenses.

ASSETS. *Assets* are items of value or use that a company owns, which usually help the company produce earnings. Assets also include properties and claims against others that may be directly or indirectly applied to cover liabilities. Each company employee is also an asset: although employees are not "owned" by the company, they help generate earnings for the business and provide valuable services for the company. Examples of other assets are cash, accounts receivable from residents, the facility buildings, the facility van, and kitchen equipment.

Depreciation recognizes the deterioration or depletion in value of an asset over time. It is determined by allocating the cost of the asset over its estimated useful life to determine the true cost of operation. Some assets may be considered to have some salvage (residual) value at the end of the depreciation period. Depreciation does not mean that an item is worthless once it has been depleted, only that the item's full cost has been allocated to its estimated useful life. Accounting for depreciation is usually based on the cost or purchase price of the asset plus installation expenses, if any. Usually the assets of a senior living community are depreciated using the straight-line method. This calculation is based on the cost less the salvage value, divided by the years of useful life.

Under the tax-based accounting method, the property is depreciated over 25.5 years, an approach that will render a higher calculated depreciation amount and in turn reduce the tax liability. The tax-based method recognizes income as it is received, or what is known as "constructive receipt." Conversely, under GAAP, income is recognized for tax purposes as it is earned. The depreciation period is 40 years, which results in a smaller depreciation amount and a higher taxable income.

LIABILITIES. *Liabilities* are a company's legal obligations to others at a given point in time, typically the end of a month. Examples of liabilities are accounts payable to vendors, loans from the bank or another company, wages payable to employees, and prepaid rent from residents.

EQUITY. *Equity* is the net worth of the company or business. By definition it is the net of assets minus liabilities.

REVENUES. *Revenues* are amounts that have been earned during a specified period or that have already been paid or to which the company is legally entitled. The term *revenue* is associated with the accrual basis of accounting. Do not confuse revenue with cash receipt, which refers to the physical collection of money from people who have rented apartments or purchased goods or services from the business. The process by which cash is received in the same period that revenue is earned is called a *cash sale*. Cash received before the period when revenue is earned is called a *prepaid item* and is categorized as a liability, because the business still has a legal obligation to provide a product or service to the resident. If cash is received after the period when revenue is earned, the business is said to be collecting on a *balance due* or *accounts receivable* item, which is an asset, because the business has a claim against the resident to pay for the services and has a legal right to collect it.

EXPENSES. *Expenses* are the costs of operating and owning a business. The term *expense* is associated with the accrual basis of accounting. Do not confuse an expense with a cash payment, which is the physical payment of money to people who have provided, or will provide, goods or services to the business. The process by which cash is paid in the same period that the expense was incurred is called a *cash purchase*. Cash paid before the period when the expense is incurred is called a *prepaid expense* and is categorized as an asset, because someone else has a legal obligation to provide the business with the goods or services requested. If cash is paid after the period when the expense was incurred, the business is said to be paying an *accounts payable* item, which is a liability, or a legal obligation to pay someone else. By paying, the business settles a claim the other party had against its assets (cash).

The costs of operating a business can be either expensed or capitalized. All expenditures for new assets and permanent improvements can be capitalized if they increase the value of the property *and* clearly have a benefit that extends three or more years *and* gener-

ally have a minimum purchase of $200 per invoice with a unit cost of at least $50 *and* are not considered repair and maintenance. Expenditures that are capitalized will not be expensed and therefore will not appear on the statement of profit and loss; rather, they become a balance-sheet asset and are subject to depreciation. Expenditures made to keep the property in ordinary, efficient operating condition, which do not add value or appreciably extend the useful life of the asset, are repair and maintenance expenses. Employees involved in requesting or approving expenditures should understand the characteristics of these expenditures in order to classify them properly as capital or expense. The circumstances surrounding the expenditure often determine whether it is capital in nature or an ordinary expense. Therefore, all requests for purchase should be accompanied by complete descriptions and justification from the department head. In most cases, expenditures that can be capitalized should be. Expenditures such as these are generally not planned for in the operations budget but are dealt with separately in a fixed-asset capitalization budget.

By knowing what information is included in the general ledger, and how to read it, you can keep track of the progress and status of your business. By reviewing the general ledger every month, you will see the final result of all the individual transactions you record, approve, or handle every month. Reviewing the general ledger can also help identify transactions that have been recorded to an incorrect account code. These errors, if left uncorrected, would misstate the results of operations at the community and perhaps its financial condition.

In any business accounting function, it is critical to set up systems that provide for a *segregation of duties*— that is, for accounting procedures to be carried out by more than one employee. Tasks should be assigned to different employees in a way that creates a system of checks and balances for everyone's work. Typically, the tasks can be categorized into three types:

1. **Custody of assets.** This function controls, has physical access to, and is responsible for a given set of company assets, such as cash.
2. **Recording of assets.** This function keeps the records of what assets the company should have on hand at a given time, based on approved paperwork and information from (3).

3. **Review and approval of assets.** This function reviews the assets on hand with (1), matches the related paperwork to the assets, and approves the paperwork and information for use by (2). It also reviews the records being kept by (2) and compares them to the assets being handled by (1).

If the records and actual assets do not coincide, the employees in each function must check their work, report their findings to each other, and resolve the problem.

Senior housing facilities can be set up with various organizational structures. Some may have an executive director, office manager or bookkeeper, and office staff, whereas others have resident manager couples who fulfill the roles of director, bookkeeper, marketing director, and so on. It is important to identify functional roles for these employees that provide the necessary segregation. Adequate internal controls must be established to protect company assets from errors and irregularities.

One of the greatest side benefits of dividing tasks in this way is that each employee involved in the monthly accounting cycle must understand the other employees' duties. Ideally, every employee should be trained to carry out the others' duties in case of illness, vacation, or turnover. Equally important, the segregation of duties can promote an atmosphere of teamwork. Each person is motivated to do his best work, knowing that his peers are relying on its accuracy and integrity and are checking their own work against it.

An *audit* is a formal review and evaluation of a company. There are two types of audits, each with a different focus or purpose. A *financial* audit is performed on a company's financial records for a specified period of time. The purpose of a financial audit is to determine whether a company's financial condition and results of operations are stated fairly in the financial statements in accordance with GAAP. An audit by an independent (external) certified public accounting firm would be considered a financial audit. An *operational* audit is also performed on a company's financial records or on general departmental operations, but its purpose is to determine whether a company has been operating according to its prescribed policies and procedures. An operational audit also evaluates whether those policies and procedures promote operating standards that comply with

GAAP. An internal audit is an example of an operational audit.

FINANCIAL ANALYSIS

Financial information analyzed varies among companies; however, return on investment and value are two key indicators of performance. In for-profit operations, these indicators are both intrinsically linked to cash flow. *Cash flow*, the actual inflow and outflow of cash, is the heartbeat of any business. It is determined by first subtracting operating expenses from gross revenues to calculate gross operating profit or loss. From gross operating profit are subtracted depreciation, amortization, taxes and insurance, and debt service to calculate net operating income, also referred to as pretax income. Finally, noncash expenses such as depreciation and amortization are added back, and out-of-pocket expenses such as principal reduction (if any) and capital expenditures are subtracted, to yield cash flow. Exhibit 2.1 summarizes the usual calculation of cash flow.

There are essentially two types of cash flow: cash flow from raising and investing capital (also known as nonoperating revenue) and cash flow from operations. The two components are combined to produce the cash balance, which may be either positive or negative. As explained earlier, cash received during the year does not necessarily represent the year's total gross revenue, as the funds (although recognized as earned under the accrual-basis accounting method) may not all be recovered from the residents or their estates. Similarly, cash disbursements do not measure total expenses for the year because some products remain in inventory at the end of the year. In other words, cash inflows and outflows may not necessarily equal the total respective revenue and expenses for the community. The company's assets (e.g., inventory, accounts receivable) and its liabilities (e.g., loans, bills payable) reveal its financial condition. This information is presented in the *balance sheet*. The balance sheet summarizes the assets and liabilities for one year, as recorded on the last day of the income statement period.

Capitalization Rates

The *capitalization rate* is an indicator commonly used to determine asset value based on a single year's cash flow before interest, depreciation, amortization, and taxes, but after a management fee (EBITDAR).

Exhibit 2.1   Income Statement and Cash Flow

	Gross operating revenue
Less	deductions and adjustments (e.g., rental allowance)
Equals	**total income or revenue**
Less	total departmental expenses
Equals	**gross operating profit or loss**
Less	depreciation
Less	amortization
Less	interest expenses
Less	other property expenses (taxes and insurance)
Equals	**net operating income (pretax income)**
Add	depreciation
Add	amortization
Less	capital improvements
Less	principal reduction
Equals	**cash flow**

Usually, the higher the capitalization rate, the greater the investment risk. Risk-averse buyers require higher initial cash-on-cash returns to attract capital because of the limited prospects for future earnings and increased property values. Generally, the higher the level of care provided in a senior community, the greater the degree of management intensity and the higher the capitalization rate. Capitalization rates are integrally composed of a number of key factors, such as loan-to-value ratio, prevailing lending rate, ratio of equity to value, and equity return. Exhibit 2.2 shows a sample calculation of the capitalization rate.

Capitalization rates can also be used to estimate the effects of revenue and expenses on the value of the community. Even a modest $50 per unit per month in increased revenue or decreased expenses yields $10,000 per month, or $120,000 per year, for a 200-unit project ($200 \times \$50 \times 12 = \$120,000$). The enhanced product value is more than $1 million using an 11 percent capitalization rate ($120,000 \div 11$ percent $=$ $1,090,909). As a general rule, every $1 savings in expenses or increase in revenue yields $10 in increased value to the community using a 10 percent capitalization rate ($1 \div 10$ percent $= \$10$). In other words, expense management by department managers has a tenfold effect on enhancing the value of the community to the owner. Conversely, managers who carelessly overspend their budgets decrease the value of the community for the owner in the same proportion.

Break-even point analyses of operating expenses only, and operating expenses plus debt service (principal plus interest), not including depreciation, can be useful in determining the number of occupied units needed to reach certain investment performance thresholds. Note that the ratios of loan to value affect the break-even point analysis relative to the level of leverage and debt service on the properties. For a new community, the first break-even point is reached when revenues cover operating expenses. Industry averages for this point range from 49 to 67 percent occupancy. Property taxes, location, and type of community also affect this margin. The second and more important break-even point is reached when operating revenues equal operating expenses plus debt service. This point is generally lower for congregate communities and increases with the level of care provided. This factor varies according to the relationship of debt service to the number of units and revenue generated from the unit mix. For a 100-unit assisted living community, this break-even point with debt service should be reached at approximately 80 percent occupancy. Projects with higher break-even points either are operated inefficiently or carry too much debt. Projects that are overburdened with debt may,

---

Exhibit 2.2   Sample Calculation of Capitalization Rate

70% Loan to value ratio × 8.75% lending rate = 6.01%

30% Equity to value × 20% equity return = 6.00%

Capitalization rate = 12.01%

Assume cash flow before debt service, depreciation, and taxes = $3,800,000

Value of community at 12% capitalization rate = $3,800,000 ÷ 0.12 = $31,666,666

An inverse multiplier of the capitalization rate yields the same conclusion:
1 ÷ 0.12 = 8.33 × $3,800,000 = $31,666,666

---

for example, be highly leveraged or expensively built. As a rule, a community operating at stabilized occupancy should have a capitalized value equal to or greater than its debt service balance. Projects that fall short of this target are probably not worth their debt service balances and will cost equity to liquidate.

Another method of calculating the value of a community is its *gross revenue multiplier.* This is derived simply by dividing the sale price by the annual gross revenue. This measure generally fluctuates with the capitalization rate. It is perceived as more reliable because gross revenues are easier to calculate than net operating income, especially considering the wide variety of operational models employed in the industry. In the preceding example, if the sale price was $32,000,000 and the gross revenue was $7,800,000, the gross revenue multiplier would be 4.1. The higher the multiplier, generally the more efficient the operation and the higher the revenue trends. Conversely, a low multiplier may indicate residents' inability to absorb increases in operational expenses.

A number of methods and ratios are commonly used to evaluate financial performance and value. The information needed to calculate these ratios is drawn from the community's major financial statements: the balance sheet, revenue and expense statement (profit and loss), and cash flow statement. These financial statements are generally prepared according to the AICPA guidelines and other GAAP. Usually the ratios are presented as percentages, and the period analyzed is usually one fiscal year but could be as short as one month. In 1990, the AICPA published

two reports that standardized the industry's accounting practices regarding the presentation of external financial statements: *Audits of Providers of Health Care Services* and *Statement of Position 90-8.* These were summarized by Fitch Investor Services and are reprinted in exhibits 2.3–2.6.[3]

Debt Service Coverage Ratio

The *debt service coverage ratio* (DSCR) measures the organization's ability to service debt from two sources: DSCR operating and nonoperating income activities, and cash flows from receipt of advance fees and deposits, less any refunds. Income-related numbers derive from the revenue and expense statement, advance fees from the cash flow statement. Thus the ratio combines dollar amounts from audited financial statements that are based on both accrual accounting and cash accounting.

The DSCR is more easily understood when it is dissected. The denominator, maximum annual debt service, is straightforward. But the numerator is known by several names, including *net available for debt service, net revenues available for debt service,* or simply *net available.*

The calculation of net available adds in actual cash from advance fees (if any), net of refunds, and subtracts noncash revenue associated with the amortization of advance fees. Thus the amortization portion is correctly excluded from net available because it involves no cash flow. This ratio accurately measures the community's ability to service its debt. A DSCR of 1.25 means that for every $1.00 in debt service, the

---

Exhibit 2.3   Calculation of Debt Service
Coverage Ratio

Excess (deficit) of revenue over expenses

Plus   interest expense

Plus   depreciation expense

Plus   amortization expense

Minus   amortization of deferred revenue from
nonrefundable advance fees (if any)

Plus   proceeds from advance fees and deposits
(if any)

Minus   refunds of advance fees and deposits
(if any)

Equals   **net available**

DSCR   **= Net available ÷ maximum annual
debt service**

---

project produces $1.25 in cash flow. Exhibit 2.3 summarizes the calculation of the DSCR.

REVENUE AND EXPENSE RATIOS
Operating Margin

The *operating margin*, also referred to as *operating profit margin*, reflects that portion of total revenues retained as operating income, and it relates solely to operations. Because CCRCs can choose how they present contributions, this ratio can fluctuate. For example, a 250-unit community, fully occupied, with $7,800,000 in gross revenue and $4,000,000 in net operating expenses, has a net income from operations of $3,800,000. The operating margin then is the ratio of $3,800,000 to $7,800,000, or 48.7 percent. The operating margin can also be calculated by subtracting the *expense ratio* from 1 $(1 - 0.513 = 0.487)$.

Operating Ratio (Expense Ratio)

The operating (expense) ratio is a useful tool for determining overall operational efficiency. It shows the proportion of operating expenses to gross revenue. By subtracting noncash items such as amortization of debt issuance expense, the operating ratio determines whether ongoing cash revenues cover ongoing cash expenses. The ratio also measures the adequacy of periodic service or monthly fees. If it exceeds

100 percent, the ratio may indicate a reliance on advance fees to cover operating expenses.

Operating expenses should include management fees, but should be net of depreciation, real estate taxes, capital improvements, and debt service. For example, a 250-unit community, fully occupied, with $7,800,000 in gross revenue and $4,000,000 in net operating expenses, has an expense ratio of $4,000,000 ÷ $7,800,000 = 51.3 percent. To approximate net operating income from an expense ratio and gross operating income, take the gross operating income × $(1 -$ expense ratio$)$. In our example, $7,800,000 × $(1 - 0.513) = $3,798,600$.

Expense ratios vary with the size of the community, underlining the importance of economies of scale. In for-profit communities of fewer than 200 units, an expense ratio of 70 percent may indicate a well-run operation; however, as the number of units increases to 250, an expense ratio of 60 percent may be more in line, and if there are more than 300 units, ratios of 50 to 55 percent are considered appropriate. Nonprofit communities have operating ratios close to 100 percent.

Total Excess Margin

The inclusion of nonoperating revenue in the equation provides a total picture of performance. Exhibit 2.4 summarizes the calculation of revenue and expense ratios.

LIQUIDITY RATIOS
Current Ratio

The *current ratio* is easily calculated by taking the community's total current assets and dividing that figure by its total current liabilities. Most lenders require at least a 2:1 ratio: for every dollar of debt or liability, the organization must have $2 of cash or assets. Ratios vary from industry to industry, and Dun & Bradstreet publishes the current ratios for a wide range of businesses. The ratio varies depending on such broad factors as composition of current assets, inventory turnover rate, and credit terms. If a community's current ratio consistently exceeds 5:1, the company has an unnecessary accumulation of funds that could indicate financial mismanagement. Conversely, a current ratio much below 2:1 could be cause for serious concern for the operation's liquidity and ability to service short-term obligations. This ratio is

---

Exhibit 2.4 Calculation of Revenue and Expense Ratios

Operating margin

$$\frac{\text{Income (loss) from operations}}{\text{Total revenues}}$$

Operating (expense) ratio

$$\frac{\substack{\text{Total operating expenses} \\ \textit{Less} \text{ depreciation expense} \\ \textit{Less} \text{ amortization expense}}}{\text{Total revenues}}$$

Total excess margin

$$\frac{\text{Excess (deficit) of revenues over expenses}}{\text{Total revenues + nonoperating revenue}}$$

---

not as useful in measuring a CCRC's cash position because its board-designated cash and investments are typically presented as noncurrent assets under the heading "Assets whose use is limited by board for capital/investments."

Other Useful Ratios

Two additional calculations, although not true ratios, are defined here because they are used in determining several ratios:

Daily operating revenues: Total revenues, minus amortization of deferred revenue from nonrefundable advance fees (if any), divided by the number of days in the period, usually 365.

Daily operating expenses: Total operating expenses, minus depreciation expense and amortization expense, divided by the number of days in the period, usually 365.

NET DAYS IN ACCOUNTS RECEIVABLE. *Net days in accounts receivable* indicates, in days, the average length of time it takes to collect accounts receivable. Senior living communities usually bill monthly fees in advance. Typically, the biggest component of receivables is Medicaid.

DAYS CASH ON HAND. *Days cash on hand* measures all cash and investments available to cover daily expenses divided by the estimated per-day operational cost. The ratio indicates an organization's

ability to withstand short-term disruptions in cash receipts. Because this limitation is commonly imposed by the board of trustees or owner, and despite their presentation as limited, these funds theoretically are available for any use, including debt service, if necessary.

AVERAGE DAYS IN CURRENT LIABILITIES. Instead of a "days in accounts payable" ratio, which measures vendor accounts payable, Fitch Investor Services calculates average days in current liabilities, because this ratio measures the average length of time elapsing before all current liabilities are met. Users should examine the working relationship between net days in accounts receivable and this ratio.

CUSHION RATIO. The *cushion ratio* measures cash deemed available in relation to maximum annual debt service. If principal amortization is not structured to produce level debt service, using maximum annual debt service prompts the user to investigate how the balloon payment will be funded. Exhibit 2.5 summarizes the calculation of liquidity ratios.

CAPITAL STRUCTURE AND CASH FLOW RATIOS
Debt Service Coverage Ratio: Revenues Only

The *debt service coverage ratio for revenues only* is directly related to the DSCR. It reflects the community's ability to service its debt, through operating sources alone. The cash received from net advance fees, a "financing" activity, is intentionally not included in this calculation. When compared to the DSCR, this ratio measures the degree to which the community relies on net advance fees to service its debt.

Debt Service as a Percentage of Net Operating and Nonoperating Revenues

Debt service as a percentage of net operating and nonoperating revenues indicates the percentage of all "cash-generating" revenue applied to the maximum annual debt service. It excludes amortization of deferred revenue from nonrefundable advance fees (if any).

Debt Service as a Percentage of Operating Expenses

Debt service as a percentage of operating expenses indicates the percentage of operating expenses applied to the maximum annual debt service burden.

Reserve Ratio

The *reserve ratio* measures the strength of an organization's available cash position relative to its long-term debt.

The next two items, although not capital structure ratios, are included here because they may be leading indicators of future capital needs:

Percentage of plant fully depreciated: Accumulated depreciation, divided by gross total property and equipment.

Average age of plant: Accumulated depreciation, divided by depreciation expense. This result is expressed in years and may indicate the possible need for future capital expenditures.

Long-Term Debt as a Percentage of Total Assets

The *ratio of long-term debt to total assets* reflects indebtedness as it relates to all assets owned. It indicates the relative strength or weakness of a community's capital structure.

Debt-to-Capitalization Ratio

The *debt-to-capitalization ratio* measures leverage and capital structure in relation to net equity or fund balance. It reflects the strength of the equity or net asset base. Exhibit 2.6 summarizes the calculation of capital structure and cash flow ratios.

Exhibit 2.5   Calculation of Liquidity Ratios

Current ratio

$$\frac{\text{Current assets}}{\text{Current liabilities}}$$

Net days in accounts receivable

$$\frac{\text{Accounts receivable (net)}}{\text{Daily operating revenues}}$$

Days cash on hand

$$\frac{\text{Current assets: cash}}{\text{\textit{Plus} assets whose use is limited to capital improvements or investments}}{\text{Daily operating expenses}}$$

Average days in current liabilities

$$\frac{\text{Total current liabilities}}{\text{Daily operating expenses}}$$

Cushion ratio

$$\frac{\text{Current assets: cash}}{\text{\textit{Plus} assets whose use is limited to capital improvements or investments}}{\text{Maximum annual debt service}}$$

Exhibit 2.6   Calculation of Capital Structure and Cash Flow Ratios

Debt service coverage ratio: Revenues only

$$\frac{\begin{array}{c}\text{Excess (deficit) of revenues over expenses}\\ \textit{Plus}\text{ interest expense}\\ \textit{Plus}\text{ depreciation expense}\\ \textit{Plus}\text{ amortization expense}\\ \textit{Minus}\text{ amortization of deferred revenue from nonrefundable advance fees (if any)}\end{array}}{\text{Maximum annual debt service}}$$

Debt service as a percentage of net operating and nonoperating revenues

$$\frac{\text{Maximum annual debt service}}{\begin{array}{c}\text{Total revenues}\\ \textit{Minus}\text{ amortization of deferred revenue from nonrefundable advance fees (if any)}\\ \textit{Plus}\text{ nonoperating revenues}\end{array}}$$

Debt service as a percentage of operating expenses

$$\frac{\text{Maximum annual debt service}}{\text{Total operating expenses}}$$

Reserve ratio

$$\frac{\begin{array}{c}\text{Current assets: cash}\\ \textit{Plus}\text{ assets whose use is limited to capital improvements and investments}\end{array}}{\begin{array}{c}\text{Long-term debt}\\ \textit{Less}\text{ current maturities}\end{array}}$$

Long-term debt as a percentage of total assets

$$\frac{\text{Long-term debt, }\textit{less}\text{ current maturities}}{\text{Total assets}}$$

Debt-to-capitalization ratio

$$\frac{\text{Long-term debt, }\textit{less}\text{ current maturities}}{\text{Long-term debt, }\textit{less}\text{ current maturities} + \text{Unrestricted fund balance}}$$

■ INTERPRETING FINANCIAL STATEMENTS

Ratios are helpful but must be used with caution. They are not in and of themselves proofs, but rather clues, providing a basis on which to form a judgment about financial performance. Suspicion of an unfavorable condition might be aroused by an unsatisfactory ratio. Conversely, the conclusion that a community is financially strong may be confirmed by compiling a series of ratios. Moreover, the significance of specific ratios varies among different forms of ownership. In analyzing a for-profit community, for example, partic-ular emphasis is laid on the operating or expense ratio. In a nonprofit community, this ratio is largely meaningless.

In their empirical analysis of continuing care retirement communities, Powell and Winklevoss caution that "the drawback of ratio analysis is that even though they may be useful for setting minimum standards, they are heavily dependent on a component that can remain constant over time (debt service), whereas other elements are increasing for inflation. This results in unusually high ratio values in future years. Therefore, taken alone, ratio analysis can present a misleading picture of the community's financial picture."[4]

Ratios calculated from a community's financial statements for only one year have limited value. They become meaningful, however, when compared with similar ratios for the same community (or company) over time, or with comparable ratios for similar companies or with industry averages. When comparing ratios externally, it is important to ensure not only that the communities are similar but also that the basis used to calculate each ratio is the same.

A trend is shown by selecting a base date or period, treating the figure or ratio for that period as 100, and then dividing it successively into the comparable ratios for subsequent periods. Analyzing trends in these ratios and in the operational revenues and expenses is useful because it identifies changes from year to year. This approach is also much simpler and lends itself to clearer interpretation than the alternative, two-step method of calculating percentage changes from year to year. See Appendix B for definitions of typical senior living metrics.

Whether proprietary or nonprofit, each owner has different financial performance expectations. The executive director and her direct supervisor should understand each other's objectives fully. An operation works best when the needs and interests of the owner are held in balance with the expectations of the residents and employees.

NOTES

1. American Seniors Housing Association, *Selected Seniors Housing Transactions* (Washington, DC, 1994), 15–16.

2. R. Delaney, B. J. Epstein, J. R. Adler, and M. F. Foran, *GAAP: Interpretation and Application of Generally Accepted Accounting Principles* (New York: John Wiley, 1993).

3. E. C. Merrigan, *Rating Guidelines for Nonprofit Continuing Care Retirement Communities: Fitch Health Care Special Report* (New York: Fitch Investor Services, 1994).

4. A. V. Powell and H. E. Winklevoss, *Continuing Care Retirement Communities: An Empirical, Financial, and Legal Analysis* (Homewood, IL: Pension Research Council, 1984), 176.

3

Management and Human Resources

The stability and consistency of a community's operation rest in the hands of the on-site employees and in the management's ability to minimize turnover. The senior housing industry is a "people" business, and operators who recognize the importance and value of long-term employees will ultimately be more successful. My roots are in the nursing home business, where there is a hierarchy among the staff that is very structured. The acquisitions program at the company for which I worked was aimed at troubled facilities, most of which experienced similar management problems. Usually it was not the owner's lack of commitment to good-quality care but rather the politics of the management on site that led to turnover in the ranks. This instability translated into problems with the consistency of care. In any operation, consistency *equals* credibility.

The employees at the bottom of the totem pole are as essential to the success of the facility as the managers. In a nursing home, these are the certified nursing assistants (CNAs). This title has always seemed a misnomer to me: if anything, the nurses assist the CNAs, who do all the physical work of caring for residents. The CNA job is without doubt one of the toughest, tantamount to indoor manual labor. It is emotionally and physically draining.

So what keeps CNAs in their jobs? In fact, there is a lot of turnover in these positions, usually more than in any other position on the property. Those who stay either are totally committed to their residents or lack the motivation to seek employment elsewhere. CNAs cannot be motivated simply by the pay they earn, but they will stay if they are given supportive management and recognition. Over time, a symbiotic and even loving relationship may develop between residents and their CNAs. Residents will tell the CNAs how much they appreciate them, comment on their appearance, and help them through personal problems. For many employees, this recognition and encouragement are valuable sources of support and job satisfaction, and they reciprocate by giving residents the best care they are capable of. It is human nature for people (especially those giving and receiving care) to bond with each other. Managers who value and nurture this bonding can enjoy lower turnover and a higher employee commitment to quality care.

HIRING PERSONNEL

The single most important decision that managers make is the hiring decision. The quality and character of the employees determines the success of the business. Most managers find hiring and firing the most difficult aspects of the job. Inexperienced managers often hire the first qualified applicant who comes along, so as not to prolong the agony of the search and interview process. In the end, however, it takes less time and effort to hire a good employee than to fire a bad one.

Employers should seek applicants who show a genuine interest in and liking for older people. Caring employees working in an atmosphere of warmth and kindness make daily operations run more smoothly. Residents tend to overlook flaws in the operation if they are surrounded by staff members who sincerely care about them. Residents will be quick to point out each and every shortcoming of the operation if it is obvious that the employees are working at the community only to collect a paycheck and do not make an effort to develop personal relationships with them.

Advertising

Help-wanted newspaper advertising is a thing of the past. Job seekers in today's market will generally first seek employment online. This way they can quickly sort available positions by job type, salary, location, benefits, or qualifications by creating an online account with companies such as Indeed, ZipRecruiter, Glassdoor, or Monster. They will be searching an abundance of other postings as well so it will be important to create a posting that will captivate their interest.

Your posting description should be imaginative, witty, clear, and concise. It should suggest that the company is growing and a rewarding place to work. Your copy should also include a statement that you listen to your staff and incorporate their ideas into your operations policies. If you want your employees to have a sense of belonging, you need to give them a voice in resident care and feel that their opinions are valued and respected. Many qualified people who are currently employed routinely scan posted positions to learn about new companies and growth opportunities and to compare wages.

Abbreviate only when necessary, as overuse of this device can make the company appear cheap. Always include contact information, such as "Ask for Molly," to give the ad a personal touch. Be careful in wording the ad, as some phrases have negative connotations for job seekers. Marilyn Moats Kennedy, in her *Career Strategist* newsletter, explains that people may read "fast-growing company" to mean "sweatshop." A "lean" organization could be interpreted as one that has "been through budget cuts, a reorganization, downsizing, or all three." And a "prestigious" firm could be one that "hopes you'll accept the afterglow from its reputation in the place of money."[1]

An advertising agency can be helpful in developing effective online postings and advertisements. Well-designed display advertisements can significantly improve response rates, and agencies routinely develop them at no charge. Once the relationship has been established, the community need only call the agency with its request, and the agency will incorporate the ad requests directly into a predesigned corporate template and send the camera-ready artwork directly to the online host.

THE INTERVIEW PROCESS

The most successful managers are those who hire and surround themselves with high-quality, self-confident people, who in turn hire the same type of people to work for them. The result is an organization built on strength and confidence from the bottom up.

Achieving this goal is not easy, however, and the interview process can be particularly challenging. In a short time, you must develop a rapport with a candidate and evaluate whether the individual is capable of performing the essential functions of the job, fitting the profile acceptable to both the management and the residents, blending into the current team, and carrying out the work in a professional and caring manner. The interviewer must create a favorable impression of the community regardless of whether the candidate is excellent or disappointing.

Interviewing to fill a management position is especially difficult. Most résumés detail accomplishments and work history but tell nothing about the candidate's people skills and management abilities. Most candidates can tell you in great detail how to do a job, but a manager needs to know how to get the job done through others.

There is no easy way to evaluate a candidate's management skills in a short interview or on paper. Nevertheless, all other management decisions pale in comparison to the hiring decision. Once made, it is not easily reversed. Other employees and the residents whom they serve are depending on the manager to make the right choice.

Preparing for the Interview

Careful preparation, along with specific training in interview skills, allows an interviewer to take full advantage of the limited time available with each candidate. To begin, she should establish a clear idea of requirements and the selection criteria for the position.

The following traits, skills, and abilities are important in employees working with seniors:

Appearance: Creates a positive first impression through appropriate standards of dress and grooming; displays a self-confident, friendly, and capable demeanor.

Initiative: Takes action to achieve goals; self-starting rather than passively accepting. Generates alternative solutions to problems and initiates action beyond the minimum called for.

Enthusiasm: Displays a cheerful, helpful, service-oriented attitude. Maintains a high level of activity.

Creativity: Generates or recognizes imaginative, innovative solutions in work-related situations. Demonstrates ability to implement an ordinary idea with extraordinary style and flair.

Maturity: Able to reflect on and learn from experiences. Projects self-confidence based on an accurate self-assessment of strengths and weaknesses. Can exercise patience and self-control in difficult situations. Demonstrates awareness of social, ethical, and legal norms in job-related activities. Able to balance work priorities and personal priorities.

Tenacity: Shows willingness and drive to work through difficulties to achieve goals, as well as perseverance in maintaining high standards of excellence.

Common sense: Exercises sound judgment, develops alternative courses of action, and makes decisions that are based on logical assumptions and reflect factual information. Calmly exercises resourcefulness when faced with an unexpected challenge.

Flexibility: Demonstrates ability to adjust readily to new and changing circumstances. Maintains adaptability in varying environments in which tasks, responsibilities, or people are constantly changing. Able to switch to a new or different way of doing something to accomplish a goal.

Warmth and kindness: Describes former peers and residents in terms of endearment and compassion. Is motivated by the development of interpersonal relationships and is a good communicator. Seems relaxed, friendly, is engaging. This is the most important characteristic for employees who will be dealing directly with residents. Residents will immediately spot and may feel threatened by an employee who is not sincere. As residents age, they feel more vulnerable, so it is important to surround them with warm and caring employees.

Communication skills: Expresses ideas clearly and appropriately and demonstrates active listening skills. Is patient when communicating with elderly people and does not interrupt when someone is talking. Written communications demonstrate appropriate vocabulary and correct grammar and syntax.

Interpersonal skills: Demonstrates ability to meet people easily and build rapport quickly. Shows consideration for the feelings and needs of others. Puts people at ease; gets along well with a variety of people at all organizational levels.

Organizational skills: Plans a logical course of action or establishes a system to accomplish goals. Properly allocates time, personnel, and resources to meet objectives and deadlines.

Work experience: Possesses relevant job experience that demonstrates interest in the senior living industry. Has demonstrated effective work relationships with peers and supervisors. Has the ability to apply and transfer insights from one work environment to another. (A pattern of dissatisfaction with working conditions, supervisors, or coworkers may indicate instability in the applicant.)

Leadership ability: Uses appropriate interpersonal styles and methods in guiding individuals (subordinates, peers, and supervisors) or groups to accomplish a task without relying on authority or position. Earns the respect of coworkers and subordinates through demonstrated results. Takes an active interest in helping others achieve their goals. Sets high standards of performance for self, and inspires others to achieve.

Education: Has completed relevant course work and achieved an adequate level of scholastic attainment. Has demonstrated similar levels of effort and motivation in achieving school- and work-related goals.

The interviewer should then familiarize herself with the list of interview candidates and thoroughly review their résumés. The key to reviewing a résumé is the ability to recognize what information is there as well as what is *not*. Omissions or unusual information on the résumé or application are signals that the interviewer may need more information about the candidate before reaching a decision. Important pieces of information to note when reviewing a résumé include the following:

- Appearance of the résumé; correct use of vocabulary, grammar, and syntax
- Level of scholastic achievement
- Degree(s) earned, or relevant course work
- Language proficiency
- Work experience relevant to the senior housing industry
- Descriptions of former positions and duties performed
- Relevant activities and interests, as opposed to "filler" intended merely to impress
- Gaps in employment or school attendance
- Reasons for leaving previous jobs
- Job-related health problems
- Availability for work

Conducting the Interview

Interviewing requires a great deal of effort, concentration, and practice. Gathering the same general background data from each candidate and remembering what each candidate said may appear a daunting task, but it becomes much more manageable when a standardized technique is rehearsed and used. The following five-step plan can form the basis for a thorough interview in which the maximum amount of information can be exchanged in a short time.

STEP 1: BUILDING RAPPORT. The first step is to put the candidate at ease and establish a warm, conversational tone. People communicate better when they feel relaxed. Interviews are stressful: most people are forced to step outside their comfort zone when talking about themselves and their accomplishments. Try to set the candidate at ease and begin to build trust. Only candidates who are comfortable with the interviewer will be willing to open up and share positive and negative information about their experiences.

Before the interview, carefully note the candidate's name and some highlights of his or her background so that you can personalize the interview questions. This personal touch will help build rapport as well as allow you to focus on relevant data.

Greet each candidate with a warm, pleasant smile and a firm handshake; look the candidate in the eye and let her know you are sincerely interested in spending time with her. Use small talk to start the conversation flowing. The important thing is to get the applicant talking about herself. Most people open up when the conversation turns to a subject of special interest or involves personal experience, hobbies, or an accomplishment of which they are particularly proud.

As soon as the candidate is relaxed, the interview can begin. By mentally preparing a transition statement in advance, you can move smoothly into the information-gathering stage without appearing abrupt. The transition statement should politely signal to the candidate that the "official" interview is about to begin.

STEP 2: GATHERING INFORMATION. Some information about a candidate, such as level of social skills or verbal expression, can be easily gathered in the interview. The next task is to dig for additional information. The purpose of the information-gathering phase is to ask questions that gather examples of past job and educational experiences related to the selection criteria, and to keep the candidate talking and maintain rapport while avoiding inappropriate topics.

Ask broadly based or open-ended questions. For example: "Suppose you begin by telling me about your last position. I would be interested in how you chose the company and what you liked best and least about your former job." (See chapter 15 for more on gathering information and asking probing questions.) A good way to let the candidate know that references will be checked is to ask him how he thinks his references would answer questions about him. Concentrate on the candidate's story, listening for significant clues, analyzing their meaning, and noting any inconsistencies or gaps that should be explored with follow-up questions.

Follow-up questions should elicit details about the information or experiences the candidate shared in response to a general question. You might say, "That's interesting. Tell me more," or "Why did you make that decision?" or "How did you react when that happened?" Even a silent pause can be used effectively as a follow-up question, encouraging the candidate to share more information in an effort to break the silence. The candidate should do most of the talking. Listen actively; avoid interrupting the candidate or changing the subject abruptly, and always be alert to nonverbal cues that may provide clues to the candidate's comfort level and veracity of her responses. (See chapter 15 for tips on improving listening skills.)

Give the candidate your complete attention, maintain eye contact, and paraphrase any unclear statements he makes. When the candidate expresses personal opinions, consider how they are expressed and whether they are consistent with the philosophy of the organization and the employee team.

Certain questions should be avoided, some because they will not yield useful information and others because they delve into inappropriate areas. Title VII of the Civil Rights Act of 1964 requires that selection criteria for job applicants be "job related." Any questions asked in a selection interview that directly or indirectly uncover information about the following areas are specifically prohibited by law: age, race, national origin, religion, marital status, dependents, child care concerns, housing, health status, type of military discharge, arrest records, sexual preference, willingness to work weekends, and any information from minority or female applicants not routinely requested of white or male applicants.

Exhibit 3.1 lists sample interview questions for candidates applying for management positions.

STEP 3: SELLING YOURSELF AND THE COMPANY. Job interviews should involve an exchange of information. Highly qualified people will require a high-quality work environment with a company that recognizes and values the individual contributions of each employee. Top people are in short supply: they are usually treated well by their employers and are comfortable in their current positions. To attract them away from competitors, an organization must demonstrate distinct advantages. Wages and salaries play only a small part in attracting people; the real motivators are the work environment and opportunities for growth.

Explain the mission of the company and note that it has grown by building on the strengths of its employees and their commitment to its mission. Success

stories build a desire to share in the company's success and motivate top candidates to want to join: examples include stories of employees who have overcome adversity and turned challenge into achievement that have strengthened the company. Ultimately, the company's reputation (good or bad) determines the type of employee who will work there. Satisfied employees are the best advertisement for new staff members.

Describe specifically the requirements and expectations of the position. The more clearly these are communicated, the more likely it is that the chosen candidate will succeed in the job. Many applicants will need a definition of assisted living or congregate housing, including a description of the services offered and the company's management philosophy. This information can help the applicant understand the job duties and performance expectations.

Finally, emphasize the considerable rewards of serving elderly people. Employees of senior living facilities are uniquely empowered to make a difference in the lives of residents. A caring staff can help seniors accept aging and cope with everyday difficulties. The reward that comes from helping people can be the single most effective motivating factor, for job satisfaction can never be bought with a paycheck.

STEP 4: CLOSING THE INTERVIEW. The conclusion of the interview is important to the candidate's overall impression of the company. Thank the candidate for his time and be encouraging but noncommittal. Tell the candidate when you expect to reach a decision, who will contact him, and whom to call if he has any questions. Verify his phone number and let him know that references will be checked.

Few gestures better reflect the high quality of the organization than the courtesy of sending a personal note. I send a note to each applicant, thanking him or her for the interview. The note usually says that the person's qualifications and background are impressive, that we are flattered that he or she is interested in working for our company, and that we look forward to the possibility of working together. Not only can this simple gesture communicate the quality of the organization, but it may also create within the applicant a desire to belong to it. Impressing an applicant in this way can strengthen the manager's negotiating position at the time of hiring while setting the stage for a positive working relationship.

Exhibit 3.1   Sample Interview Questions for Management Candidates

I. Education

1. How did you become interested in this field?
2. What courses did you particularly enjoy or excel at?
3. What courses were a challenge for you?
4. Did you participate in any clubs or organizations?
5. How long did it take you to complete your degree or certification?
6. How has your education prepared you for this position?

II. Experience

1. How has your experience prepared you for this position?
2. At this point in your career, are you satisfied with what you have accomplished? Have you realized the career goals that you set for yourself?
3. What are your most important career accomplishments?
4. Have you ever been promoted?
5. What features of your previous jobs have you liked?
6. Describe your best boss and your worst.
7. What is the best piece of constructive criticism that you ever received? What did you do with it?

III. Motivation

1. What interests you most about the position we have? What interests you least?
2. What are your short- and long-term planning objectives?
3. Apart from benefits and compensation, how would you look to gain from or develop in this role?
4. How would you describe success?

5. What is the most important decision you have ever made?
6. What is the biggest disappointment you have suffered recently?
7. What do you look for in a position?
8. Why do you want to leave your current position?
9. What kind of references would you receive from your former employer?
10. What would you like to do better? or What do you struggle with?
11. As your new boss, what should I learn from your former boss on how to motivate you?

IV. Personality

1. What is the greatest risk you have ever taken?
2. What do you look for in the people you hire?
3. How would your coworkers describe you? Your subordinates?
4. Describe the professional profile of someone whom you admire. What are some of their professional skills that you would like to incorporate into your own professional style?
5. How do you communicate impartiality to your staff?
6. How do you create personal and professional boundaries?
7. How do you find time to think and plan strategically each week? When do you call for help?
8. What professional accomplishments are you most proud of?
9. What keeps you up at night worrying about in your work life?
10. Do you have any questions for me?

If the candidate has been eliminated from the selection process, explain why. There are many legitimate reasons for declining applicants, including the following:

- The applicant is qualified for the position, but other applicants may be better suited to the team.
- The applicant's skills do not meet the requirements for the position.
- The applicant has insufficient education or experience for the position.
- The applicant provided false information on the application or résumé.

STEP 5: EVALUATING THE CANDIDATE. Evaluate all the information collected to determine whether the candidate possesses the traits necessary to succeed in the position. The evaluation process draws on information from the résumé and interview and from former employers and coworkers. The hiring decision is often a gamble; there are many more marginal applicants than top-quality people looking for jobs. Take the time to make an informed decision, for a decision made in haste can create conflict within an established team and be time-consuming to reverse. In addition, a bad hire can reflect poorly on the manager and embarrass the company.

It is generally better to hire someone who is slightly underqualified for a position and can then be trained and molded than to hire someone who may be overqualified for the job and may feel that he is settling for less than what he wants or deserves. It is easier to motivate someone who is feeling challenged in the job than someone who feels bored.

The best predictor of future performance is past behavior, and reference checks are the most reliable way to verify impressions and authenticate the information the candidate has presented. Do not make up your mind about a candidate before checking references, even if you feel pressure to do so. Incomplete reference checks can put the organization at risk of hiring a problem employee and cause the interviewer to pass up others who deserve consideration. The candidate should be asked to provide the names and phone numbers of at least one subordinate (if the position entails supervision), one peer, and one supervisor. One measure of the quality of an employee is how that person treats people at all levels in the organization. Managers who treat subordinates and supervisors differently may be inconsistent in how they perform the many functions of their jobs.

Formulate questions before contacting an applicant's references. Questions asked of a candidate's subordinate should pertain to sense of fairness, job knowledge, attitude toward employees and management, supervisory skills, and interest in subordinates' career growth. Questions for a peer might address teamwork, involvement in company politics, demonstration of willingness to share credit for accomplishments, and the candidate's success in the job. The nine tough questions in exhibit 3.2 are adapted from *Robert Half on Hiring*, by Robert Half, the founder of one of the largest recruiting firms in the United States.[2]

Checking references is a time-consuming and often frustrating process in today's litigious business environment, for many employers hesitate to be candid in giving references, fearing a lawsuit by a former employee. And even if employers are forthcoming, it is not always easy to interpret their comments, especially if they do not confirm the interviewer's impressions of the candidate. Most people have established long-term behavior patterns: do not assume you can manage an unsatisfactory applicant into a good employee. Most behavior problems follow people from one job to the next; if they had difficul-

---

Exhibit 3.2   Nine Tough Questions for a Candidate's References

1. How does this candidate compare to the person who's doing the job now? Or, what characteristics will you look for in his replacement?
2. If this candidate was so good, why didn't you try to rehire her? Or, why didn't you try to induce her to stay?
3. When there was a particularly urgent assignment, what steps did she take to get it done on time?
4. None of us is perfect at everything we do; please describe some of his shortcomings.
5. Have you seen his current résumé? Let me read you the part that describes his job with your organization. (Stop at each significant point and ask the reference for a comment.)
6. Not all employees like all other employees. With what kinds of people did she have difficulty?
7. On average, how many times a month does he take off for personal reasons or sickness? How many times a month did he come in late or leave early?
8. Who referred her to your company? (Could it have been a relative or a customer or client?)
9. When she was hired, were her references checked thoroughly? Who checked these references, and what did her references have to say?

---

ties with former employers, they may have the same (or worse) difficulties with you.

Do not expect all information to fit perfectly. Most people are not specific when offering comments about an employee; ask them to explain any broad generalization. If you hear only glowing accounts of an employee's past performance, ask the source to cite specific examples to support those accolades.

When hiring employees who will have direct contact with seniors, try to speak with residents she has worked with, the president of the resident council, or an unrelated senior to test perceptions of the candidate's attitude and approach toward elderly people. Seniors are generally candid and can provide the most important perspective—that of the customer.

In an industry that brings employees into contact with vulnerable elderly people, it is essential to hire trustworthy staff and to conduct background checks. The Criminal Offender Record Information System

(CORI) includes records and data compiled by a criminal justice agency that relate to the nature or disposition of criminal charges, arrests, pretrial proceedings, other judicial proceedings, sentencing, incarceration, rehabilitation, and release. The Criminal History Systems Board restricts access to this information to individuals or businesses for which it has been determined that the public interest in disseminating such information clearly outweighs the risk to security and privacy. This category includes senior living communities. This information is collected and controlled by each state, although federal databases also exist. After going through a certification process, a management designee can access the system for a fee per employee to screen current and prospective employees and volunteers who may have unsupervised contact with elderly or infirm people in their homes. Consistent use of the CORI system helps the management minimize the risk of criminal activity among employees. Employees should be notified that all staff members who work with residents in the privacy of their units are subject to a CORI check, and new hires should be notified at the time of the interview.

Given the challenges of recruiting, selecting, and screening potential employees, hiring former employees or promoting from within is often the best and safest choice. The individual is already well known to the organization, and rewarding top performers with promotion boosts company morale. Recommendations from friends and acquaintances can also yield qualified candidates, although it is wise to check references regardless of who recommended the candidate.

Finally, do not be afraid to reject all your candidates and start the process over: wait for the right candidate, and sooner or later she or he will come around. It is far better to be slightly shorthanded or ask other department heads to pitch in than to hire the wrong person for the job. The residents will understand; after all, they are paying for, and expect, the best.

In many areas of the country, the competition for qualified and competent staff members outstrips the competition for prospective residents. It is a good idea to develop a one-page summary fact sheet outlining the employee benefits offered by the company. It is also helpful to develop a brochure that attractively presents the benefit plan.

For new hires, the benefit plan should be perceived as part of the total compensation package.

One good way to convey this impression is to develop a compensation summary worksheet for each employee that calculates the dollar value to the employee of each benefit. It can be prorated for part-time employees. The prospective employee can see that, even if the starting wage may be lower than that of competing companies, the total value of the compensation package reflects a much higher dollar figure. These summary sheets should also be prepared annually for all employees when raises are announced to remind them of the value added in the benefit package, or to minimize dissatisfaction resulting from changing benefit plans.

Once a job offer has been accepted, send the newly hired candidate a letter to confirm the terms of employment, along with the compensation summary worksheet. The letter should welcome and encourage the new employee and confirm the title, salary, commencement date, and review schedule. It should also state the direct supervisor's name and include a job description to be signed in duplicate and returned. Finally, the letter should restate the company's objectives. For example, "I am looking forward to this new partnership and to the significant contribution that I know you will make to our operations. Let's work together to make [the company] the preferred provider, the choice employer, and the standard by which excellence will be measured in the senior living industry. If you have any questions or need clarification, please feel free to contact me. Otherwise, please sign and return the second copy of this letter to confirm your acceptance of this offer. Welcome!"

Sometimes even the best research will not avert a problem after an employee has been hired. In such a situation, you might want to call a few of the references again: "Remember me? I'm Ben Pearce. I called you about six weeks ago in connection with a reference that you gave regarding Joe Slow, and we hired him." Ask the source for clarification about the employee's problem. When confronted with a specific complaint, the source is likely to be more candid and offer some suggestions on how to manage the issue. At the very least, the source will think twice before offering such an enthusiastic endorsement in the future.

PERFORMANCE EVALUATIONS

Giving employees feedback on their performance is fundamental to good management. The evaluation process provides an opportunity to assess an employee's performance from a manager's point of view, and the manager's ability to manage from the employee's point of view. It creates a setting in which managers and staff members can overcome objections, voice concerns, and discuss opportunities, goals, and expectations. The result should be a positive exchange of information leading to a clear-cut set of goals and objectives for continued staff development. As managers, we are empowered to be leaders and teachers, providing specific guidelines and opportunities for growth and exerting personal influence on our organizations.

In practice, however, the evaluation process is often fraught with anticipation and anxiety for everyone involved. Annual reviews provide managers and employees with the opportunity to review and evaluate the process, allowing greater understanding of its importance. Yet managers often conduct a performance evaluation with one goal in mind: to get through it without having to tell an employee how they really feel.

Any meaningful evaluation process must be ongoing. Each employee is entitled to regular and consistent feedback. Even a distinguished performer should receive feedback on areas of possible improvement and be given goals and objectives for continued development. The process should regularly note and evaluate themes or trends in an individual's performance, highlighting those that are positive, planning how to correct those that are not, focusing on future growth, and establishing priorities.

If the supervisor has proactively managed the employee's performance throughout the year by providing recognition and support for accomplishments and redirection when needed, the evaluation meeting should be the culmination of this process and should be a positive experience for both parties. It is not the time for surprises.

Performance evaluations are useful not only as an annual assessment tool but also as a means for managers to clarify their expectations. Often performance issues arise because employees become mired in details and lose sight of their priorities. The performance evaluation can help redefine the essential priorities of the position. Moreover, performance problems often indicate some bigger issue. The performance evaluation is one of the best tools at the manager's disposal to identify the fundamental problem and get things back on track.

Negative performance evaluations, or the fear of them, usually result from poor management. An inexperienced manager may avoid confronting performance issues, hoping things will improve. Procrastination leads to a deterioration of the situation and creates resentment. Breakdowns in communication between the supervisor and the employee almost always degenerate into conflict, ultimately leading to a hopeless situation that can result in the employee's termination. Managers must not be allowed to "fire problems away." It is easier and cheaper in the long run to manage performance than to start from scratch with a new employee. Managers should be taught to look for solutions to problems.

Evaluations of people working for more than one supervisor should be conducted by the supervisor of the department in which they spend most of their time. Input from the other supervisor(s) should be sought and used during the review process. The department head and the executive director should review every evaluation form before the supervisor discusses it with the employee. In this way, the executive director can understand the strengths and vulnerabilities of all the employees and help each supervisor clarify expectations for the staff. The executive director can also reemphasize the importance of the evaluation process and coach the supervisor on how to achieve the desired results.

▆▆▆▆ GUIDELINES FOR PERFORMANCE APPRAISALS

Like most management skills, constructive evaluation requires preparation, concentration, and practice. Summarizing information about an employee's strengths and areas for improvement is for most supervisors an agonizing task. Most of our time is spent handling the day-to-day issues that arise and performing the essential duties of our position. Rarely do we take time to communicate with our employees regarding how they feel about the job: their perceptions about work flow, residents, other employees, and the company. Yet the appraisal process can be a welcome respite from the daily grind and one of the most effective uses of a manager's time. Performance appraisals should be carefully planned and should encompass the following key components: (1) preparation, (2) discussing the appraisal, (3) giving feedback, (4) listening, (5) establishing agreement, (6) discussing improvement in performance, and (7) closing.

Step 1: Preparation

The appointment should be made well in advance so that the supervisor and employee have ample time to prepare for the discussion. It is a good idea to distribute a self-appraisal form that provides the employee an opportunity to evaluate her or his performance and begin to set future goals. The employee should return the completed form to the supervisor before the meeting.

Review the employee's personnel file before writing the appraisal of job performance. Pay particular attention to areas for improvement that were previously noted. Be prepared to review accomplishments and to discuss any negative areas. Striking a balance between positive and negative feedback demonstrates the validity of the process and the manager's fairness.

The supervisor should anticipate and be able to answer several questions from the employee:

- How am I doing?
- Where do I go from here?
- What are my major skills?
- In what areas do I need to improve?
- What do I need to do to improve?

Step 2: Discussing the Appraisal

Schedule the meeting in a private place free from interruptions. Allow enough time so that neither party feels hurried. Avoid interrupting the appraisal to take care of business. After an appointment has been set, it should not be postponed, and the meeting should start on time, thus communicating to the employee the importance of the process and demonstrating respect.

Begin the meeting with a discussion of the purpose and objectives of the performance appraisal. Emphasize that the process is not intended simply to give the employee a report on his or her performance but also to open lines of communication. You may need to take some time to put the employee at ease. Most people find it difficult to talk about performance; the evaluation process is at best intimidating. The supervisor should set the stage for a relaxed discussion.

One way to begin is by discussing the performance of the department in general and areas of potential growth. Ask informally how the employee feels about the job: what does he think about the department, the supervisor, and coworkers? In this way, the employee can begin to feel comfortable talking about himself.

To discuss the evaluation form, you may want to review each item on a *blank* evaluation form, making sure that the employee understands all the criteria. Then allow the employee to discuss his views or to say what each evaluation criterion means to him. Sometimes it is easier to ask the employee for his own evaluation of how he is doing relative to the criterion. If the employee feels that he is not there to be criticized, he will tend to be more objective and honest with the supervisor—and himself. But if he thinks he is going to be disciplined as part of the evaluation process, he may become defensive and even argumentative. This is the hard way to evaluate performance. It is easier to be fair and honest with employees, showing concern and a genuine desire to look for solutions, than to provoke an argument during which neither party listens and nothing is accomplished. If the supervisor has done her job throughout the year by giving continuous feedback to the employee, then the evaluation process should be simply a summary of solutions and corrections, along with recognition for positive contributions. The employee should, likewise, feel free to share his views and help the supervisor understand how to manage the department and its employees more effectively.

Do not discuss merit increases during the appraisal. Although increases are based on performance, increases should be communicated at a later date, with approval from the management. A supervisor who promises an increase without approval may jeopardize her credibility in the eyes of employees.

Step 3: Giving Feedback

How you give feedback to an employee is just as important as *what* you say. If the style of the supervisor's feedback makes the employee defensive, then little will be communicated, and no improvement is likely. Employees often want to "cut to the chase" and determine their final rating. Instead, the supervisor should methodically cover each area, building justification for the outcome. Explain the expectations of the job as specifically as possible. It is up to the supervisor to take the guesswork out of good performance. Most people want to do a good job, but to do so they need and deserve to know what excellence is.

Characterize an employee's work in terms of the established performance standards. When commenting on interpersonal matters, *never* evaluate personality.

Criticizing someone's personality is unproductive and almost always evokes defensive reactions. Most people cannot change their personality, and an employee will recognize that if his supervisor finds fault with his personality, his long-term prospects with the company are limited. Behavior is manageable; personality is not.

The performance appraisal should present a balanced view of the employee's performance. Give feedback about strengths as well as weaknesses. Never withhold high ratings if they are deserved, for they build self-confidence and encourage people to strive even harder. Good news inspires employees to do even better, and effective managers will gain employee commitment by helping employees feel like winners. At the same time, be honest with the employee. It never helps to gloss over real problems by offering only praise: this is the reason that managers seeking to terminate a problem employee are often surprised to discover outstanding performance evaluations in the employee's personnel file. Most people are aware of their vulnerabilities, and they deserve feedback that will enable them to overcome them and grow as professionals.

Step 4: Listening

Listening is the key skill in performance appraisals. The very act of listening communicates to the employee that her opinions are valued and worthy of consideration. A manager who does not seek the opinions of employees is a fool. After all, they are doing the job; who better to advise the management on how it might be done better or more efficiently?

The most obvious way to get the employee talking is to begin by asking *what, how, where,* and *why.* For example, "How do you feel about improving _____?" Open-ended questions and follow-up questions solicit information on attitudes, commitment, and understanding of the job. The supervisor in turn needs to demonstrate some flexibility and sincere interest.

Some tangible evidence of acceptance is helpful in encouraging the employee to speak out. Nod, smile encouragingly, and punctuate the employee's statements with "Yes," "Good idea," or "I see." Reassurance is particularly important if the employee is saying something that may cause him anxiety.

Paraphrasing is another useful method of encouraging others to talk and demonstrating that the supervisor is listening. Restate in your own words what you think the employee is saying. Capture the es-

sence of the thought and repeat it. Usually the person will pick up on the restatement and continue talking, giving more information.

The ideal time to be silent is after you ask a question. The employee knows it is his turn to talk. If the employee pauses before responding, you know he is trying to decide what to share. Silence is also useful when the employee stops speaking. Wait a few seconds before going on; the employee may be hesitant about telling you something important.

Step 5: Establishing Agreement

Listening without arguing helps people accept feedback. If you disagree with the employee on a particular point, clarify the areas of disagreement and summarize. If the employee disagrees with the observation, let him voice his feelings. Make every attempt to resolve the conflict by giving specific examples of performance. Look first for small things on which both parties can agree in order to build consensus.

Focus on the issues. In the face of criticism, many employees strike back, attacking a manager's style and personality. Try to resist the temptation to become defensive. Do not allow the employee to redirect the focus to community problems not relevant to the employee's personal performance.

Do not allow yourself to be backed into a corner by an employee. If you are too quick to give in on one point, the employee may pick at others. But if the employee raises a valid concern, be prepared to admit the misunderstanding and correct it. Ultimately, the purpose of the evaluation is to clarify expectations and manage the employee's performance in a fair and consistent manner.

Step 6: Discussing Improvement in Performance

The employee should be involved as much as possible in identifying areas needing improvement. Be careful not to intimidate her by focusing on too many areas at once. It is preferable to set priorities and develop action plans for the most important areas, which you can identify by asking, "What is the negative impact on the operation if nothing is done to improve the situation?" Focus on the issues most visible to the residents and other employees or those that affect the quality of the services rendered.

A success plan should be specific and stick to the issues. The plan should define and clarify the expectations for the job. It should illustrate what an employee needs to do to succeed in the job, and paint a clear picture of what success looks like rather than document failures. The plan should be clear and specific enough to reduce the expectation to a choice: the employee can either choose to follow the plan and succeed in the position, or choose not to follow the plan, a decision that can be used to justify termination. The plan should establish specific goals and target dates for achieving them.

The law protects employees from discrimination and wrongful termination. The federal Equal Employment Opportunity Commission (EEOC) will provide employees with free counseling and arbitration if they file a complaint. The first thing an EEOC investigator will ask is whether the employee was treated fairly. A record of proactive action plans that confirm the management's efforts to influence the employee in a positive manner before termination and demonstrate that the employee *chose* not to respond can help avoid a negative EEOC determination or legal action. Employers who get into legal trouble with employees usually have either failed to communicate expectations or made a bad hire in the first place. It is simply good business to treat people fairly.

Performance appraisals should never be used to put pressure on an employee, to find an excuse for discharging someone, or to bully someone into changing their behavior. Such actions will cause employees to fear the process rather than perceive it as useful. The management should motivate employees to deliver good service and equip them to do so, rather than threaten them if they do not.

Step 7: Closing

The closing of the performance appraisal meeting is as important as the opening. Conducting it properly will maximize the possibility of improving performance. It should entail the following steps:

- Ask the employee to recap his understanding of the major topics of the review and plans for achieving them. This gives the supervisor the opportunity to determine whether the employee has understood the points communicated.
- Ask the employee for his overall feelings about the review. If they are negative, encourage him to say more. You do not have to agree: merely granting the

employee the right to express negative feelings can be helpful in dissipating them. Many organizations allow the employee's responses to the appraisal process to become part of the record. This practice is useful for managers to understand what personal barriers may be present which may prevent managing the employee to more positive outcomes.

- Ask the employee to sign the appraisal form. If the employee refuses to sign, the supervisor should remind him that his signature merely confirms that the appraisal discussion occurred and does not indicate agreement with the points raised.
- End the review on a positive note. Everyone benefits from a well-executed performance review: the employee, the supervisor, the residents, and the company.
- Most important, make a commitment to follow up and participate in the employee's success. The management's commitment to making this process worthwhile, positive, and honest will be reflected in the overall success of the company.

COMPENSATION

Before determining wage scales and calculating merit increases, the management needs to survey local wages and employment rates. It should first decide how competitive it wants to be in the labor market. Does it want to pay at the high end of the scale, as do many start-up operators or troubled facilities, or at the low end, trading on its good reputation, desirable location, or stability? Paying a competitive wage is critical if the community wants to attract and retain employees.

Management should also strive for consistency in its pay scales. If entry-level wages are standardized, overall wage administration will be perceived as generally fair. Few things foment more employee dissatisfaction than the perception of favoritism or inequity in compensation rates. Standardization of wages also helps avoid legal complications and labor relations issues, such as disputes over equal pay for equal work.

The most important source of information is the community's primary competitors. Collect wage and salary data on each position in the community, from dishwasher to administrator. The best way to collect this information is to have the bookkeeper from your community place a call to the bookkeeper of each competitor. The bookkeeper should explain that he is conducting a wage and salary survey of communities in the area and offer to share information with them. Usually, the other bookkeeper will share information if the arrangement is reciprocal, but if he is hesitant, offer to have the executive director call the competitor's executive director. Request information on entry-level hourly wage, the size and frequency of incremental increases, shift differentials, employment inducements, and benefit levels. Compare the information to the current rate and actual average rate for each position in your community. Also consider factors influencing the competitors' pay scales, such as labor unions and business and product quality. Once entry-level rates have been established, there should be no exceptions. Adjustments for current employees may be appropriate and can be handled through the performance-evaluation process so that they are tied to performance rather than market conditions.

Other sources of information on compensation include online website postings such as Indeed or ZipRecruiter, the state department of wage and labor, and trade associations such as Argentum.[3]

Although it is important to pay competitive wages, work environment and community reputation are also key factors in job satisfaction. Top-quality employees rarely leave to go to a competitor for a few dollars more if they are satisfied in the job and believe the management treats them fairly and values them.

Mature communities that are well managed and consequently enjoy low employee turnover often need to establish maximums for hourly positions. It is standard practice in the industry to set this limit, often referred to as the "red circle," at 25 percent above the established minimum. The maximum rate is then increased if the minimum rate is increased, to avoid wage compression. When employees reach the maximum, other forms of incentive should be available. These may include the following:

- An annual bonus based on performance. This can be equivalent to the budgeted percentage increase for the community, but it is paid in a lump sum, while the base rate remains constant.
- Additional vacation or personal days.
- Company-paid health insurance or dental insurance premiums.
- Company contributions to retirement plans.
- Creative scheduling.

Calculating Merit Increases

It is helpful to establish guidelines for outstanding, competent, and acceptable performance and to use ranges, not a flat percentage (e.g., 4 to 6 percent for "competent"). The high end of the scale should be set to place the individual's salary at an appropriate position in the salary range with respect to length of service, performance, and the salaries of other employees in the same or similar positions.

Employees with less than 12 months of service should receive a prorated share of the annual merit increase. This strategy helps avoid wage compression and promotes fairness. For example:

"Jane Doe" is a concierge. She has been with the company for 10 months. Her present salary is $12.00 per hour. She has been rated as a competent employee and will receive a 4 percent increase. The computation is as follows:

$12.00 per hour × 0.04 (percent of increase) = $0.48
$0.48 ÷ 12 shares = $0.04
$0.04 × 10 shares = $0.40
(based on 10 months of service) per hour increase

A computer spreadsheet can be developed to prorate employee raises based on the date of hiring. The total compensation increases can then be calculated by department or for the entire community for comparison to the budget. Usually flat percentages are used to adjust the total payroll budget of the community for annual merit increases. The prorating method enables the management to allocate the total merit-increase dollars available in a way that rewards longevity and performance proportionately.

Annual increases at midyear minimize the cost to the community. Giving employees a 3 percent annual raise in July will cost the project only 1.5 percent for the fiscal year. This impact is further reduced by prorating raises for new hires.

EMPLOYEE OPINIONS

Soliciting employees' opinions about the operation is essential to good management and communication. No one knows better than the employee how her job might be done better, and employees have valuable perceptions about the management, training, resident satisfaction, benefits and compensation, and the company image. Collecting and analyzing employee opinions can not only help measure employee satisfaction but also communicate to middle management the company's expectations of how they should act toward the staff. Many companies use feedback from employee surveys to help manage dissatisfaction and reduce turnover. Employee turnover is the single highest cause of resident and family dissatisfaction. Residents and families come to trust and rely heavily on long-term employees with an intimate knowledge of their clients' preferences and needs. Such employees are the basis for the quality of care in a community.

Employee turnover tends to be higher in large facilities, as the management is not usually as aware of employee dissatisfaction in large groups. Turnover also tends to increase with the level of care. Employee burnout, stricter regulatory environments, management turnover, and pressure to perform all take a toll on longevity. Some nursing homes experience 90 to 100 percent turnover annually; in senior living communities, rates of 40 to 60 percent are more typical.

Employee turnover is usually calculated by dividing the total number of terminated employees in a given period (typically 12 months) by the sum of the total employees at the beginning of the year plus new hires. For example, if you have 100 employees at the beginning of the year, and you hire 50 new employees and terminate 25, you would have 17 percent turnover (25 terminations/[100 new hires + 50 beginning] = 17 percent), a good record by industry standards.

Companies that solicit regular feedback from employees often find that managers communicate better with the staff and treat them with more respect. The process communicates to the staff that the management values their opinions. Employees who feel they have some influence in the overall success of the community are more likely to think of themselves as part of a team and to feel they are helping to build something rather than just working shifts and collecting paychecks. Feelings of accomplishment can never be bought with a paycheck. Employees at all levels need to feel a sense of purpose when they come to work.

Surveys should be conducted at least annually (or more frequently if problems develop), and the management should expect 100 percent employee participation. The management should call a general meeting of the employees to go over the survey instrument and explain the importance of participation. The surveys should be distributed during a neutral time of year. When asked to evaluate something, most of us tap into our short-term memory, so a recent event, such as a wage increase, may positively or negatively skew the results. Because the survey is intended to summarize employees' opinions over a given period (the time elapsed since the last survey), they should be cautioned not to evaluate only their most recent encounter with the management. Furthermore, employees should be asked to ensure that their completed survey reflects their own opinions and not what they may have heard from other employees or from residents. Surveys can be distributed via an online service such as SurveyMonkey and sent to each of their email addresses. If they do not have an email or access to a computer, the business office can make arrangements for them to have web access at the facility with a laptop computer or tablet device. Encourage the employees to fill out the survey as soon as possible to discourage collaboration, and offer them a small incentive to complete their survey within 24 hours. Staff should be reminded that surveys will be tabulated by the website to guarantee the participants' anonymity and confidentiality.

The survey instrument should be designed with two objectives. First, it should solicit opinions on such matters as job satisfaction, supervision, management, perceptions of resident satisfaction, compensation and benefits, company image, and overall satisfaction. Second, it should reinforce the company's philosophy of supervision and management. The choice and wording of the questions communicate the company's mission and values. Provide a translation for those for whom English is a second language. It sends the wrong message when employees whose opinions are supposed to be valued must struggle to understand the survey.

A survey of any nature raises the expectations of the population surveyed. Employees offer their input on the assumption that the management intends to respond positively, quickly, and thoroughly to the issues and concerns raised. Some companies are reluctant to disseminate the results of surveys, fearing that some specific results may add fuel to the arguments of special-interest groups and affect employee morale. If the management is not willing to publicize and act on the responses, it is better not to conduct the survey at all. Conversely, positive results from an employee survey can be a powerful tool for recruitment. Negative responses exceeding a predetermined threshold should automatically trigger a plan of correction, which the department head and her direct supervisor should formulate within 30 days of the tabulation of the survey. Plans of correction that are SMART—specific, measurable, attainable, responsive, and time-measured—are most effective. This should not be an exercise that simply identifies existing problems and proposes general recommendations that are "ongoing." Department heads should call all their employees together to brainstorm so that everyone can be part of the solution. Plans of correction should describe the area in need of improvement in specific terms, detail a solution, assign a responsible party, and set a completion date. Employees who are encouraged to participate in the process have a greater tendency to own the results.

The results of an employee survey should never be used to discipline managers; rather, they should be used as a tool for training and education. Managers must embrace the process rather than fear it or use the feedback to retaliate against employees. The management should familiarize supervisors with the potential effect of survey results on productivity, profitability, and service.

■ MANAGEMENT

Employees are most productive when they are led, not threatened. The amateur manager sees employees as tools to perform critical functions in the business; the professional manager recognizes that the success of the business lies in the hands of its frontline staff members. The front line *is* the bottom line.

Today's successful business leaders reflect a paradox: they are tough as nails and uncompromising about their value systems, but at the same time they care deeply about and respect their employees. They are able to articulate a clear and broad vision of what their operation will look like when it runs well, while paying obsessive attention to detail.

In his book *Loyalty Rules!* Fred Reichheld points out that loyalty is the hallmark of great leadership. The long-term rewards of employee and customer loyalty ultimately outstrip even the most spectacular short-term profits. Loyalty, however, can be earned only when leaders put the welfare of their customers and employees ahead of their own interests.[4] Managers must evaluate decisions based on their effects on

customers (residents and their families), the employees who serve them, and owners. If the solution is one-sided, then loyalty may be compromised. Balance is the key: while sometimes a solution may favor one group over another, it is important that all groups feel that the management is treating them fairly.

Most organizational inflexibility is caused by people who have power and are unwilling to give it up. The professional manager is willing to listen and create an environment in which employees play an active role in decision making and have a stake in the success or failure of the operation. Table 3.1 differentiates the amateur manager from the professional manager.

Today's professional manager is a facilitator who understands basic human problems. She recognizes the value of the employee team and encourages everyone's participation. Her focus is positive and solution-oriented. The professional manager is "hands on" and looks for opportunities to develop the strengths of employees, rather than ways to assign blame when things go wrong. She defines excellence specifically for employees, and charts successes rather than failures. By teaching employees the essential elements of

Table 3.1 Characteristics of Amateur and Professional Managers

Amateur	Professional
Police officer	Cheerleader
Enforcer	Facilitator
Judgmental	Understanding
By the book	Flexible
Do it or else	Team builder
Closed-minded	Open-minded
Hypercritical	Supportive, rewarding
Negative focus (what is wrong)	Positive focus (what is right)
Seeks to blame	Seeks solutions
Hands-off	Hands-on
Hires the "right" person, and if they can't do the job, finds someone else	Developer of human potential; plans to ensure the success of the staff
Disciplines employees frequently	Uses a systematic approach to ensure employees' success
Generates fear or anxiety	Builds self-esteem
Reacts	Responds
Poor communicator	Friendly and approachable
Assumes	Ensures
Unclear about standards	Outlines specific expectations
Settles	Asks questions, probes
Waits for problems to arise	Follows through
Insecure	Confident

success and outlining the resources and expectations needed to do the job well, the manager ensures better performance. The professional manager then becomes a performance developer (see exhibit 3.3).

Psychologists have demonstrated that expectations alone can influence the behavior of others: if we have high expectations of our employees, they generally live up to those expectations. On the other hand, if we expect our employees to perform poorly or give us problems, they probably will.

The job of a manager is to influence subordinates, and some of the most miraculous rescues in the business world have been the result of positive expectations set by the management. Conversely, negative expectations can lead to failure: during the Depression, rumors of financial bankruptcies were self-fulfilling and led to the ruin of the country's economy at the New York Stock Exchange, where investors' beliefs about how a stock would perform influenced its value and ultimate performance. In business, as in other areas, expecting excellence can actually produce it.

A manager's expectations are transmitted by four critical means of communication:

1. **Climate:** Nonverbal messages from the manager or company leaders affect employee motivation and self-perception.
2. **Feedback:** Managers generally (subconsciously) give positive reinforcement to employees of whom they have high expectations and negative or limited feedback to those of whom they have low expectations.
3. **Input:** The high-expectation employee often receives the resources and a description of the expectations that are needed to do the job well, whereas the low-expectation employee receives little direction or information.
4. **Output:** High-expectation employees are given more opportunities to offer opinions and more assistance in finding solutions to problems.

▰▰▰▰▰ MOTIVATION AND REWARDS

Adequate financial compensation is a necessary but not sufficient condition for good employee performance: you cannot buy dedication with a paycheck. Motivation can and must be planned and managed. Motivated employees are more dependable, self-confident, produc-

---

Exhibit 3.3   Fundamentals of Management

1. Frontline staff must have the authority to make decisions as they relate to customer satisfaction issues.
2. Frontline staff must be encouraged to think and act independently without fear of the consequences of making a bad decision. Create a work environment in which employees motivate themselves.
3. Job content and expectations must be spelled out clearly and reinforced constantly until the employee can understand the philosophy. People work best when expectations are clear, freedoms are spelled out, and consistency is the norm.
4. Managers must understand basic human problems and be sensitive toward all the emotional forces that motivate staff.
5. Managers must act as cheerleader, facilitator, coach, and confidant. They should see themselves as a resource for their employees and look for ways to help them be more effective.
6. Only through constant encouragement and support will the manager be able to build the level of self-confidence in the staff that will let them feel free to serve the customers as if they owned the business themselves.
7. Managers must articulate a clear vision of exactly what the business looks like when it is running well.
8. Measurable plans must be developed for the realization of that vision based on balancing the needs and interests of the owner(s) with those of the employees and the customers they serve.
9. Managers must build consensus among the staff and create a sense of urgency.
10. Managers should not seek to impress those for whom they work, but those who work for them. Results will always speak for themselves.

---

tive, satisfied, and team-oriented. Most important, the motivated employee stays in the job longer and performs better. Motivation is more than being nice to people, complimenting them, and creating a friendly work environment: it means giving employees continuing opportunities to learn more, to test their knowledge, and to achieve personal growth and advancement—and expressing recognition of employees who rise to those challenges. Guidelines for motivating employees are listed in exhibit 3.4.

Sources of dissatisfaction include low pay and benefits, poor working conditions, poor supervision, lack of job security, perceived corporate instability, unfair policies and administrative practices, perceived inequities in pay, lack of recognition, lack of social relationships, and low status. Although some of these factors may be beyond a manager's control, she does have the power to determine the tone of her relationships with her staff. The manager who treats employees with indifference and operates the community from behind closed doors will create a sense of fear and intimidation. Senior managers often look down on employees, and it is hard to see things eye to eye when you are looking down on someone. Abuse of status and power by a manager can create dissension and destroy team spirit.

Provided that salary ranges and benefits are competitive, the biggest motivator for employees is to be *appreciated,* recognized, and treated with respect. Employees who are rewarded for strong performance are more productive, satisfied, and stable. Awards for performance need not be financial. Noncash incentives such as merchandise, travel, recognition, and status can be as effective as cash in motivating and rewarding employees. Employee focus groups within senior living communities across the country have confirmed this basic truth. Equally important, employees expect and are motivated by supervisors who manage people effectively and set the right example for the staff. In his book *1001 Ways to Reward Employees,* the management specialist Bob Nelson explains, "Employees find personal recognition more motivational than money.... Yet it is a rare manager who systematically makes the effort to simply thank employees for a job well done, let alone to do something more innovative to recognize accomplishments."[5]

Recognition flows down from the top of an organization, and its source is self-confidence. People feel empowered by recognition: it builds self-esteem and confidence. Managers often feel that they lack the time and creativity to come up with ways to reward and recognize employees. Yet those who look for opportunities to do so will themselves be rewarded by employees who take pride in their work and believe they have a stake in the operation's success. When this confidence and commitment are shared by frontline employees, they form the foundation for exceptional service to residents. Building confidence, however, is a

continuous process: when the source runs dry, blame often replaces recognition and mediocrity once again becomes the norm.

IRAC

Often employee dissatisfaction comes from a lack of role clarity. It is up to management to delineate each team member role in key management areas and if their role is to be simply informed (copied on this issue), to recommend (input into decisions considered),

---

Exhibit 3.4   Motivating Employees

- Create a proactive work environment; recognize employees for their strengths and have tolerance for their areas of vulnerability.
- Generate a sense of belonging and team spirit among the group to pull together and accomplish goals.
- Promote the building of relationships with residents and their families.
- Demonstrate that management is "hands-on" and not afraid to roll up its sleeves and participate in the work.
- Talk to employees, ask questions, and listen.
- Discourage ego trips and turf building.
- Learn that everyone is responsible for making the operation run well. Managers who say "It's not my job" might as well say "I quit."
- Keep employees informed and involved in the overall operations of the community.
- Build self-esteem among employees and empower them to recognize problems and take steps to solve them as they arise. Create an atmosphere that encourages employees to take risks without fear of reprimands when honest mistakes are made.
- Respect employees' intelligence and opinions; seek out their ideas.
- Understand basic human problems and be sensitive to all the emotional forces that motivate people.
- Encourage laughter. Organizations that create a level of urgency mixed with the right amount of humor learn to take themselves only seriously enough to get the job done. Companies that create an atmosphere in which people enjoy their work and each other are far better positioned to be successful than competing firms run by taskmasters.

to approve (decision authority), or to consult (request input that may or may not be used in decisions). An IRAC (inform, recommend, approve, consult) document can be used to specifically define roles and authorities so that duplication is avoided and responsibilities are clear. IRACs can be created for accounting, marketing, wellness, and the community as a whole.

STRATEGIC PLANNING

In addition to operating the community to balance the needs and interests of ownership with employees, families, and vendors, the seasoned executive director must allocate some time to moving the entire project forward as a business. Many executive directors become entangled each day in the problems at hand and may lose sight of the long-term objectives of the project they are managing. Each year a strategic plan should be developed and reviewed quarterly to identify long-term goals and objectives rather the day-to-day demands of their position. A thorough assessment of the community's strengths, weaknesses, opportunities, and threats (SWOT) should be undertaken so interested parties can discuss where the business needs to improve overall. The SWOT is used as a game plan for strategic evaluation and prioritization at each community. It is designed to identify major objectives to be accomplished for the year ahead according to the strengths, weaknesses, opportunities, and threats each community is facing to achieve its full potential. The analysis identifies specifically how management is going to accomplish the strategic objectives, who will be held accountable for achieving the objectives, and when each objective is to be completed.

This tool is reviewed quarterly by the executive director and department heads with the vice president of operations.

- Strengths: Characteristics of the community that give it an advantage over competitors.
- Weaknesses: Characteristics of the community that place it at a possible disadvantage relative to the competitors.
- Opportunities: Elements in the environment that the community could exploit to its advantage.
- Threats: Elements in the environment that could cause trouble for the community.

This tool is a great way to chart what needs to be done in areas such as referral building, family and employee satisfaction, differentiation from competitors, operator branding, building lead volume, physical plant needs, leadership development, and financial management. It can also be used by the executive director to demonstrate that not only has the community staff kept all the routine operations going and solved ongoing problems, but together they have accomplished so much more in measurable results to create a better business model. A sample SWOT and strategic plan can be found in appendix A.

The job responsibilities of an executive director are complex. They are not only entrusted with the management of the physical asset, but they must also be adept at balancing the needs of ownership with the needs of the residents, the staff that serve them, with family members, and even vendors and referral sources. Appendix D provides a handy checklist of the minimum responsibilities for the executive director position and details what should be done daily, weekly, monthly, quarterly and on an annual basis.

Managers must be able to define excellence and communicate specific expectations to their staff. Most employees want to do a good job: the more clearly a manager can show what a good job entails, the better equipped employees will be to work toward that goal. Walt Disney put it best: "You can dream, create, design, and build the number one place in the world, but it takes people to make it happen."[6] If there is not a big difference between what you offer and what your competition offers, there had better be a big difference in the way you treat people.

NOTES

1. Quoted in *Wall Street Journal,* September 13, 1995.
2. R. Half, *Robert Half on Hiring* (New York: Crown and New American Library, 1986).
3. Argentum, https://www.argentum.org.
4. F. Reichheld, *Loyalty Rules!* (Boston: Harvard Business School Publishing, 2001), 2–3.
5. B. Nelson, *1001 Ways to Reward Employees* (New York: Workman, 1994), xi.
6. Quoted in Disney University Professional Development Programs, *The Disney Keys to Service Excellence* (Lake Buena Vista, FL: Walt Disney Company, 1995), 4.

4

Safety, Risk Management, and Privacy

Managing a senior living community entails not only operating the facility and supervising the staff to maximize productivity and resident satisfaction but also ensuring that the community complies with federal, state, and local laws intended to protect the rights and safety of staff and residents and the confidentiality of residents' medical information. In addition, the community should take steps, in cooperation with its insurers, to minimize the risks of injury or damage to residents, staff, and property and the community's exposure to liability if incidents do occur. This chapter reviews the principal regulatory and insurance requirements faced by most communities and the appropriate procedures for handling and reporting incidents.

EMERGENCY AND DISASTER PLANS

All senior living communities should have an emergency and disaster response and communication plan. The plan should cover medical emergencies such as choking, heart attack, and shock; police emergencies such as robbery and vandalism; fire emergencies; engineering emergencies such as a catastrophic building system failure; natural disasters, such as tornadoes, hurricanes, and earthquakes; and medical contingencies that are not considered emergencies. Many of these plans have now been adapted to cover infection prevention and control planning (IPCP) response and recovery. In most communities,

the executive director is responsible for emergency planning. Advice on developing a comprehensive emergency plan is available from local emergency management services as well as from organizations like the American Red Cross.

The person who discovers the emergency is responsible for calling the emergency services and giving her name and the location and nature of the incident. This person stays on the line for instructions from the emergency dispatcher. The concierge should then initiate the communication plan and place an emergency group call to the appropriate department heads.

WORKERS' COMPENSATION

Workers' compensation is a state-mandated program under which employers are required to pay all the medical bills and a portion of lost wages to employees injured on the job. Large employers that self-insure pay these claims as a direct expense to their operations; smaller concerns typically purchase insurance, with premiums based in part on their claims history and job classifications.

The Workers' Compensation Rating Bureau determines the payroll classification and thus the insurance rates for different types of work. Take care when selecting a class code for a position to avoid classifying it at a higher rate than necessary. Slight differences in classification can mean big savings on rates. For example, in Tennessee, class codes 9052 (Hotel—All other employees, salespeople, and drivers) and 9058 (Hotel—Restaurant employees) carry a rate of $3.92 and $2.89 per $100 payroll, respectively, compared to code 8835 (Home health/home care employees), which has a rate of $5.96. To calculate your own rate, take your estimated annual payroll for the employee, divide that number by 100. You then multiply that number by the premium rate for the class code to find the total cost of workers' compensation insurance for that employee.

Experience rating is mandatory in most states for all but the smallest incidents. The experience rating is a method of modifying a standard workers' compensation insurance premium by comparing a company's actual loss experience to that deemed normal for the type of business. When a business is first established, the experience modifier is set at 1.00. It is then adjusted up or down depending on the company's claims experience. A history of frequent claims can drive the experience modifier up to 1.3, which translates to a 30 percent increase in the premiums paid by the employer for the same coverage as competitors. Conversely, if the claim frequency is lower than that of competitors, the experience modifier can drop below 1.0. A modifier of 0.80 means that the employer pays 20 percent less than competitors. In a 100-unit community, this can translate into an annual savings of $9,000 in premiums alone, not to mention time loss, overtime coverage, and excess claims. The experience rating is calculated on the basis of a three-year rolling average, ending one year before the effective date of the policy period. This means that if the management implements effective strategies to lower claims, it will be two years before the premium is reduced. Therefore, it takes a long-term commitment by the management to make such initiatives pay off. The National Workers' Compensation Council is the main rating organization that disseminates workers' compensation experience modifications.

The experience rating plan is designed to give more weight to the frequency of loss than the severity. For example, fifteen $3,000 claims would have a greater effect on the rating than one $45,000 claim. Loss experience has two components: *primary losses* and *excess losses*. Losses of $5,000 or less are considered primary losses and are assessed at face value, whereas any loss above this amount is considered an excess loss. The excess loss amounts are capped by the applicable state's per-claim accident limitation. The larger claims are capped so that they will not have too great an effect on the experience rating. A single large loss may be anomalous, and it would not be fair to penalize a policyholder for three years because of one incident. The management has more control over the frequency than the severity of losses. But frequent small losses can often lead to a severe loss, and they are penalized accordingly. Problems with loss frequency are easily identifiable.

Workers' compensation is a manageable expense. A proactive and well-managed workers' compensation program can save a community thousands of dollars in claims (and premiums) that can be spent on employee compensation and other more productive expenditures. These programs should promote safety awareness, reduce injuries, manage the recovery process, and minimize the expense of returning employees to work. Employers who promote safety consciousness minimize costs and disruption of their operations through time lost. Safety and loss control must be part of everyday operations rather than ad hoc responses to an incident.

An effective workers' compensation program emphasizes critical, measurable results, such as days without time-loss injuries. To be effective and to gain employee support, it must demonstrate the management's concern for the welfare of its employees and not be presented or perceived merely as a way to control costs. It includes education, wellness programs, community-sponsored fitness events, safety committees, and routine inspections of the physical plant. Incentive safety programs and contests among teams of employees are good ways to heighten safety awareness. Contests should be creative, goals should be within reach, and awards should be presented at least quarterly to keep the program fresh and on everyone's mind. An awards ceremony can be incorporated into all-employee meetings at which the management recognizes the efforts of winning employees and reinforces the program's objectives.

Preemployment screening can be an effective tool in injury prevention. Candidates should be asked to demonstrate the ability to handle the physical demands of the position for which they are applying. If the position involves lifting, they should have demonstrated the ability to do so in previous positions. It is a good idea to contact the state workers' compensation office to review a candidate's previous claim history. It is illegal to discriminate by not hiring individuals with previous injuries, but knowledge of previous injuries may indicate a need for additional safety training to prevent future injuries.

Occasionally employees use workers' compensation claims to cope with personal problems or to avoid income interruption due to job-performance issues. All employees should be educated on the disadvantages of claiming workers' compensation. Becoming injured as a result of an unsafe act is simply not worth the time off. Workers' compensation for time lost does not start until the sixth day, except in cases of severe injury; therefore, employees need to use up their sick days before receiving compensation. Also, many employees are unaware that the compensation rate is only two-thirds of their usual hourly wage. (However, because workers' compensation benefits are not taxed, the typical employee can end up receiving 80 to 90 percent of his previous take-home pay.) Finally, workers' compensation is a benefit designed to protect those truly injured. If the company suspects a fraudulent claim, it may seek a legal remedy that could be expensive to the employee.

Economic trends can affect employees' use of workers' compensation. According to insurance specialists, during a recession, employees become fearful that they may be laid off and are more likely to report injuries that prevent them from coming back to work. In effect, going out on workers' compensation becomes a way of guaranteeing a paycheck in hard times. As the economy improves, those fears subside, and employees are more willing to return to the job quickly. This same trend is seen in individual communities that may not be making financial projections: employees concerned about potential cutbacks by the management may file workers' compensation claims.

Procedures for filing claims are governed by the Workers' Compensation Act of 1991. The important distinction is between time-loss cases and medical-only cases. To qualify as a time-loss case, an injured employee must be incapacitated for a period of 5 calendar days and is eligible for compensation from the 6th day of disability forward. The employee must be incapacitated and unable to earn full wages for 21 days to be eligible from the first day of disability. In other words, if the employee is incapacitated for more than 5 days but less than 21 days, he or she is entitled to benefits for only those days in excess of 5 days (rules vary in some states).

In about half of the states, the company can specify the health care practitioner whom employees consult for care following the injury. Employers can identify local physicians with a record of more conservative treatment and recommend them to injured employees. The object is not only to avoid doctors who might overprescribe tests and treatments but also to find those interested in returning people to the job.

It is a good idea to refer any injured employee initially to a clinic with whom the management has previously made arrangements. The physician should be provided with a job description for the particular employee and advised whether or not the employer will allow a return to light-duty work. The physician should be willing to contact the employer immediately after seeing the employee to advise on the employee's condition and disability. The management should make every attempt to return the employee to work, with appropriate limitations, as soon as possible. The cooperation and accessibility of the initial treating physician can be valuable in this effort.

The management should conduct a thorough investigation with witnesses and coworkers to ascertain the circumstances of the incident. In some cases, if unsafe practices by the employee caused the accident and resulting injury, the compensation may be reduced by 50 percent. Therefore, any violation of policy or procedure should be thoroughly documented.

When workers are hurt, the management's communications can significantly affect the course of claims. The community should designate one person as claims coordinator, the liaison to all injured employees. This coordinator can then call homebound employees frequently and make sure they are receiving their checks. The object of this attention is to keep communication channels open and let the employees know that the company misses them and is eager to see them return.

Employees who are returned to light-duty work after an injury will feel useful and valued by their employer. Light-duty work generates positive emotions that aid the healing process. It also allows employees to stay in touch and feel connected to the work routine. The program should be managed by someone with sensitivity and an ability to recognize an employee who does not want to come back to work for either personal or personnel reasons. These employees invariably allege reinjury so that they can collect benefits and stay home. Once an employee is assigned light-duty work, the rehabilitation process should be monitored as closely as if he or she were on temporary disability, and a date for return to full duties should be set. The employee, physician, and physical therapist should all be strongly encouraged to meet that date.

A successful light-duty program requires the support of the local medical community. Physicians will release patients to light duty if they know that a well-managed light-duty program exists, and they will be less likely to order three or four days of bed rest for an employee who may simply want time off from work. Some companies have invited local physicians to review their light-duty programs on-site, to help them make informed decisions about returning employees to work.

If the employee claims to have been injured at work and requires medical treatment by a physician but is incapacitated for less than five days, the claim is a medical case only, and the employee is not eligible for time-loss benefits. Such claims should also be thoroughly investigated through a check of the accident site, the injured employee's report, and witness verification. Accidents requiring only in-house first aid should be similarly documented, cross-referenced to similar accidents, and reported to the safety committee. They should be reported to the insurer if the incident is unusual or possibly not work-related.

When the employee is released to work without limitations, the physician should put this in writing. The employee's previous position should be offered to him; if it has been filled, then a comparable position should be offered at the same rate of pay (if available). If the employee refuses this offer, he or she should be asked to sign a statement of refusal to accept such employment, or the company should confirm the offer and refusal in writing by mail to the employee.

Clearly, preventing accidents is the key to minimizing workers' compensation costs. Educating employees on proper body mechanics and the serious injuries they can sustain in their positions can help keep them aware of the risks. To remain effective, however, this training must be paired with employee-centered, proactive management. Employees should understand the direct benefits to them of a safety program and recognize that the costs of absenteeism and workers' compensation ultimately hurt everyone.

RISK MANAGEMENT

The operations of senior living communities are exposed to a wide range of risks. To analyze and minimize these risks, operators must determine what standards of care apply or should apply and to which they may be held. Senior living communities are an operational hybrid and differ from other types of business, such as rental apartments or condominiums, for which landlord-tenant laws have developed and evolved over time. They are similar to other types of housing and service providers for specific populations with special needs and vulnerabilities, such as health care facilities, nursing homes, and group homes for elderly people. They also possess many of the characteristics of the hospitality and residential housing industries.

Standards of performance specific to senior living may include state regulations and other statutes and regulations, including landlord-tenant, consumer protection, fair housing, and antidiscrimination laws. Recent laws governing the confidentiality of patient information also specify performance standards for health care providers. (For more information on the Health Insurance Portability and Accountability Act of 1996, see below.) Other standards to which the senior living community may be held include accepted clinical and professional practices, evolving industry standards, and even representations and promises (oral or written) made in connection with marketing efforts and materials, residency agreements, resident handbooks, service plans, and representations by community employees.

Risk management is as much a mindset as a science. Operators must be as committed to implementing and managing risk-control policies as to marketing the building. Poor risk management will empty a building faster than good marketing will fill it. One widely publicized incident of resident abuse or molestation can effectively negate thousands of dollars of advertising.

Effective risk-management policies and procedures can be developed by working with a loss-control professional. Such services are generally available through an insurance provider, for once the insurer has underwritten a policy covering a community, it is clearly in their best interest for that community to minimize risks. Most national carriers have a full-time loss-control department that works with communities to design risk-management programs. The goal of any loss-control program is to identify risk and then engineer an effective means to reduce or eliminate the chance of loss or exposure.

Loss-control programs are designed to mitigate risk. The following areas are typically covered in a loss-control audit:

- Accident prevention
- Emergency planning
- Evacuation procedures
- Fire prevention and protection
- Handling hazardous materials
- Hazardous waste disposal
- Analyzing loss and identifying trends
- OSHA hazard communication
- Smoke and fire safety programs
- Vehicle safety
- Infection control

Contracts with outside service providers often include a section dealing with insurance and/or indemnification. Such contracts must be reviewed to consider their overall impact on the risk-management program. The review should cover:

- Certificates of insurance
- General contracts
- Indemnification
- Insurance requirements
- Limits on liability
- Management agreements
- Personal care management agreements
- Procedures and responsibilities
- Service agreements

In the skilled-nursing environment, regulations have been developed to protect the interests of the residents and ensure the delivery of proper and appropriate care. In many ways, the regulations themselves are specific enough to minimize risks to the resident associated with the delivery of care. This is clearly not the case in assisted living. As residents age in place and as competition drives providers to stretch the definition of assisted living, the commu-

nity will be exposed to the complications of meeting residents' increasing health care requirements. This trend will inevitably expose the typical assisted living provider to increased risk. Until legislators regulate assisted living, the management must develop its own procedures to manage this risk, and they would be well advised to prepare a comprehensive risk-management program proactively, as a preventive measure, rather than retrospectively, following a serious incident that might have been prevented.

Shared Risk with Negotiated Risk Agreements

Senior living entails the right of a resident to choose services and negotiate the risk associated with his or her choices. Providers serve both themselves and their residents best when they discuss limits on care and risk management at the onset of residency and negotiate a formalized risk agreement.

Senior living providers should respect and recognize a resident's right to make choices regarding lifestyle, personal actions or behaviors, and the personal service plan. Providers and residents' families must recognize that in some cases a resident's decision or action may involve an increased risk of personal harm and may therefore conflict with a provider's responsibility to meet the established standards for senior living services, care, and supervision. Here the concept of informed consent comes into play; such consent can be secured through risk-sharing agreements.

Risk-sharing agreements should be simple and understandable to residents and the employees who serve them. The community should develop protocols to explain why a certain decision or action may pose a risk and suggest alternatives for the resident's consideration. Residents who are competent to do so should be encouraged to discuss these decisions with their families so that all understand the risk associated with those decisions. If, after consultation, the resident still wishes to pursue an action or refuse service that may involve increased risk of personal harm and conflict with the provider's responsibilities, the provider should take the following steps:

1. Describe the action or range of actions subject to negotiation.
2. Negotiate a risk agreement acceptable to the resident that meets all standards for the safety and

comfort of the community as well as any applicable statutory and regulatory requirements.

3. Follow a resident's preferences over his or her family's preference, unless the family has been granted legal powers of decision making.

4. Record the agreement, the provider's proposed alternatives, and the provider's role, if any, in mitigating the risks in a document signed by the resident and the provider.

5. Implement any mitigation efforts to which the provider has agreed.

6. Outline a time frame within which the risk-management issue will be addressed with the resident once it has been identified and a risk agreement developed.

7. Review the decision documented in the risk agreement with the resident if the resident's mental or physical condition changes substantially after the agreement is signed, renegotiating and re-signing the agreement when appropriate.

The provider should develop a policy statement that indicates that risk-management agreements are not intended to abridge a resident's rights or to avoid liability for harm caused to a resident by the provider's negligence. They are simply a format within which to document the resident's decisions regarding the provider's involvement (and the limits thereof) in attending to personal care needs. Operators who use shared-risk agreements to cover such contingencies as falls, elopement, and skin breakdown can use them to mitigate legal consequences in the unlikely event of such a problem arising, and to reach an agreement with the family on reasonable limits of care. A thorough analysis of "negotiated risk" is often debated as to whether or not negotiated risk includes waiver of a facility's legal liability. There are variations in interpretation from state to state. Waiver of liability generally arises in terms of inadequate care, rather than offering residents an ability to exercise functional freedom while understanding potential negative outcomes related to their activities. This has been interpreted that the agreement was intended by the facility and family to enable residents to reside in a noninstitutional assisted living setting even though they may have care needs that would normally require them to reside in skilled nursing. It is important for the operator to clinically assess each resident to determine what may or may not be an appropriate level of risk that they (and the family) are willing to accept to offer a continued quality of life while keeping the resident safe from physical harm. These agreements do not allow the operator or the family to skirt discharge requirements outlined in the respective state's regulations governing care delivery at the licensed site.

Insurance Coverage

Typical insurance coverages for senior living communities are outlined in exhibit 4.1. No amount of insurance, however, can replace prevention, operational policies, and staff training. The management or owner needs to develop comprehensive protocols and procedures to maximize the effect of the coverage that is in place.

Most, if not all, hospital professional liability policies (including assisted living) are written as *occurrence policies.* An occurrence policy has lifetime coverage for the incidents that occur during a policy period, regardless of when the claim is reported. These provide coverage even when a claim is made after the policy period in which the incident took place. For example, if someone fell and suffered injuries, and then, a year after the policy term ended, the family chose to file a suit and the company filed a claim, the claim would be covered. With a *claims-made policy,* coverage is provided only within the term of the policy period, unless a "tail" is purchased. These policies are usually written for special cases and always require the company to purchase a tail. The tail extends coverage beyond the policy term and is usually expensive, (amounting to one full year of the then-current premium) to provide the customer with an incentive to renew the policy.

All department heads should understand common causes of loss and the underlying concerns they create. Slips and falls are the most common types of loss and typically are the result of a hazard on the premises. These types of loss can be avoided with constant upkeep of the building. If an emergency call system is maintained for the residents, the system must remain fully operational. Such systems are delicate and can fail without notice. The most troublesome risk in facilities where private units have locked doors is the increased chance that residents could fall while alone. This could lead to an invasion-of-privacy issue if the

---

Exhibit 4.1   Typical Insurance Coverages

- Property coverages
  - → Buildings and personal property
  - → Loss of business income and rental income
- Boiler and machinery
- Crime coverages
  - → Employee dishonesty and cybercrime
  - → Forgery and alteration
  - → Money and securities—inside and outside
- Commercial general liability
  (occurrence form—no deductible)
- Health care facility professional liability
  (occurrence form—no deductible)
- Employee benefits liability
  (claims-made form—no deductible)

Additional Coverages
- Workers' compensation
- Umbrella liability
- Business auto policy
  - → Owned vehicles
  - → Nonowned, hired car liability
- Business electronic equipment
- Employment practices liability
- Directors and officers liability
- Fiduciary liability
- Group health, life, disability, and dental

---

management wants to enter an apartment from which there is no response.

Most people think of abuse or molestation as a deliberate act of violence toward a resident, such as striking or other mistreatment. But the insurance industry has broadened the definition of abuse to include situations of extreme negligence. For example, a resident in a dementia care unit who used a wheelchair gained access to the rear loading dock of the facility, which was supposed to be locked. The loading dock was deserted, and the ramp was in the lowered position. The resident went speeding off the ramp and sustained serious injury. The state attorney general's office investigated this incident as a possible case of abuse based on the extreme negligence of the facility.

For communities that accommodate residents with dementia, wandering residents create exposure to another form of risk. There must be a clearly defined agreement with the resident and his or her family or responsible party stipulating that this resident, unlike the typical senior living resident, cannot come and go unattended. Otherwise, it is possible that if the management attempts to keep the resident on the premises for his or her own safety, the community could face exposure to a personal-injury suit for false imprisonment.

Most states emphasize the rights of independence, dignity, and privacy. The residency agreement or resident handbook should state that staff are permitted to enter a resident's apartment for emergency services and response (as well as for routine maintenance and the opportunity to show the resident's apartment to prospective tenants if notice to vacate has been given). Visits for daily care or housekeeping should be scheduled in advance, and staff should knock before unlocking the door.

Communities that advertise security in their marketing materials must have procedures in place to guarantee it. Even the implication that 24-hour staffing will ensure a more secure or safe environment may expose the community to lawsuits. In a senior living community in Massachusetts, a criminal gained access by pressing the front door buzzer until someone let him in. There was no receptionist on duty in the building. Although the community employed security staff, no one was scheduled for this particular shift. An elderly resident who was expecting a visit from the maintenance department had left her door ajar, and the criminal used this opportunity to rape and rob her. This horrifying event shows the importance of enforcing strict security measures at each community. The following measures can help control access to the building:

- All visitors, without exception, should be required to sign in at a centrally located reception desk.
- A well-organized key-control system must be in place. Each unit's key should be coded to avoid showing the room number and should be kept in a locked area with minimal access.
- The property should be well lit inside and outside.

Most communities offer transportation services to their residents as one of the basic amenities. Investigate thoroughly all employees who will be performing this service. Research applicants' personal driving records and criminal histories.

The use of independent contractors is common in the senior housing industry and usually increases with the level of care. Generally, anyone on the premises to provide services creates an exposure to risk. If one of the residents is injured or abused by the actions of one of these providers, and the community referred this person to the provider, the community may be involved in the resulting lawsuit.

The management should be able to answer "yes" to each of the following questions:

- Has the management investigated the past performance of all independent contractors to ensure that they are professional and reliable?
- Does the management have references or referrals to back up this information?
- Does the management maintain files with a current certificate of insurance evidencing the contractors' professional liability insurance?
- Is the contractors' professional liability insurance company of good standing and solvency, with an AM Best's rating of A or better?
- Do the contractors carry sufficient limits of insurance (preferably $1 million per occurrence)?
- Is the community named as an additional insured on the contractors' policies with respect to their work at the community? The community must take great care to obtain evidence that contractors carry insurance with adequate limits.

Residents often hire companions or outside contractors such as home health agencies to perform a variety of services in addition to the services they purchase from the community. In fact, some communities do not provide personal care services and contract all such care to outside contractors. The actions of outside contractors can also expose the community to risk. Communities are strongly encouraged to have the resident or responsible party sign a disclosure statement and waiver before allowing the contractor to deliver any service at the community.

The waiver should certify that the contractor is an independent contractor to the resident, is entering the community solely at the request of the resident to perform services for the resident, and has not in any way contracted with, been solicited by, or agreed to perform services for the community or any of its partners, employees, officers, directors, affiliates, agents, successors, and assigns. It should also state that the contractor has not represented to the resident that the facility's owners are in any way involved with or in control of the contractor's business, that the owners have endorsed the contractor or the services to be provided by the contractor to the resident, or that the owners have control over or charge of or are responsible for any aspect of the services performed by the contractor at the facility. The contractor must be validly and properly licensed by any and all applicable regulatory bodies to perform the services for the resident. The contractor must certify that the contractor has procured such comprehensive general liability insurance and, if applicable, workers' compensation and employer's liability insurance as the contractor believes is necessary to protect the contractor adequately and that the contractor shall not be covered by any of the owner's insurance.

The contractor should be provided with and acknowledge receipt of the rules and regulations of residence as set forth in the residents' handbook and should comply with these rules and regulations and cause its employees and agents, including other employees who may work for the contractor within the building, to comply with these rules.

The agreement should also require that the contractor accept the facility in its "as is" condition and specify that the owners have made no representation or warranty regarding the condition or maintenance of the facility, nor the safety or suitability of the facility for the purposes contemplated by the contractor. In this way, if the contractor becomes injured other than through the negligence of the community, the contractor has limited remedies.

Finally, the contractor should release the owners from and waive any and all claims, damages, fines, penalties, losses, costs, and expenses (including but not limited to attorneys' fees) against the owners or management that arise from or are in connection with the services performed at the facility. The contractor should also agree to indemnify the owners or management from any claims relating to the services performed by the contractor or any of its employees or consultants. Such obligations should not be construed to negate, abridge, or reduce other rights or obligations of indemnity that would otherwise exist, whether in contract, at law, or in equity.

Incorporating these acknowledgments into agreements can remind residents of their obligation and responsibility for their own contractors and insulate the community from legal risks from contractors not directly hired or controlled by the community.

In most senior living communities, the in-house operation will want to capture as much as possible of the market for private personal care delivered to the residents. Allowing free access to the residents by outside home health providers seeking to increase their private-pay billable hours will reduce this source of profit and fragment the delivery of good-quality services to the residents. The community management will, of course, be held responsible in the eyes of the families, the state, and the press for any problems (or negligence) associated with the delivery of that care, regardless of who was responsible.

Reporting Incidents

All incidents resulting in injury that include more than the typical slip and fall should be documented and reported to an insurance company. These include incidents resulting in fractures, dislocations, serious bleeding, medication error, head injury, verbal or physical abuse, or any unusual occurrence. In making the report, keep to the facts, state only the obvious, and avoid drawing conclusions. Exclude any assumptions from the incident report, because they can often be used against the management in court. Differentiate between incidents and accidents. All accidents are incidents, but not all incidents are accidents. An incident can be simply an unusual circumstance or behavior, up to and including an accident, in which someone may be hurt. A good rule is that if the incident is worth talking about, it is worth documenting.

The resident record is often the best line of defense in litigation, and it serves as the main communication tool for continuity and evaluation of services. Standards for documenting, handling, and protecting the resident record will help ensure that information is available, clear, and valid. During litigation, plaintiff attorneys scrutinize records for any evidence of tampering, which would render the documentation questionable. Inconsistencies in record keeping can discredit the entire resident record. Improperly made changes to or entries in this record could lead to allegations of a cover-up and create doubt in the minds of jurors. Thus, the integrity and preservation of resident records are imperative.

After an incident, all pertinent records should be gathered, analyzed, and locked in a secure area. These records—including the incident report, internal investigatory notes, and any statements taken from witnesses—should be kept separate from the resident's standard file. Any contact with the resident's family or their lawyer must be carefully approached and documented to avoid compromising the defensive posture of the community and its employees. Procedures for receiving and reporting a summons, suit, or subpoena should be clearly defined in order to avoid penalties for default or other legal consequences. If a summons and complaint are forwarded to the community, the date on which these documents are signed for determines the date by which a response to the allegations must be filed in court to avoid penalties for default. One individual, typically the executive director, should be responsible for notifying insurance carriers, claims management, defense attorneys, workers' compensation authorities, and other involved parties, as well as for the method of notification established.

It is critical for the members of the community to understand their duties as an insured in the handling of incidents at the property. What to report, when to report, and how to report are all important factors in complying with the "duties of an insured" clause in the liability insurance contract.

Take the following immediate measures at the time of an incident:

1. Provide medical care and first aid. Any injury to the head should be immediately assessed by a registered nurse or by a member of the emergency medical services.
2. Call all emergency personnel whose services may be required (e.g., emergency services, utility companies, elevator service company). Document the time of call and response time.
3. Call the resident's or visitor's family and personal physician to report the occurrence. Note the time and record the details of the call.
4. Conduct a thorough internal investigation to ascertain the facts and circumstances of the incident, and identify witnesses. If the police are conducting an investigation on-site, insist that a member of the management accompany them.
5. Call the community's insurance agent to report the incident.

WHAT TO REPORT. Most state regulations provide an online portal for reporting serious incidents. Facilities are required to report incidents/accidents, illnesses resulting in death, or hospitalization to next of kin immediately, sponsors within 12 hours, state regulators in writing within 5 to 10 days of incident/accident (these notification time requirements vary by state). Reports should be made to the insurance agent for anything of a serious or unusual nature. It is much better to over-communicate to the insurance company on minor incidents and learn from their reporting guidelines than to fail to report an incident that could blow up later. They will open a case file for the incident and track it. If nothing further develops, they close the case; if something does develop, such as a request for records or a summons notification, the insurance company must be notified.

WHEN TO REPORT. Employees who witnessed the incident should complete an incident report before leaving work at the end of their shift. As soon as you have the facts of the incident, report it to the insurance company. You want your insurer to get involved early to investigate the facts while they are still fresh in everyone's mind and to decide with you how to proceed. Most incidents never become claims, but for the few that do, you will want to tap the resources and experience of your carrier to help handle them. It is critical to report serious incidents to the insurance company; failure to do so can potentially invalidate facility insurance coverage.

HOW TO REPORT. The sample incident report in exhibit 4.2 provides all of the information required by most insurance carriers. Most carriers have their own incident forms, however, so be sure to check with yours first. The more you can tell your carrier in the report, the easier the investigation will be. Be factual: report only what you know to be true. Do not theorize about the occurrence, for speculation can often lead to the wrong conclusions.

Investigating Incidents

After an incident, first stabilize the victim, then conduct an investigation immediately. Every passing minute allows for disturbances, intentional or unintentional, that may lead investigators to incorrect conclusions. Even a professional investigator from the insurance company cannot reconstruct an accident accurately several days later. There is no substitute for a prompt and thorough investigation by the management.

The integrity of the accident or incident scene must be preserved, as it contains much of the tangible evidence that will lead investigators to the proper conclusions. A photograph can record the positioning of the furniture, the presence or absence of obstacles, the clothing worn by the injured person, the lighting, the presence of housekeeping equipment, and other factors that may help investigators determine the cause and contributing factors. A sketch of the scene can also include the position of a fall, or of bedding, clothing, or furniture that may have been involved. Remember that the first person on the scene is usually a member of the community staff, followed by a member of the management; thorough documentation of the scene will lend them credibility in any subsequent legal action.

Before conducting the investigation, make a list of questions to cover. For example, in the event of a fall, the list may include inspecting the scene, interviewing residents and staff members, reviewing a resident's medications for potential side effects that could cause instability, and reviewing her care or service plan and any scheduled interventions immediately preceding the incident.

Listing all the potential witnesses (residents and staff) and collecting all the relevant documents helps narrow the investigation. Reviewing staffing schedules, time sheets, assignment sheets, and visitation records as well as the master logbook helps determine which staff members may be appropriate subjects for interviews.

Conduct the interviews as soon as possible so that the incident is fresh in everyone's mind and staff members do not have the opportunity to discuss the incident with other staff or family members. The longer these interviews are delayed, the less accurate reports will be. Ask the staff members to document exactly what they witnessed and sign and date their statements. Key documents can help corroborate testimony. These documents can also generate critical questions and reveal any inconsistencies. Resist the temptation to draw any conclusions until all of the evidence has been systematically evaluated.

On completion of the investigation, summarize all the interviews and documents reviewed. Organize

---

Exhibit 4.2   **Sample Incident Report**

Name of community: _____

Address: _____

Date of incident: _____ Time of incident: _____ Date of report: _____

Name of injured individual: _____ Male/female: _____ Age: _____

Please check: ❑ Resident   ❑ Visitor   ❑ Other

Address (room number for resident; full address for visitor): _____

_____

Entrance date into community: _____

Physical/mental status currently: ❑ Ambulatory   ❑ Nonambulatory   ❑ Alert   ❑ Disoriented

❑ Other (explain): _____

Place incident occurred: _____

Nature and description of incident: _____

_____

Injury sustained?   ❑ Yes   ❑ No   If yes, describe: _____

Hospitalized?   ❑ Yes   ❑ No   If yes, where? _____

Name(s) of witness(es): _____

_____

9-1-1 called: ❑ Yes   ❑ No   Time: _____

Resident's family notified of incident: ❑ Yes   ❑ No   Time: _____ Date: _____

Family reaction (understanding/supportive versus angry/accusatory): _____

Personal physician notified?   ❑ Yes   ❑ No   Time: _____ Date: _____

Name of physician: _____ Examined by physician? _____

Physician report regarding findings/treatment/change in functional ability:

_____

_____

Final disposition: _____

_____

Report prepared by (signature and date): _____

Personal care director (signature and date): _____

Executive director (signature and date): _____

---

the salient facts in chronological order or in chart format. This step will clarify the chain of events that may have led to the incident as well as highlight any gaps in the evidence.

Sometimes even the most thorough investigation remains inconclusive: perhaps a rational explanation simply cannot be found. Occasionally pressure from the management may lead the investigator to speculate. Yet it is far better to accept that you do not and may never know the cause than to make one up. Remember that investigations are aimed at *fact finding*, not *fault finding*. People will be more likely to share accurate information if they trust that you are not out to blame them or retaliate against them. In addition, misinformation that is later proved false can subject the entire investigation to criticism and improve the opposition's case in the event of a lawsuit.

Before summarizing the findings, consider the purpose and audience of the report. It should lead the reader to conclude that the investigation was thorough and impartial, and it should include factual evidence to support any conclusions reached. The more impartial the report, the better it will serve to justify the conclusions. Prepare an outline to document the investigation process, using the list described above as a guide. Note how the causes of the incident were discovered and emphasize the logic of the findings. A thoroughly prepared report can not only protect and limit the management's liability but also build credibility. It can also be used to develop plans and recommendations to prevent recurrences.

Frequently a community will receive its first indication that a claim or suit is contemplated when the family of a resident (or their attorney) requests a copy of the resident's file. Simply responding to this request without requiring the proper authorization papers will compromise the confidentiality and integrity of the file. When this type of request occurs, notify the insurance carrier. The insurer will then direct its adjuster or company-assigned defense counsel to handle the requests of the plaintiff's attorney. Information released will be strictly limited to that required to fulfill the purpose stated on the authorization. Authorizations specifying "any and all information" or other such broadly inclusive statements are generally not honored by defense counsel. They understand that the release of information that is not essential to the stated purpose of the request is specifically prohibited, and they will do everything to protect your community and residents from the release of confidential information.

All incident reports should be reviewed by the nurse and safety committee. The incident should be evaluated to determine if it could be avoided in the future, and if so by implementing and monitoring appropriate interventions for that resident. All interventions added should also be documented in a revision of the resident's care plan (see chapter 17) immediately and each time there is a change in the resident's condition. Any changes to the resident's care plan should be communicated promptly to care staff and the family or responsible party.

PRIVACY AND THE HEALTH INSURANCE PORTABILITY AND ACCOUNTABILITY ACT

The federal Health Insurance Portability and Accountability Act of 1996 and its implementing regulations (45 CFR parts 160–164) (HIPAA) set forth standards for protecting the privacy of individually identifiable health information (i.e., protected health information, or PHI). Pursuant to HIPAA, the covered entity (provider) is required to enter into business-associate agreements with all of its contractors, agents, and related and unrelated third parties that perform a function or activity on behalf of the covered entity that involves the use or disclosure of protected health information. These privacy rules were created to protect a resident's (patient's) privacy relating to certain privileged health care information routinely collected by senior living communities and other health care providers.

Essentially, confidential information may be distributed on a need-to-know basis with only the minimum amount and to the minimum number of individuals necessary to meet the service needs. Business associates to whom information is provided must not further disclose this information and must apply safeguards of their own to prevent unauthorized use or disclosure of this confidential information. Now with electronic medical records and communication, extra precautions must be taken with any information released as it is all too easy to send protected HIPAA information carelessly.

Most health care providers have created a simple contract addendum with which to inform their business associates how they intend to comply with HIPAA regulations. The regulations, which became effective on July 13, 2006, remain in effect until all of an individual's protected health information is either returned to the individual or destroyed. Because most states require that residents' files and charts be kept for at least five years, HIPAA regulations are often in effect long after the resident has been discharged.

II

Resident Services

Concierge and Reception

5

The concierge position is one of the most important in a senior living community. Not only is this the hub of activity and communication for the residents, but the concierge is also usually the first contact for guests and prospective residents. All too often, the sales staff has invested many telephone contacts in a prospect, finally convincing her to come for a tour, only to have her ignored or kept waiting in the lobby. It is rare, indeed, that prospects are impressed enough with the "sticks and bricks" to confirm a sale: what persuades them are relationships and solutions, and those take a personal touch. It is important to get off to a good start, especially with the typical reluctant prospect who may be looking for any excuse to delay the move to a senior community. All guests and visitors should be greeted with a warm smile, a cheerful and friendly attitude, and an air of professionalism and confidence that will convince them that the community will deliver on the good quality it promises.

The primary responsibility of the concierge is public relations, both internal and external. Individuals working at the front desk should be hospitality-oriented professionals who can manage multiple tasks simultaneously and thrive in a fast-paced and challenging environment. They should project calm, friendliness, and efficiency in person, on the phone, and in written communication. The concierge is typically the one person in the community who has daily contact with the residents. In addition, the concierge is usually the first person to whom a resident turns with a problem, request, complaint, or question. The concierge should therefore possess a high degree of patience and an understanding of the senior population and be able to provide prompt, courteous, high-quality service at each encounter. Happy and satisfied residents are a key ingredient of marketing and a source of good referrals.

The concierge must create and maintain an atmosphere of warmth, personal interest, and positive emphasis as well as a calm environment, despite the daily chaos of this highly charged position. The successful concierge possesses a high degree of patience and an understanding of the senior population, welcoming them as though they were visitors to his own home. He can choose behavior to suit every encounter with the public, and this behavior should be a cloak for all his personal problems, prejudices, and feelings. He should be primed always to be in decision-making mode to solve problems and manage the traffic at the front desk.

Communities that have experienced outbreaks of communicable diseases are turning to the concierge or reception as the first line of defense. This position has now been charged with screening all visitors and staff that enter the building for symptoms. Symptoms include fever, cough, shortness of breath, body aches, and temperature higher than 100.4 degrees. They must also verify in writing if the visitor has been out of the country, tested recently for COVID-19, come into contact with anyone testing positive, or had any symptoms in the last 14 days. The concierge position is also used to maintain a tracking worksheet of residents and employees with any disease symptoms, and monitor any changes in the course of the disease and the outcome of the individual. These are requirements recommended by the CDC and state health department officials who may periodically verify these records, and screens are routinely taking place. Prior to releasing the visitor into the community, the concierge will ensure each individual is treated with at least a 70-percent alcohol-based hand sanitizer.

The concierge or receptionist not only greets visitors and residents but also serves as the conduit between the residents and the community staff for communication of needs and policies. In addition, the concierge often monitors the emergency call system and building security. Many operators also ask the night-shift reception staff to perform administrative support services, including typing or spreadsheet maintenance for department heads, light accounting (such as summarizing meal credits), or special projects that can be done on a laptop or by hand. They can also assist with marketing tasks, such as the collation of direct mail pieces. Because of the importance of the concierge position to the overall success of the community, guest and telephone protocol are discussed here in detail.

GREETING GUESTS AND HANDLING INQUIRIES

I once visited a senior community and, while waiting for a tour by the sales director, noticed a small sign behind the reception desk that said "Our Reputation Is in Your Hands," an obvious reminder to the reception staff of their importance in creating a positive impression. The receptionist should immediately greet every person entering the lobby. Whenever possible, he should address the individual by name. When speaking on the telephone and unable to speak to a guest in the lobby, the receptionist should acknowledge the visitor with eye contact and a smile, nod, or wave. All visitors should be made aware that the receptionist knows they are there and will assist them as soon as possible. After greeting the visitor and determining her needs, the receptionist should contact the appropriate staff member to assist her. The concierge staff must therefore know who all the administrative and marketing personnel are and their exact responsi-

bilities. Visitors should be offered a seat and, if possible, refreshments, and they should not be kept waiting; if the appropriate staff member will be delayed for more than 10 minutes, somebody else should be contacted to assist the visitor.

The concierge's telephone manner is as important as in-person contact. The concierge position should have established standards for greeting callers, acceptable hold times, and accurate recording of information and taking messages. The staff should keep in mind that *each phone call is a potential sale.* You never know who is on the other end of the phone: everyone should be treated with the same courtesy. Although not every caller is a prospective resident, any caller may have a family member or friend who is. The caller might be influential in the larger community or an area business owner whose opinion of the community is critical to its success. Advertising, marketing, outreach, and print media are all expensive. The money and time spent to make each sale is far too great to be negated by a cranky person answering the phone.

In dealing with prospective residents, the concierge should provide only basic information in response to inquiries: requests for more detailed information should be directed to the sales staff. This will lessen the possibility that incorrect or outdated information will be given out. Sales staff are also better equipped to evaluate callers as prospects and persuade them to visit.

STAFFING

Staffing levels for a concierge or reception desk depend on the level of care provided at the project, the property configuration, the emergency response system, and the number and expectations of the residents. Usually the reception desk is staffed around the clock (24 hours per day, 7 days per week = 168 hours, or 4.2 full-time employees [FTE]). In assisted living communities, however, the front desk is usually staffed 12 hours per day (7:00 a.m. to 7:00 p.m.), with night calls forwarded to the nursing station. In some larger communities (with more 300 units), a second person may be necessary to assist residents and guests during the busy afternoon and evening shift. This second person can work from 3:00 p.m. to 11:00 p.m. and also serve as the manager on duty to avoid the need for a night maintenance person. This manager on duty, or night manager, should be trained in emergency maintenance and elevator operations, certified in cardiopulmonary resuscitation (CPR), and trained in handling resident emergency calls. In addition, the night manager should respond to and assist in emergency situations, monitor evening activities and programs, and respond to residents' needs.

There are a number of ways to provide coverage for the concierge during breaks, lunch, and bathroom visits. The desk should never be left unattended: the most vocal resident or family member will inevitably have a problem just when the concierge goes to get coffee. During the day, the desk can be covered by administrative or activity staff. At night, the laundry staff may be the best substitutes. The night shift is the best time to run the community laundry operation, as there is an ample supply of hot water and less distraction, so the staff can be cross-trained to cover the front desk during breaks and even staff absences.

Several key employees should be trained on the finer points of operating the front desk. Usually the office manager or resident relations director supervises this function. In smaller operations, the office manager should work one shift per week at the desk to maintain contact with the residents, understand the workload of the employees, and monitor the overall communication of the building. This can save up to $6,000 per year in staffing costs while demonstrating to the residents and other employees the management's commitment to creating a team environment by sharing the workload.

The higher the level of care, the more night staff the community will employ. Rarely does one find night reception staffing in assisted living or skilled nursing facilities; this function is usually performed by transferring the phones to the nurses' station. One assisted living community transferred its phones to an answering service that could page the night aides if necessary. If the emergency call enunciator is located on the assisted living floor or can be tied into the paging system, and if regulations permit, it eliminates the need for a nurse to sit at the desk at night. Other systems can be adapted to send an emergency alert by computerized voice through a two-way radio held by the night-shift employees.

Resources

As the concierge desk is "communication central," a well-organized resource file helps the staff to answer questions knowledgeably and competently. The file should include directions to and from the property, airport, local restaurants, sports facilities, and downtown by way of local, recognizable arteries, along with copies of a local map that can be handed out. Reviews of restaurants sorted by cuisine type may also be useful to residents and their guests. Most better hotels have a database of information about major restaurants so that printouts can be distributed to guests. The area chamber of commerce usually offers a complete listing of local places of worship, community resources, and other useful information on its website. These pages can be printed out and kept on file for quick access by residents, family members, and guests. In addition, it is helpful to maintain a list of local pharmacies and grocery stores that offer a delivery service, along with cab companies, tour operators, major attractions such as the museum or aquarium, hospitals and nursing homes, emergency numbers, and so on. Also useful is a copy of entertainment listings and weekend events from the local newspaper. Some communities also keep maps for walkers and joggers and information on attractions within walking distance of the property. Keeping local bus schedules and directions to the nearest stop can ease pressure on the transportation department. The concierge desk also will coordinate off-site transportation for the residents using Uber or Lyft, making arrangements and then billing back the resident's account monthly (see chapter 7 for details).

Logbooks

The concierge should keep several different logbooks. These should be hardbound books with sequentially numbered pages to keep a continuous, unalterable log. A log of all entries and exits through the lobby can be useful: it can track residents, staff, and deliveries; note comments made by residents or changes in their behavior; and record emergency alarm activation. All visitors should sign in and out of the logbook in order to track families and vendors. This record enables the supervisor to track resident patterns and staff workload and follow up on residents' questions and incidents. A computerized work-order log and system accessible at the concierge desk allows the maintenance department to track and prioritize requests from staff and residents while ensuring that they are filtered through one central location (see chapter 13 for more on the work-order system). The activity sign-up log records residents' reservations for group tours and local trips on the community bus. Another essential log is the transportation appointment request book, this is best accomplished using a computer-based calendar that has the ability to share appointments with families, activity staff, and the driver. This enables residents to schedule their requests for transportation by automobile on a first-come, first-served basis. The concierge should be aware of all daily activities and upcoming events and any scheduled changes. Finally, the concierge should maintain the reservation calendar for guest accommodations.

Deliveries

Many local pharmacies, dry cleaners, grocery stores, and eateries provide delivery services to senior communities. The residents should be asked to notify the concierge or reception staff of expected deliveries so that assistance can be provided if possible. The concierge should accept the package and notify the resident. All deliveries should be entered into the visitor's logbook. The concierge should not accept furniture or other large deliveries on a resident's behalf.

If the resident plans to be away and cannot accept a large delivery, the concierge can arrange to give delivery people access to the resident's apartment but only with advance written permission. A staff member should remain in the apartment with the delivery person until the delivery is completed. Normally these consist of durable medical equipment, hospital beds, or oxygen concentrators or tanks. The concierge should not accept COD packages or grocery deliveries in the resident's absence.

It is the resident's responsibility to pay for items on delivery. Although checks may be held at the front desk, the concierge should not be permitted to hold residents' cash for delivery payments or any other purpose. Delivery people should not be permitted to transact business on the premises unless authorized by the management at the resident's request. To avoid accusations of loss or damage, the concierge should not be permitted to hold residents' incoming or outgoing dry cleaning at the desk. If a resident is expecting a delivery, it's best to ask them to wait in the lobby for the driver to arrive.

The management should not provide bell services such as parcel delivery or assistance with groceries on request, nor should the concierge provide such assistance as a favor to residents. Items can either be taken under supervision to the resident's room by the delivery person or stored near the front desk to be delivered to the resident's apartment at the end of breaks or by the drivers between runs. The concierge should not accept perishables or valuables, as the community may be held responsible for any losses. Some communities provide small wheeled carts or wagons for residents to transport their packages and groceries to their rooms themselves.

Shipping companies usually refuse to deliver items to residents' apartments, and storage and handling of such deliveries may become burdensome: residents have been known to run businesses out of their apartments, with continuous parcel deliveries to the front desk! In such cases, arrangements should be made with the residents to deliver the parcels for a small fee. Residents should be encouraged to be as independent as possible, even if they complain about it. The exercise is good for them and helps offset additional staffing costs. If residents are unable to handle these tasks without assistance, another level of care may be more appropriate, unless of course their disability is temporary.

Guest Suites and Overnight Guests

Most communities have furnished suites that are available for use by residents' guests on a short-term and first-come, first-served basis. The resident host is usually held responsible for the guests' behavior and all charges they incur. There is usually a charge per night for the use of guest suites that is competitive with the rates at local hotels; most operators include continental breakfast. A list of charges should be available at the concierge desk or in the resident relations office. Often residents like to treat their guests, and this can be done discreetly by adding the charge to the next month's bill. If guests insist on settling their accounts themselves, they may write a check to the property accountant when they check out.

During their stay, communities typically allow guests to eat meals in the dining room at the current meal rates. Usually a certain number of meals per month are included in residents' monthly fees. Residents who do not eat all these meals may want to apply meal credits to their guests. This should be strongly discouraged. Operators do not adjust their purchasing or staffing if residents miss a few meals; the same overhead applies whether they are present or not. The fact that there is some economy of scale to mass-producing meals and other services allows for the profitability in the operations. A guest meal that costs $8 to $10 to produce and serve can be offered to a guest for $12 to $15. No payment for meals should be accepted in the dining room.

Reservations should be made for the guest suite and for each meal by contacting the concierge and the dining room. All guests should be encouraged to wear a mask while transiting within resident areas during communicable disease outbreaks. Children should be permitted in the guest suite only when accompanied by an adult and properly supervised. Most insurance policies cover accidents that befall both residents and their guests, but such precautions do little to appease angry residents who feel that their facilities are being abused and their home has been invaded.

Check-in time for guest suites should be after 1:00 p.m. and check-out by 11:00 a.m. to allow housekeeping and kitchen staff time to tidy the apartment and deliver the arrival amenities, such as cookies or a fruit bowl. Amenities are an inexpensive way to please guests and impress the residents they are visiting.

The resident relations department and the housekeeping supervisor should develop a list of supplies and furnishings for the guest rooms and apartments. The list should include bath linens and amenities, bed linens and pillows, clock radio, notepads, telephone instructions, room service menu, clothes hangers, kitchen equipment (including place settings and flatware, glasses, coffee maker, pots and pans, tea kettle, water pitcher, kitchen utensils), paper goods, arrival amenities, television set with remote, smart phone charging station, and so forth. It is also a good idea to include an information packet that contains a welcome letter, floor plan of the building, menu, and brochure. In most states, the operation of the guest suites falls under the jurisdiction of the Inn Keepers Act, and a copy of this, along with the emergency exit path and directions, must be posted in a conspicuous location, usually on the back of the door.

Residents should be encouraged to invite friends or relatives to stay in their own apartments. For security purposes, they should be required to notify the concierge when guests are staying with them, and overnight guests should sign in at the concierge desk on arrival. Residents should not, however, permit guests to stay with them for any extended period: friends or relatives who move in while they are "between jobs" can be difficult to extricate without permanently affecting the management's long-term relationship with the resident. A person living in a resident apartment for more than 30 days should automatically be considered a second occupant and should be charged as such on the next month's statement. Most residents' agreements and the Americans with Disabilities Act allow operators to maintain the age requirement for these types of property. Some communities charge a "companion fee" for a resident's private duty aide who spends 18 hours or more per day at the property.

Answering the Emergency Call System

In many senior communities, each unit is equipped with an emergency call device that activates a signal at the front desk. Whenever a resident's pull cord or call light is activated, the staff should consider the situation an emergency. Residents must be instructed on arrival in the community and their apartment that the pull cords are for use in emergency *only* and are not to be pulled for room service, for maintenance requests, or because their housekeeper is late or they cannot find their glasses. They must also be instructed on the community's emergency procedures and the completion and disposition of an emergency information card (see chapter 6).

When an emergency signal is activated, the resident's apartment should immediately be called to determine the nature and urgency of the request and to reassure the resident that help is on the way. The concierge phone system must have a separate trunk set-up to deal with emergencies, in case all the rollover lines are busy. The community operations manual should detail the appropriate procedure, along with the emergency numbers to call. The paramedics should be met at the community entrance nearest to the resident's apartment and escorted there. Another trained staff member should stay with the resident until help arrives. The concierge should, if possible, stay at the concierge desk to coordinate emergency response. If the facility's smoke alarm activates the emergency alarm, the concierge should call 9-1-1. Most alarm systems are connected directly to the fire dispatcher, but these have been known to fail.

SECURITY

As seniors age, they often experience a heightened sense of vulnerability that is manifested in their call for additional security measures and (usually) more staff. Security is an increasingly important issue for property owners and managers, not only because crime is on the rise in many areas but also because, according to data compiled by a Massachusetts security analysis firm, apartment owners and managers are increasingly being held responsible for crimes occurring on their properties. Forty-three percent of all reported suits were brought in Texas, New York, California, and Florida. Most of these suits involved cases of rape, robbery, and assault and battery. The average jury verdict and settlement amounts are rising. Just over 78 percent of all cases receive awards of less than $1 million; however, some have been as high as $3 million. A number of recent legal developments have made it easier for plaintiffs both to sue and to win.[1]

Twenty-four-hour concierge service, an emergency response system, the use of security cameras, or simply locking a building at night do not constitute security services. Operators must not claim to provide security unless they have trained security personnel on staff or contract for regular patrols of the hallways and grounds. Otherwise, it must be made clear to the residents and their families that, although the management attempts to screen visitors and guests, the property does not employ security staff.

Staffing a Security Department

Appropriate staffing of a security department depends on such factors as a community's size and configuration and crime statistics in the neighborhood. The size of the force can range from one night watchperson (10 hours per day, 7 days per week, or 1.75 FTE) to 24-hour security at a guard station (24 hours per day, 7 days per week, or 4.2 FTE) plus night patrols around the property (1.75 FTE). Additional temporary security staff may be necessary from time to time to protect the residents and staff from potential workplace violence or to guard construction projects or additions. Twenty-four-hour security staffed with qualified, experienced employees, along with benefits, insurance, communication, and supplies, can add many thousands of dollars per year to the operating budget. Like most services, once it is implemented, full-time security is not easily dispensed with.

Thorough multistate background checks should be conducted on candidates for security positions. According to law enforcement agencies, the security profession often attracts individuals who have been deemed inappropriate for employment in public service and are looking to the private sector for work in an enforcement capacity. Although operators may be exposed to risk without a security staff, they may also be inviting trouble when they hire one. An excellent solution to the problem may involve the local police department. Some communities take advantage of their significant local political influence to persuade the chief of police to schedule regular patrol visits by uniformed officers. Although this scheme may not provide much of a deterrent, it reassures residents. At the very least, operators can encourage the local patrol officers to stop by daily for coffee and fresh muffins.

Usually, security cameras that cover the parking areas, loading dock, and employee entrance and are monitored by the concierge provide adequate routine coverage. In my experience operating communities across the country, the worst problems have involved stolen or damaged cars in the parking lot, one disgruntled employee who had to be physically removed from the property, and one drive-by shooting. All these incidents were effectively handled by the local authorities. Two cars were even stolen while a security guard was on duty checking room flags! My contract valet parking attendant was once robbed at gunpoint, but the event was recorded on camera, and the police later apprehended the perpetrator. Security cameras have become very sophisticated and inexpensive while providing high-quality stored recordings in a cloud-based server for easy retrieval by date and time.

Security employees can be asked to perform housekeeping duties in the common areas and the lobby. Applicants should be told that the position may include some of these tasks and asked whether they are comfortable performing them. Depending on the facility, these duties might include cleaning carpet, changing light bulbs, polishing brass and furniture, and updating information boards. In addition to performing their regular patrols, some operators ask the night security staff to check the "I'm OK" door flags.

"I'm OK" Program

Senior living communities employ a number of systems to check daily on the status of each resident.

Both electronic and manual systems are available, and both work well if correctly managed. The door-flag system is one of the best. Each apartment door frame is fitted with a small, oval, clear Plexiglas tag about three inches long with a hole drilled at one end, attached near the top of the door. The tag is loosely attached to the frame so that it rotates freely around the hole. When the tag is rotated up against the door and the door opens, the tag drops down. Equipped with a roster of all occupied apartments, the security guard can then determine if the resident has opened the door; if marketing, housekeeping, or maintenance has visited a vacant apartment; or if other entry has been made. The occupied apartments with flags still up are then checked out, usually by 10:00 a.m. All flags are reset each night.

Electronic systems that use electronically programmed keys can track each time a door is opened with a key. Specifically coded keys can be issued to the resident, housekeeping staff, maintenance crew, and anyone else who needs to enter an apartment. The system can be programmed to search all entries to and exits from occupied apartments and print out a list each morning of "no activity" doors. The morning concierge can then call to check on residents. This system is also effective for determining who entered an apartment if something is declared missing; it can also be hardwired to the emergency response system. The key readers in the locks do fail at intervals and require trained personnel to replace them or override them manually. In addition, as with any electronic system, they can be vulnerable to power surges and spikes. Battery-operated card-reader lock systems with memory are also available, but unfortunately the batteries all seem to fail at once, and their replacement can be expensive, as well as inconvenient for residents who may be locked out.

Another useful daily check-in system being installed in communities features a lighted button, adjacent to the pull cord in the bedroom, that the resident simply pushes on arising each morning. This action sends a check-in signal to the monitoring system. A central computer then prints out a report listing the apartments that have not checked in so that the concierge staff can call the residents. The system can also monitor the unit and outside doors; it can be disabled at the resident's request. Other systems, such as one that uses a button by the resident's phone that is tied to lights on a central board at the front desk, are equally effective. Still others are incorporated into resident management software programs and apps that can track resident whereabouts using a wristband or pendant. Some of these programs allow family members to track residents throughout the facility or trigger a warning if the resident wanders off the premises.

Manual systems can be used for any size population but are best suited to communities with fewer than 200 units. The most effective manual system accounts for residents in the dining room at mealtimes. A resident roster is printed each day and posted at the entrance to the dining room: residents check off their names as they enter or leave, or the dining room manager or host checks them off. The list of absentees first goes to the concierge to be updated to account for people who are known to be away; then it is passed to the dining room staff to check whether the resident opted for room service or did in fact appear in the dining room. After dinner, the evening concierge calls any residents who are still unaccounted for. Under this system, residents should be encouraged to call the concierge if they will not be coming down for a meal.

NOTE

1. Norman D. Bates, "Major Developments in Premises Security Liability," Liability Consultants, 1999. The company can be contacted at 131 Coolidge St., Suite 202, Hudson, MA 01749, phone 978-310-7403, https://www.liabilityconsultants.com.

6

Resident Relations and Health

The residents of a senior living community can be a source of both job satisfaction and anxiety. Managers of these communities are uniquely positioned to make a difference in the quality of people's lives. For people who have been living independently, the transition to a community lifestyle and increasing dependence on others can be traumatic, and seniors deal with this trauma in a variety of ways. Many begin the process in denial, then exhibit anger and hostility, followed by bargaining and ultimately acceptance—just as they might experience a bereavement. In fact, they may be experiencing one of the most disruptive losses in their lives: the loss of their home, and with it much of their independence. For many, this loss can threaten their very identity.

Although most residents accept and adapt to their new environment after a few months, others find it more difficult. As people age, they become more resistant to change, but the aging process itself necessarily involves change, some of it sudden, unwelcome, or both. No one ever chooses to be widowed, need a hip replacement, or face difficulty with simple tasks such as preparing meals. For some, adapting to these changes can be painful.

This chapter outlines some of the approaches managers can take to prepare new residents for life in the community and help them through the adjustments demanded by their new lifestyle and advancing age. The more clearly managers can explain what residents can expect of their senior living experience, the fewer surprises and difficulties they and their families will encounter. And when problems do arise, a positive, straightforward approach to their solution can save time, frustration, and money.

RESIDENT HANDBOOKS

A well-written, concise, and thorough resident handbook is essential for presenting the policies, services, and amenities of the community and offering other general information, as well as for outlining the management's expectations of the residents. The resident handbook is also an integral component of the residency agreement and is often considered a legal document. It should include at least the following components: a welcome letter, a list of important telephone numbers, a description of services, community policies and procedures (including policies regarding the use of public areas), emergency and safety information (including security procedures), rules and regulations, and a community map and building floor plan. The resident packet may include additional forms that are required by the state or your insurance company. These documents may include authorizations for photos or release of information, negotiated risk agreements, emergency preparedness procedures, resident rights, HIPAA policy, permission to transport, or pet addendum.

The Welcome Letter

Signed by the executive director, the welcome letter should offer a warm and friendly introduction to the community. It should explain that the community's residents care about each other and pursue lives of growth and fulfillment, and that the community is designed to enhance their lifestyle by providing services that promote individual well-being. The welcome letter should also give the purpose of the handbook: to provide information about the community's operations and services and the management's expectations of the residents. It should affirm the importance of resident feedback and outline the procedures for offering comments. Finally, it should state the open-door policy of the management and their personal commitment to maintaining a caring, financially viable, and smoothly running community.

Important Telephone Numbers

Included here should be telephone numbers for emergency services, hospitals, pharmacies, the front desk, executive offices, dining room, marketing department, beauty shop, bank, and other on-site businesses. Some communities also include a list of residents' telephone numbers.

Services

This section should offer a short description of all services offered by the community and specify whether they are included in the monthly service fee or incur additional fees. Residents often press the management to stretch services: specifying the extent and limits of services clearly in the resident handbook can help avoid disputes and ensure consistent and fair treatment for all residents and employees.

Policies and Procedures

This section should address operational policies and procedures that directly affect the residents, such as those governing use of residents' apartments, apartment changes, apartment modifications, locks and keys, storage, billing, deliveries, privately employed personnel, parking, pets, smoking, and tipping, and conduct of guests. It should also state the management's expectations of residents and their guests and describe how residents can derive the greatest benefits from the services offered and help ensure that things run smoothly in the community.

In particular, the management should clearly state the policy on use of the grounds and public areas, emphasizing the benefit of having common areas and shared amenities that allow residents to socialize with others and enjoy special activities. The handbook should make it clear that although the residents should consider these areas as extensions of their apartments and an integral part of their home, these areas are used by all residents, and that family members and guests may use them only when accompanied by residents. It should describe the function of each public space, along with any associated rules or restrictions. Residents should be asked to help keep the common areas in good order so that everyone can enjoy them.

Emergency and Safety Information

This section should provide a clear and detailed description of procedures to be followed in an emergency, along with a description of the community's fire alarm and emergency call system. Each resident should be provided with a map showing an evacuation route to the emergency exit nearest his apartment and the location of the nearest alarm station and fire extinguisher. The handbook should explain how the fire alarm and sprinkler systems work. It should state that residents will be required to participate in regular fire drills and evacuation practices. In addition, it should give details of the procedure for dealing with medical emergencies and provide the emergency services telephone numbers.

The procedure for contacting the police department should be specified, along with a description of the community's security measures, key-control policies, and visitor access procedures. If the community has an established program to check on each resident daily, such as an "I'm OK" program, it should be described here.

RESIDENT SATISFACTION

Residents define the quality of the facilities and services of a community as the difference between what they expect and what they get. If their expectations are met or exceeded, they will view the community as a good-quality operation. Conversely, if the community fails to meet their expectations or deliver on its promises, residents will not recommend the community to friends and may even become hostile to the management.

Exceeding expectations is often simply a matter of doing little things properly. Communities that ensure that all employees are service-oriented and empowered to handle small problems for residents as they arise often exceed the residents' expectations.

New residents often move into senior living communities with negative expectations. Those with little prior exposure to these communities may expect them to be restrictive, cold, and institutional. The staff should be trained to recognize the forces that shape residents' expectations. Some communities even provide sensitivity training in gerontology to equip employees at all levels to understand the aging process and to be sensitive to the emotions their residents may experience.

High-quality service is defined by personal attention, dependability, consistency, promptness, and competence. Residents need not always get everything they ask for, as long as they receive a prompt, courteous, and competent response to their requests. Managers should understand that a beautiful building complemented by an extensive service package does not guarantee resident satisfaction: in fact, the nicer the property, the greater the residents' expectations for service.

Ensuring resident satisfaction requires commitment from employees at all levels. Moreover, it is directly affected by employee-management relations. Managers seeking to improve the level of resident satisfaction in their operation must first ensure employee satisfaction. Contented employees are better equipped to serve residents with a positive and cheerful attitude. Conversely, happy residents are easier to take care of and less demanding, helping to create a positive work environment.

A critical component of the satisfaction cycle is employee turnover. Long-term employees learn the personal needs of the residents. For example, even though Mrs. Cameron orders ice cream for dessert every night, Rose, her server, knows that she is lactose-intolerant and serves her low-fat frozen yogurt as a substitute. Housekeeper Beatrice knows that she must be extremely careful with the seashell collection of Mr. Crane's deceased wife. If long-term employees become dissatisfied and leave, they take with them this personal knowledge of the residents' preferences, which is critical to resident satisfaction. The well-intentioned new replacement for Rose will, of course, serve Mrs. Cameron ice cream as she requests, thereby causing her discomfort and dissatisfaction. The management must appreciate the importance of keeping its employees in their jobs and communicate to them their value to the operation.

Resident satisfaction is dynamic, not static. The resident evaluates both the process and the outcome. For example, residents will accept a marginal food product temporarily if they receive consistently good service, and vice versa. But the perception of a poor overall product cannot be overcome by good personal relationships—at least, not for long. Nor will a good product outweigh poor treatment. If the management fails to deliver both good products and good service, dissatisfied residents will become part of the problem. To create the high level of resident satisfaction necessary to earn resident endorsements, the management must understand and even shape the residents' expectations.

RESIDENT OPINION SURVEYS

Opinion surveys have long been the principal measure of resident satisfaction. A well-conducted survey can identify problems and usefully quantify the residents' assessment of the service package. I limit the discussion here to resident satisfaction surveys, as other survey tools are discussed in detail in other chapters. Among the most important factors in conducting a meaningful survey with a high response rate are frequency, design, distribution and collection, interpretation of results, and follow-up.

Frequency

Most communities conduct an annual survey of resident satisfaction, and this is generally sufficient. Communities that inundate their residents with surveys place a burden on the residents, who may become reluctant to respond. In the end, those who do return the surveys may represent only a minority of chronic complainers, rather than the resident population as a whole. If the management demonstrates a willingness to respond to resident feedback, residents will be more tolerant than if the survey process is perceived as a routine exercise or a token attempt by the management to convince residents that their opinion matters. If the survey results reveal a high level of dissatisfaction in a given department, then an abbreviated follow-up survey of that department may be useful after steps have been taken to correct the problem.

Design

Resident opinion surveys should be designed to quantify satisfaction and dissatisfaction with the community's services and amenities: essentially, to show how well the management's promises to residents are fulfilled. Surveys should also measure how well an organization is functioning internally.

Survey instruments will evolve over the life of the community. In a newly established community, the management may want to conduct a comprehensive survey that evaluates residents' experiences from their initial visit with marketing staff to the orientation process, responsiveness of staff, dining-room service, food quality and quantity, frequency and variety of activity programs, condition and cleanliness of apartments and common areas, landscaping and curb appeal of the property, frequency of transportation, and communication by, fairness of, and confidence in the management. It is also a good idea to ask the residents if they think the staff are treated fairly and are happy in their work: if employees are not happy, the residents are often among the first to know. Finally, the survey should ask whether residents would recommend the community to their friends, and if not, why not.

After the community has reached stabilized occupancy and the residents' expectations have taken shape, a shorter survey may be appropriate. It might ask residents to rate the overall performance of each department as *excellent*, *good*, *fair*, or *poor*.

In the wording of survey questions, care should be taken not to set the management up for failure by phrasing questions in ways that create expectations of perfection. For example, a question that asks the resident to check the appropriate ending for the statement "The food is delivered promptly to my table: *always*, *seldom*, or *never*" can imply that it is the management's obligation always to deliver food promptly—a standard that may not be realistic or expected even in fine restaurants among leisurely diners. Rather, if it is worded "My meals are usually delivered to my table within a reasonable period of time: *yes* or *no*," the statement implies that residents should expect and tolerate occasional operational problems that might delay their meals.

To guarantee a good response, the survey should be kept relatively brief. Most residents will fill out a two- or three-page survey; if the survey exceeds five pages, the response rate may drop to less than 50 percent.

The appearance of the survey is also important. Surveys should be professionally copied (at a copy or reprint shop), in double-sided format to use fewer pages, and they should be set in large print for the benefit of visually impaired residents.

Distribution and Collection

For the survey to be objective and useful, it must represent the opinions of the majority of residents. Distribution and collection of the survey should be managed accordingly. Every resident should receive an individual copy (including residents who share apartments), and it should be emphasized that everyone's opinion is valued. Some communities offer incentives to residents to complete the survey, ranging from a free guest meal to "I've Been Heard" stickers or buttons. Many operators are now going to online survey instruments such as Survey Monkey. A simple survey can be crafted and saved with an online account to create a highly professional and "independent third party" looking document. These are then sent via email to residents and/or families. Surveys can be collected and analyzed with a number of tools and produce charts or graphs with statistical comparison against prior surveys. These can be customized with logos and colors and even provide a survey URL. Data can be exported (CSV, PDG, PPT, SPSS, or XLS) for further analysis and presentation. A copy of the survey can also be printed out and hand-delivered to residents who are not tech savvy, and results can be input manually by the concierge.

A well-managed survey process can yield up to an 80 percent response rate; if the process is left to chance, a 40 percent response is more typical. Although it is important to identify areas of dissatisfaction, surveys with a low response rate can be misleadingly negative. Their results may not accurately represent all residents' opinions, and they can lower employee morale. Residents who are dissatisfied and claim to speak on behalf of all the residents will be the first to respond. Those who feel that everything is fine will usually not bother to fill out and send in the survey unless specifically requested to do so. Residents who are happy with the way things are generally do not fill out the survey, so in the interest of a balanced result every resident should be continually encouraged to complete the survey until 80 percent is achieved.

Surveys should be conducted when there is not much happening in the community that could sway the results. When asked for an evaluation of something, most people tap into their short-term memory: consequently, recent positive or negative occurrences, such as a successful resident event or a fee increase, may disproportionately influence the results.

Before the survey is distributed, the management should call a meeting of the residents to go over it and explain the importance of everyone's participation. Residents should be asked to base their responses on their impressions over the entire year, not only on their most recent experience with each department. Furthermore, residents should be asked to be certain that their surveys represent their personal experiences and opinions and not what they may have heard from other residents. The management should also conduct individual floor meetings and select resident wing or floor captains to collect the completed surveys from the residents in their part of the property. The surveys should be returned in sealed envelopes to the floor captains, who should check them against a list of residents.

Finally, before distribution, the survey should be reviewed with employees (especially the housekeeping staff) to ensure that they understand its purpose and importance. Results should be tabulated off-site, either at corporate headquarters or by a consultant, if for no other reason than to guarantee the participants' anonymity and confidentiality.

The survey should be distributed along with a cover memo explaining its purpose and importance. The cover memo in exhibit 6.1 provides an example.

Interpretation of Results

The response rate to the survey determines its validity. Response rates of 60 percent or less, while providing some useful information, do little to offset negative perceptions. Response rates greater than 80 percent represent a majority of the respondents and are statistically valid. When questions ask respondents to rate facilities or services by categories such as *excellent*, *good*, *fair*, or *poor*, the responses should be tabulated according to the same categories.

Exhibit 6.1   Sample Cover Memo for Resident Survey

Dear Resident:

Your happiness and satisfaction are critical to us. I hope that every day our staff is doing everything they can to make your move to our community a rewarding experience. We invite you to take a moment to review how well we are meeting your needs, and we also welcome suggestions for improvement.

Please complete the following questionnaire, seal it in the attached envelope, and return it to your resident representative. Your comments and observations are vital to us and will help shape our services and amenities. In addition, we will be using your responses in part to evaluate our staff at your community. So even if you feel everything is fine, please complete your survey and send it in so that your opinion can be properly recognized. If the survey is difficult for you to read, or if you have a question, ask your housekeeper or any management representative for help.

We also would like to take this opportunity to thank you for the many referrals you have given us; clearly, a fully occupied community is in everyone's best interest.

Thank you for taking the time to share your impressions with us.

Very truly yours,

Benjamin W. Pearce
President

The survey results should be tabulated in a spreadsheet format so that an overall score can be determined. Most online survey platforms offer a report menu to create customized results. An unfavorable change in the residents' opinion of any department that exceeds 10 percent could indicate a problem to be addressed. The management should not settle for anything less than 90 percent of the residents indicating satisfaction and a willingness to recommend the community to their friends, for resident endorsements are the cheapest and most effective form of advertising.

More important, the management should carefully evaluate the differences, both positive and negative, from one survey to the next to determine whether progress has been made in correcting residents' perceptions of previously identified problems. The wording of questions should remain consistent in successive surveys to allow comparisons that might identify trends. Changes in the percentage of residents' responses from favorable to unfavorable or vice versa may occur for a variety of reasons, including but not limited to the survey response rate, changes in staffing, attitudes of the leaders of the resident council, differences in residents' perceptions of value for money following a significant monthly fee increase, or a real change in the quality of services or products.

Managers of multiple properties can compare their resident-satisfaction results using a quality index (QI) system, which measures an individual community's service ratings against company-wide service ratings. It is similar to the method used to calculate the consumer price index. All QI scores are based on combined favorable responses: *excellent* plus *good*, or *yes* percentages for the yes-or-no questions on the survey. For example, satisfaction with housekeeping in community A may be compared to that across all communities, as shown in table 6.1.

The average of all *excellent* and *good* responses is set at a baseline of 100, and the QI scores are measured against this baseline. Community A's score of 107.2 indicates a level of resident satisfaction with housekeeping considerably above the average levels for other communities. In general, scores above 100 indicate acceptable performance, whereas scores below 100 show a need for attention. The farther above or below 100 a score falls, the higher or lower the relative level of resident satisfaction. The long-term objec-

Table 6.1	Sample Quality Index Rating	
	Housekeeping: All communities	Housekeeping: Community A
Excellent	43.3%	47.2%
Good	48.2%	50.9%
Total	91.5%	98.1%

Note: Index score for community A = (98.1% ÷ 91.5%) × 100 = 107.2.

tive for the company is to bring all QI service ratings close to the score of 100 for all communities. Using this system, corporate operations managers can easily identify problems in specific communities.

Follow-up

Unless residents are convinced that the management will act on the results of the survey, they will not respond. In addition, if the management fails to respond to problems revealed by the survey, it may damage its credibility with the residents and their families. Any combined *excellent* and *good* or *yes* response level lower than 85 percent, or any increase in combined unfavorable *fair* and *poor* or *no* response level greater than 10 percent, should automatically trigger a plan of correction, which should be formulated by the department head and her direct supervisor within 30 days of the tabulation of the survey.

This response should not be an exercise that simply identifies existing problems and lists solutions that are "ongoing." Department heads should call all their employees together to brainstorm so that they all can be part of the solution. Plans of correction should describe the area in need of improvement in specific terms, detail a solution, assign a responsible party, and set a completion date.

Some communities are reluctant to publicize the results of their surveys, citing fears that some specific results may fuel arguments by special-interest groups among the residents and affect employee morale. A survey of any nature raises the expectations of the population served. Residents offer their input on the assumption that the management will respond positively, quickly, and thoroughly to the issues and concerns raised. If the management is unwilling to commit to providing survey results to the participants and acting on them as quickly as possible, it is better not to do the survey at all. Conversely, the dissemination of positive results from a resident survey can go far toward counteracting the negativity of vocal and chronic complainers.

The results of a resident survey should never be used to discipline a manager, as an excuse for discharging an employee, or to coerce an employee into a behavioral change. Such measures will cause employees to fear the process rather than regard it as a useful management tool. The management should familiarize supervisors with the survey results and coach them on increasing their individual contributions to productivity, profitability, and service. The management must motivate employees to deliver good service and equip them to do so, rather than threaten them if they do not.

A positive survey response—90 percent satisfaction or better—shows that the management is obviously exceeding residents' expectations. Such a response is even more impressive if the community is also meeting its budgetary goals. The staff's ability to balance these often-conflicting objectives consistently is clearly a reflection of their professionalism and commitment to building value in their operation.

■ HANDLING COMPLAINTS

The business of operating senior living communities is unique in that the customers are to a large extent a captive audience. They can't just go away or be appeased with a gift coupon or free meal. Managers need to satisfy them permanently or clearly communicate the limits of what can and cannot be done for them.

In part because of these unique circumstances, residents may be reluctant to bring their complaints to the attention of the management: indeed, the management is often the last to hear residents' complaints. Usually residents will first mention the issue to their families; next to be told are other residents, then the line staff, and ultimately the management. Such complaints spread like wildfire through a community, especially if they involve gossip or the actions of the management.

Problems don't just go away. Managers who avoid dealing with issues as they arise run the risk of their escalation. Left unchecked, they can require massive amounts of money and unproductive time to resolve. Studies have shown that:

■ For every resident who bothers to complain, there are 24 silent unhappy residents. Yet if residents do complain and the complaint is resolved quickly,

90 percent will recommend the community to their friends.
■ The average "wronged" resident will tell 8 to 16 people, each of whom may tell 5 others.
■ It can cost five times as much to attract a new resident as it takes to keep an existing one happy.

Complaining can have positive consequences: it can open lines of communication, identify real and solvable problems, dispel rumors, and build resident satisfaction and referrals. The retailer Marshall Field aptly summarized the importance of constructive complaints when he said, "Those who complain teach me how I may please others so that more will come. Only those hurt me who are displeased but do not complain. They refuse me permission to correct my errors and improve my service."[1] The Technical Assistance Research Programs Institute conducted studies of the handling of consumer complaints in the United States. The researchers found that one in four customers of the average American organization is dissatisfied enough to consider taking their business elsewhere. Yet only 5 percent actually register a complaint; the other 95 percent would rather switch than fight. According to TARP, consumers overwhelmingly believe that "complaining won't do any good; no one wants to hear about my problem." The TARP report concludes that this pessimism is well founded: more than 40 percent of the consumers were unhappy with the action taken to resolve their complaints. It is important for managers to learn to hear and resolve complaints respectfully and in ways that minimize the wear and tear on themselves, residents, families, and employees.

A firm and confident approach to interaction with a resident will be more positive and productive than an ambivalent one. If the management has a reputation for quick, courteous responses to complaints, residents will be more ready to present their grievances calmly and rationally, and their behavior will serve as a model for other residents with problems.

Why People Complain

A complaint is not always a criticism. Moreover, it is not always easy to identify the real problem behind a complaint. A resident's complaint may be a minor problem compounded by difficulties in adjusting to the community; such difficulties may be further complicated by feelings of rejection and guilt.

Most seniors who have retired are on fixed-incomes and have become conditioned to austerity. When first introduced to a modern senior living community, many react negatively to a lifestyle that they consider lavish. Many hope to pass on their life savings to their heirs; they may have lived frugally in their own home or apartment and feel guilty about spending money on themselves. Therefore, they may be vigilant about how the management spends their money and quick to criticize any perceived waste, incompetence, or substandard service.

Family members may also experience guilt about influencing a parent to move into a senior living community. Many are forced by busy careers, geographical distance, and other family commitments to seek professional care for their aging parents. Because of the enduring negative stereotypes of senior living communities, family members may experience feelings of guilt at having "abandoned" their parents. Such feelings may contribute to anger toward the management if they feel that a resident is not being appropriately treated in the community.

Some residents recognize their families' feelings of guilt and may consciously or unconsciously exploit them. Indeed, residents can be much harder on their families than they are on the management, prefacing their complaints with "I told you this place wasn't right for me," and expecting family members to become personally involved in solving their problems. This behavior occurs more frequently among new residents, who may feel lonely, than among more established ones. Complaints to families tend to decrease with time, as residents adjust to their environment and make new friends.

Family members who complain to the management are usually passing on their parents' complaints to them. In handling such complaints, managers should point out that their parents may be experiencing difficulty adjusting to their new lifestyle and that the complaints may be a manifestation of other, broader issues. They should remind family members that everyone must support the resident and be patient.

Family members who relay their parents' complaints to the management usually do so without the parents' knowledge or approval. They should be assured that the management will do everything reasonable to resolve their parents' issues discreetly. But they should encourage their parents to report concerns directly to the management as they arise and to express complaints in specific terms so that appropriate solutions can be found.

Managers should also realize that some complaints have ulterior purposes. When a resident tells her family, "I've told them about it and they never do anything," it might mean that the management has already turned down the request, perhaps because granting it would be inconsistent with community policy. Residents may sometimes seek special treatment or try to differentiate their situations from those of other residents. Any success in convincing the management to bend the rules for one individual might be considered a triumph to be flaunted before other residents. The management should take great care to ensure that all residents are treated fairly and equally.

Of course, not all complaints are rooted in family dynamics or emotional turmoil. Residents can become upset for a variety of reasons. In working to resolve their problems, it helps to understand possible causes or contributing factors. For example, residents may become upset for any of the following reasons:

- They have an expectation that has not been met. Someone in the organization may have promised them something that was not delivered or has changed. They may have made an erroneous assumption about what the community would provide. (It is critical that sales representatives avoid making promises that do not reflect operational reality: *never overpromise or underdeliver.*)
- They may already be upset for reasons beyond anyone's control. They may feel tired, sick, stressed, frustrated, abandoned, or afraid that their personal autonomy is eroding with age.
- Someone on the staff may have been rude, indifferent, or discourteous to them. They may have been given conflicting information by different staff members, or acted on incorrect information from a staff member. They may have been embarrassed about doing something incorrectly or had their integrity or honesty questioned.
- *They may have a valid complaint.*

Responding to Complaints

Although managers cannot control the behavior of residents or anyone else, they can adjust their own behavior to avoid an escalation of conflict. In addition to the lists in exhibits 6.2 and 6.3, which give specific approaches to use and steps to take in defusing arguments and responding to complaints, this section offers some guidance.

Don't react to difficult situations, *respond*. We *react* when our immediate instincts take charge; we *respond* when we listen, consider the alternatives, and develop a workable solution to a difficult situation. See exhibit 6.2 for some tactics on engaging the resident proactively.

Above all, listen carefully. Focus on not only what the resident is saying but also how she is saying it. The resident may not *say* she's angry, but her voice conveys it loud and clear. Listen carefully for emotions as well as facts. Take great care not to patronize a resident who is in error, as she may already feel vulnerable in her new environment.

Residents can quickly discern whether you are paying attention. If they were mildly agitated before, inattention can push them to anger. Repeat or paraphrase what you understand the resident to have said. Sometimes hearing you say it makes it sound worse than the resident believes it is, and he will back down a bit. At the very least, he will know you are listening.

Residents want empathy. Tell them you understand how they could feel that way. Validate their concerns by admitting that others have felt the same way. Finally, offer an explanation that has been acceptable to others: "What they have found is that two separate dining times can create a more intimate setting and better service." The "feel, felt, found" technique acknowledges residents' feelings, validates their concerns, and offers solutions based on experience.

Be consistent in your responses. The residents will test the consistency of responses, and consistency equals credibility. Sometimes the hardest thing for a manager to do is to say no and mean it. It may seem much easier to give in to a resident's demands to get him off your back, but you may pay for it later. Giving favorite residents special treatment will be transparent to most residents and staff; it is never worth the short-term benefits. It is usually better to say no to a resident's request if you are not sure you can accommodate it. This will buy you some time, perhaps enabling you to resolve the problem in the resident's favor and surprise her. If you merely say you will "look into it," there is no closure. You are accepting the responsibility to follow up personally

---

> **Exhibit 6.2   Response Tactics**
>
> - Listen carefully and clarify before you respond.
> - Engage the resident. Face him and look him in the eye.
> - Adopt an open, not defensive, body posture; show your concern.
> - Avoid being condescending or impatient.
> - Never argue or interrupt a resident; let him get it all out. He may just be blowing off steam.
> - Be sincere and show empathy.
> - Eliminate distractions.
> - Use a pleasant tone of voice.
> - Be solution-oriented.
> - Don't take things personally.

---

and risking further animosity if you cannot offer a solution.

Avoid responding to insults or taking criticism personally. Upset residents may call you names, curse, or say other unpleasant things about you, your coworkers, or your organization. If you allow yourself to become upset by this behavior you may lose your objectivity, and you must remain in control if you are going to find a solution to the situation. It is natural to feel attacked personally when a resident is abusive or accusatory. He is lashing out at whatever is nearest—in this case, you. More often than not, you did not cause his grievance; remind yourself of this. If a resident says, "You messed up my order," he probably means, "My order didn't arrive in a reasonable amount of time, and the kitchen is disorganized. Whoever is responsible for this is in big trouble, and you're the one who is going to hear about it."

Avoid becoming defensive. When the management becomes defensive, the customer becomes frustrated, and the problem may escalate. Look for things you can agree on, and attempt to validate some of the concerns. Exhibit 6.3 provides a step-by-step approach that can create an atmosphere for a successful resolution to a complaint.

Of course, sometimes the mistake may have been your fault. We all make mistakes. Experience teaches us to recognize them when we make them again! It will often disarm residents if you take responsibility and apologize.

Don't be afraid to say, "I don't know" or "I don't have the answer right now." Tell the resident, "That's

---

Exhibit 6.3   Handling Complaints:
A Step-by-Step Response

- Disarm the resident with a calm response.
- Isolate the resident from other residents or guests.
- Verbally cushion the resident's behavior by softening your approach in order to calm the resident.
- Use the *feel, felt, found* approach.
- Apologize for the situation.
- Assure the resident that you want to help.
- Probe to identify the specific problem, not just the symptoms. Ask the resident to elaborate on sweeping accusations.
- Paraphrase the resident's concerns to clarify your understanding.
- Find something in the resident's remarks with which you can agree.
- Avoid being defensive and making excuses.
- Show the resident that you value this information and appreciate her candor in bringing the problem to your attention.
- Ask how she would like you to respond or specifically resolve her concern.
- Explain available options; offer choices.
- Summarize actions to be taken—yours and hers. She may be part of the solution.
- Thank the resident for bringing the matter to your attention.
- *Follow up!*

---

a good question. I'll find an answer for you and get back to you tomorrow."

Don't be afraid to acknowledge problems. Never cover up anything.

Residents who are upset may demand immediate action. They want the manager not to "look into it" but to do something *right now*. They may want compensation, restitution, or someone to take the blame, and so may demand the reprimanding or even termination of a staff member. In such cases, assure the resident that corrective action will be taken, to show that you understand the seriousness of the concern. Sometimes the resident just wants to know that some action has been or will be taken, so that no one will have this problem again. Most of all, residents want attention and to be listened to. If they feel neglected or ignored, they will go to great lengths to make their points.

Dealing with Difficult People

The steps outlined above will enable managers to resolve most complaints. Occasionally, however, a resident may seem more difficult to please. Fortunately, residents who have a difficult time adjusting to the community are the minority, and solutions or interventions can be found that will work for them. But employees and other residents sometimes label them "chronic complainers" or "difficult" residents. Employees need to recognize that these are not bad people, only people whose behavior is challenging. Behavioral problems usually have an identifiable cause, such as stress, medical problems or physiological imbalance, anger over the loss of a spouse, family or financial problems, or simply rejection of the normal aging process. Some people internalize these problems, whereas others direct their feelings outward and exhibit hostility to the world around them.

Residents who may be temporarily upset are not necessarily difficult people. When a reasonable person gets upset, he or she may react inappropriately. Chronically "difficult" people, by contrast, have a psychological need to gain attention by disruptive and negative means. They are hard to communicate with and may have lived their entire lives this way, moving in a vortex of anxiety from one place and encounter to the next. They seek satisfaction through validation and solicit the support of others. Sometimes residents use any excuse to prove they are right, whether or not they actually are. A resident may have a chip on his shoulder or hold deeply rooted prejudices that are expressed in arguments and complaints. If this behavior continues, residents and staff members alike will begin to avoid contact with the difficult resident, which can make matters worse. He may soon find himself sitting alone in the dining room or with new residents, until they also become weary of the negativity.

Some people will be unreasonable no matter what you do. Usually they make up only about 1 percent of the resident population. In extreme cases, some communities may temporarily refuse service to difficult residents in the main dining room, delivering their meals to their apartments instead. This alternative can protect the other residents' rights to the quiet enjoyment of the community's common areas. It usually also has a moderating effect on the difficult resident's behavior, as isolation can be unpleasant and embarrassing.

When Complaints Escalate

Residents who are not satisfied, or who become frustrated with the management's inability to resolve their concerns reasonably, may seek validation from other residents. In extreme cases, such situations can deteriorate into conflict. When lines of communication break down, residents will seek alternative ways to make their points. They may attempt to organize other residents by circulating a petition, posting a bad review online, seeking legal advice, or even reporting their complaint to an ombudsperson or to state regulatory authorities who may be required by law to investigate. Some extreme situations may lead to litigation. Large quantities of money and energy can be spent because someone was unwilling to listen to a minor complaint.

Resident petitions can set a dangerous precedent because they circumvent and invalidate the normal methods of communicating and solving problems. It is within a resident's rights to circulate a petition, but the management should make every attempt to resolve a resident's concerns before a petition gains momentum. If residents report being intimidated by others into signing a petition, it is appropriate for a manager to speak to the persons responsible. But the management should never give the impression that it is afraid of a petition or is attempting to derail it; rather, managers should address the issue and clarify the situation or policy, or call the residents together and make a presentation on the subject. Most residents understand and accept standard business practices. Corporate management responsible for multiple sites must be careful not to accept the role of arbitrator, a decision that may compromise the executive director's authority to manage the community. Whenever possible, the decision of the executive director should be final.

Forestalling Complaints

The most effective way to handle complaints is to prevent them. Proactively manage your residents' expectations and opinions. Reinforce the feeling that the residents are part of a thriving community by distributing flyers and memos about community affairs, providing formal communications on important issues, and sharing good financial and other news about the community. Recognize the residents' contributions to the community's success through resident-appreciation events, awards for volunteers, photographs and features in the community newsletter, and displays of photographs of special events. Share pertinent information with residents through flyers and memos about community affairs, accomplishments of the owner(s), formal responses to important issues, and good news about marketing accomplishments or details on the new-resident referral program.

A suggestion box can be valuable in managing complaints and feedback. Residents who complain, either at meetings or in less formal situations, should be encouraged to document their specific concerns in a contribution to the suggestion box, along with signed suggestions on how things could be improved, so that the management can follow up. They should also be urged to recognize the value of positive reinforcement by offering praise for jobs well done, not only complaints. Residents whose suggestions are ignored may resort to posting a negative review online to make their point. Once these are posted, they are there permanently even after the resident's issue is resolved, unless the resident takes them down.

The management should respond to all suggestions submitted by documenting the suggestion and providing an appropriate response, perhaps in a report distributed monthly to the president of the resident council. In this way, as residents' concerns are identified, the management can offer specific solutions to derail the criticism that "nothing ever happens if you complain." Suggestion-box responses from the management should be kept on file and consulted on issues that may resurface.

Resident and family issues can also be dealt with immediately. To avoid escalation, a family's observation can be solicited at any time, day or night, and before they leave the building. Create a family feedback system that enables a visitor to scan a QR code sticker (Avery 22805 print-to-the-edge 1.5-inch square labels) on each resident's door frame that immediately populates an email to top company management. This lets them voice their concerns while they are still at the community. It is never a good idea to let a disgruntled family member go home and stew about something they didn't like. They can now easily report about an exceptional employee or moment of excellence they witnessed, request a maintenance work order, let nursing know about any unmet care needs, or anything else they would like to say. This system is a simple and effective way to provide residents and their families a direct conduit to top management so that their voice is heard. Often the simple act of voicing one's concern can actually relieve family anxiety and avoid misunderstandings which can cause problems down the road.

Residents with grievances occasionally confront the management publicly such as in resident meetings. When this happens, it is important to validate the resident's concerns but to separate her from the group to prevent uproar. Resident meetings can get out of hand quickly when angry residents maneuver the management into a defensive posture. It is like the dog and the mail carrier: if the carrier shows fear, the dog will give chase!

Come to resident meetings with an agenda and stick to it. There should always be something special on the agenda, such as announcing the employee of the quarter or offering some resident recognition, to add a positive note to the meeting (you might want to save this item for last). Asking residents for ideas is always well received. If things begin to get off track, schedule the topic for another meeting to allow yourself time to research the situation. Another good way to encourage participation in family meetings is to conduct them in a Zoom call. This is an online video meeting platform that has become widely accepted since the COVID-19 outbreak forced many people to isolate at home. The meeting can be announced via email with an invite and an attached PDF document agenda. Often the families come up with great suggestions at these meetings that are easy to implement, such as issuing the family a report card detailing the latest in their loved one's condition. Families have asked if they could wear a name tag with their relationship to their loved one added, so the staff and other families can learn to recognize them. Others asked for a doorbell or text number they could use to get out of the building after their visit rather than tracking down a staff member. The more communication, the better the partnership that operators can have with families.

The use of these tools as a communication conduit will depend solely on the management's response. One of the largest and most successful food stores is the family-owned Stew Leonard's Dairy, in Norwalk, Connecticut. The sales volume per square foot is about 10 times that of conventional grocery stores. Obviously, the Leonard family are on to something. One secret of their success is their obsession with customer service.

Near the front door is a suggestion box where customers are encouraged to share their comments, suggestions, and complaints. Each morning the contents of the box (an average of 100 suggestions per day) are emptied out and typed up. By 10:00 a.m. the comment sheets have been photocopied, distributed to all department managers, and posted and left on tables in the employee break areas, so that everyone knows how well the company is doing in the eyes of its most important managers—the customers.

It doesn't end there. Within 24 hours, someone on the store's management team—often someone named Leonard—has followed up with a phone call to thank the customer for the comment, explore the details of the suggestion, or discuss ways to resolve the problem. Within 48 hours, there's a letter to the customer in the mail. Customers who take the initiative at Stew Leonard's find out quickly how highly their input is valued.

RESIDENT COUNCIL

No business can succeed without the support of its customers. Residents can be both a manager's greatest ally and her worst nightmare. They are paying large sums of money for the services they receive; it is only reasonable that they should have some voice in how the services are delivered. Many communities have found a resident council to be the best way to give residents that voice while restraining the influence of special-interest groups. The council should play *an advisory role only* and not participate directly in the management of the community. After all, residents are paying the management company for professional supervision. Residents trying to do that job will only complicate the management's efforts to control costs and increase revenues.

A resident council by definition should represent the interests of the entire resident body. Its members should be selected by a democratic process on the basis of demonstrated objectivity and interest in representing the resident body as a whole. It should not be a popularity contest; residents should be advised to screen candidates carefully to avoid potential conflicts of interest. The council should never be perceived as a rubber-stamp committee that only sings the management's praises. It should understand the importance of balancing the objectives of the owner(s) and the expectations of the employees and the residents they serve. The operation will run best when everyone's needs are addressed.

The resident council should be made up of no fewer than five residents. Some communities elect a president and a secretary plus a representative from each floor, building, or wing. The management should set up procedures for electing members of the resident council, establish initial bylaws, and recommend standing rules of procedure. Although community needs may differ, the following suggestions will facilitate the creation and clarify the role of a proactive resident council.

Electing Members

The term of service on the council should be limited to two years. To prevent the formation of special-interest groups, council members should not be allowed to run for immediate reelection. To ensure both continuity and objective representation, terms should be staggered. Each year the council should have at least two new members, depending on its size. A nominating and elections committee should prepare a slate of at least two candidates for each vacancy on the council. In addition, residents not on the committee should be allowed to nominate any number of additional candidates by petitions signed by a number of other residents—say, 12. The committee should verify that each nominee has indicated a willingness to serve. The names of the candidates should appear on the ballot in alphabetical order (which is generally perceived as fairer than a random order).

The elections committee should establish an annual schedule for the election. An all-resident meeting should be held to introduce the candidates and explain the process. The election should be by sealed ballot: the candidates who receive the greatest numbers of votes will be elected. Ballots should be placed in residents' mailboxes on a specified date and returned to the ballot box (kept at a convenient but secure location, such as the receptionist's desk) by another specified date, usually one week following distribution. The ballots should then be counted at a meeting of the nominating and elections committee. In case of a tie, a runoff election should be held using the same procedures as in the first election.

When the candidates elected to the council have been determined, the remaining candidates should be listed according to the number of votes received, and this list should be retained for the following year

and used to fill unexpected vacancies on the council. If any member is unable to complete a term of service, the council should name as a successor the person at the top of the list. To prevent wounded feelings and grievances, actual numbers of votes for each candidate should not be announced.

Council Bylaws

The bylaws should establish the name of the organization, usually the "Resident Advisory Council of [community name]." They should also establish its purpose: to bring to the attention of the management any concerns and questions brought forth by the residents and to act in an advisory capacity to the management on behalf of the residents. The bylaws should specify the number of members, terms of service, and the policy for replacement of members who cannot complete their terms. They should specify a policy on attendance at council meetings: for example, three unexcused absences might result in a letter giving the dates of the absences and advising the member that she will be dropped from the council. Absences should be considered excused when the council president is notified in a timely manner before the meeting. The president should be elected for a term of only one year and be eligible for another term only after a one-year break in service. The officers of the council should be defined and confirmed by an affirmative vote by a majority of all council members.

The bylaws should establish the duties of the officers.

PRESIDENT
- Preside at all council meetings
- Develop an agenda for monthly meetings
- Report to all resident meetings on the work of the council
- Appoint, with council consultation, chairpersons and members of committees
- Chair the nominating and elections committee
- Serve as ex officio member of all other committees
- In the absence of the secretary, appoint a secretary pro tem

SECRETARY
- Record in the official minutes actions taken at council meetings and distribute copies to council members and the management

- Act as custodian of council minutes and related notices, communications, and reports
- Act as custodian of the official documents of the council, including the bylaws and rules of procedure
- In the absence of the president, call the meeting to order and preside over the election of a president pro tem

Meetings should be held monthly unless otherwise provided for by the council. A majority of all council members should constitute a quorum. Special meetings can be called with advance notice by the president, at the request of the management, or by three members of the council. Written notice should be given stating the business to be conducted, and the meeting should discuss only that specific business. Each member is entitled to one vote, and any member may abstain from voting. Motions are passed by a majority vote of those members present and voting at the meeting. The president or, in her absence, the secretary should call meetings to order. An agenda should include introduction of guests; reading, correction, and approval of minutes of the previous meeting; reports of the president, secretary, and committees; unfinished business; and new business. *Riddick's Revised Rules of Procedure* can be used to govern council proceedings unless otherwise provided in the bylaws and the standing rules of procedures.

There should be two standing committees: the nominating and elections committee and the employee appreciation fund committee. Other ad hoc committees may be created to address specific issues, but their number should be limited. Some communities establish committees for each service department, but such a structure may create peer pressure to find things to report on, even when a department is running smoothly, and may cause department heads to feel they are being scrutinized by residents looking for problems where none exist.

Employee Appreciation Fund

The management in senior living communities usually discourages employees from accepting tips and may have a policy expressly prohibiting tipping, in order to discourage employees from favoring some residents. In addition, tipping might disproportionately favor dining room and housekeeping employees: it takes the combined efforts of all employees, including those behind the scenes, to deliver resident services. As an alternative, the resident council usually establishes an employee appreciation fund to distribute gratuities to all employees. Residents often ask the management for guidance in determining employees' eligibility in order to ensure fairness.

Although the management can assist residents in administering this fund, it must be clear that this is an undertaking of the residents and is not sponsored by the community. This distinction is important because the federal and state tax authorities are likely to view any disbursements by the community to employees as compensation requiring the necessary withholding and employer matching taxes. The fund should be held in a separate non–interest-bearing bank account using the name and Social Security number of the executive director as the primary contact. Setting it up as a non–interest-bearing account avoids income-tax implications and reporting requirements. Residents can then make gifts payable by check to the account. A general notice can be given to the residents outlining the purpose of the fund, the deadline for contributions, and the methods by which eligible employees are selected and the funds distributed.

Department heads should be ineligible for awards from this fund if they are eligible for other bonuses or performance incentives. The executive director should never receive anything, and only sales staff who are not paid commissions should be included. Ultimately, it should be left to the residents to decide who receives awards, but it is in the residents' best interests to recognize those employees who directly serve them. Usually the resident council collects the funds for distribution two weeks before year-end holidays. Some communities have a summer collection as well. Other communities have established a "Christmas club": contributions are made monthly to the fund and then distributed at the end of the year. This approach is helpful for residents on a tight budget, who may find it difficult to come up with a lump sum at a time of the year when they may also be buying gifts for relatives.

To ensure fairness, the collected funds should be distributed to the employees based on total hours worked during the award period. For example, if awards are distributed annually, the amount collected should be divided by the total hours worked by all eligible employees during the past 12 months.

To calculate the dollar distribution, multiply the per-hour figure by the total hours worked for each employee (to a maximum of 2,080 for a full-time employee). Awards are thus prorated for part-time employees and more recent hires. Most communities require the employee to be employed actively at the time of distribution and for at least three months previously to be eligible.

The suggested contribution for residents will vary depending on the affluence of the community. The resident council might aim to collect $365, or a dollar per day for the preceding year, from each resident; some communities may choose a more modest contribution, such as $10 per month. Although some residents may not be able to afford this level of contribution (resident contributions average about $150 for most communities), all gifts are appreciated. In one large, affluent continuing care community, the fund accumulated more than $140,000: when divided among the 200 employees, this amount resulted in a nice holiday bonus (especially for the long-term employees). I have even heard of a distribution of $1,200 per employee from a large campus community. Usually the funds are distributed in cash, in sealed and labeled envelopes. The management should remind employees that this distribution is considered tip income and should be reported to the IRS. The management should expect some employee resignations after the funds are distributed, as employees planning to leave often wait for this bonus before announcing their departure.

RESIDENTS ON GOVERNING BOARDS

Residents nearly always request representation on governing boards. In some states, the law requires resident representation on the boards of continuing care retirement communities (CCRCs). In addition, some legislators support giving residents voting status on boards. Governing boards of CCRCs are realizing the value of resident participation for the success and acceptance of their policy initiatives.

The voting status of a resident board member can be a sensitive issue. Residents who participate on boards without voting rights may be viewed as "token" representatives by other residents. This situation can create animosity between resident representatives and the residents, for having responsibility without authority can place the nonvoting representatives in an awkward position. Residents may insist that they be represented by vote to formally establish their position on critical issues; in that case, however, if they are outvoted, they may demand equal representation. The danger of this situation comes when a conflict of interest arises on initiatives, such as increases in monthly service fees, that may not be well received by the general population but may be necessary to ensure the financial stability of the project. Nevertheless, boards are increasingly recognizing the rich resources of skill and experience among their residents, which can be tapped to facilitate the problem-solving and long-term planning processes.

MEDICAL CHALLENGES

The quality and longevity of a resident's life can be measurably improved through companionship and preventive care. As stewards of the elderly people living in senior communities, managers cannot escape the obligation to assist residents in facing the inevitable medical challenges that will shape their lives. Many seniors who inquire about living options are seeking a supportive environment that will enable them to continue to function independently as they grow older. A caring community can do more than simply support individuals with special needs: it can help them to flourish. Seniors who continue to live in their home after the loss of a spouse tend to focus on the things they cannot do anymore—their limitations. This attitude can lead to chronic depression and despair, which in turn can lead to an earlier death. Time and again I have seen residents who had moved into senior communities chronically depressed, or with extensive medical complications, out on the dance floor after six months of companionship and activity. Herein lies the primary motivator for many employees, who are uniquely empowered to help residents claim back their lives.

The Centers for Disease Control and Prevention estimates life expectancy for an infant boy born in the United States in 2021 to be 73.5 years, and that of a girl 79.3 years.[2] The average entry age of seniors in CCRCs today is about 78 years; for congregate communities, about 81.5 years; and for assisted living communities, 82.5 years. Residents who are 80 years old today have significantly exceeded their life expectancy at birth, which for those born in the 1910s was 50.2 years for men and 53.7 years for women.

More than 25 years have been added to the life expectancy of infants in the United States since 1900, largely owing to our improving ability to combat infectious diseases.

In his book *How and Why We Age*, the gerontologist Leonard Hayflick differentiates between life expectancy and active, healthy, or functional life expectancy.[3] Active life expectancy ends when a person's health declines to a point at which she loses independence in matters of daily living and must depend on others for some form of care. Most Americans over the age of 65 are healthy and live productive lives, but with increasing age, health generally deteriorates and the need for care increases. One study found that 45 percent of those over the age of 85 needed help with one or more basic activities of daily life.

There's a saying: "Age is a thing of mind over matter—if you don't mind it, it don't matter." For many old people, however, taking the attitude that "it don't matter" can mean ignoring or denying age-related health complications, which can lead to serious consequences. The best thing that seniors can do to optimize their later years is to understand and identify potential common problems while they are still treatable. Residents should be encouraged to establish a course of preventive checkups and screenings with their primary care physicians. The following tests and procedures are based on guidelines recommended by the American Heart Association and the American Cancer Society:

- Immunizations: Flu shots can be helpful in preventing complications brought on by common viruses. Also COVID-19 vaccinations and booster shots will likely be an annual recommendation by the CDC, especially considering its ability to mutate into different strains.
- History: Health history should be taken every two and a half years after age 61 and annually after age 75 for healthy individuals.
- Mammogram: A mammogram is recommended once between the ages of 35 and 40 to establish a baseline and then every two years until age 50. Thereafter, an annual test is recommended.
- Stool slide tests: This is an analysis of the stool to search for hidden traces of blood, the appearance of which could signal cancer or some other disorder in the digestive tract. Tests are recommended annually for everyone over 50.

- Urinalysis: This test is recommended annually as a general screening for the function of many vital organs.
- Blood tests: Full blood tests should be done every two and a half years.
- Pelvic examinations: All women over the age of 40 should have a pelvic exam annually.
- Electrocardiogram (EKG): The American Heart Association recommends a baseline EKG at ages 20, 40, and 60.
- Physical examinations: The American Heart Association recommends an annual physical after the age of 75. The American Cancer Society recommends an annual screening for cancer after the age of 40, especially for cancer of the thyroid, testicles, prostate, ovaries, lymph nodes, and skin.

Many operators establish preventive care programs. During weekly meetings of department heads, the agenda should include reports from employees of any observed changes in resident status. Employees of key departments, such as housekeeping, should be trained to recognize health changes in their residents and to report them promptly to their supervisors. They should be made aware that residents may conceal health problems for fear of being asked to transfer to a more supportive environment. In fact, many health problems, when detected early, can be managed by a physician, enabling residents to continue to function independently and live in greater comfort. See also chapter 17, "Assessments and Interventions," for details on identifying and tracking resident health status and offering interventions.

At the first sign of a change in health status, the executive director should approach the resident for a consultation. In extreme cases, it may be appropriate to notify the resident's family members or physician immediately. It is advisable to establish a dialogue concerning physical, physiological, or gerontological issues, keeping them informed and soliciting their support. Working with the family or their support network in turn helps elicit cooperation from the resident in dealing with age-related challenges.

It may be appropriate to schedule quarterly or semiannual meetings with the family and key department heads to monitor the status of some residents. Never wait until a resident's condition becomes unmanageable before involving the family or physician.

These meetings can be a valuable source of information on the level of the resident's or the family's satisfaction, health and dietary concerns, and affordability issues. No one likes surprises, particularly if they may entail a confrontation with a loved one in denial. As with any problem-solving exercise, issues are best dealt with as they arise, with attempts to build consensus among all interested parties.

Common Health Complaints

For people over 65, the top three causes of death (accounting for about 75 percent of deaths) are heart disease, cancer, and cerebrovascular disease (stroke). Thus it is helpful for managers to recognize the symptoms of these and other common disorders of elderly people, including dementia, incontinence, and substance abuse.

HEART DISEASE AND STROKE. Cardiovascular disease is the leading cause of death in the United States and other developed countries. Atherosclerosis, a thickening and hardening of the walls of the coronary arteries, is the most common form of heart disease. This condition begins early in life and may in later years result in a heart attack (myocardial infarction), angina, or a stroke. Symptoms of heart attack include pain in the chest, shoulder, or jaw lasting more than two minutes. Vomiting and sweating frequently accompany the pain. People may also experience a sudden state of confusion or change in mental status, or simply feel breathless. Some people experience small heart attacks that are symptomless and show up only on EKGs. Heart disease can often be prevented with a simple change in diet to reduce cholesterol, combined with a regular exercise routine. The American Heart Association has a wealth of educational materials that are easily accessible.[4]

Risk factors for stroke include hypertension, heart disease (including coronary artery disease), a previous stroke, smoking, obesity, high cholesterol levels, consumption of large amounts of caffeine, cancer, and infection. The incidence of stroke is directly correlated with blood pressure: higher blood pressure can force small blood clots to the blood vessels of the brain or heart, causing a stroke. Up to 50 percent of all strokes occur in people with a history of previous stroke or transient ischemic attack (a so-called ministroke).

CANCER. Cancer is an insidious disease that can present itself as a tumor (as with colon and breast cancer), as a skin lesion, or as a condition of the blood (such as leukemia). It can be fatal, but in many cases can be cured with early detection. Some gerontologists believe that the increased incidence of cancer with age is the result of an immune system less capable of detecting and destroying cancer cells in elderly people. The "seven danger signals of cancer" as developed by the American Cancer Society are: (1) a change in bowel or bladder habits; (2) a sore that does not heal; (3) unusual bleeding or discharge; (4) a thickening or lump in the breast or elsewhere; (5) indigestion or difficulty in swallowing; (6) an obvious change in a wart or mole; and (7) a nagging cough or hoarseness.[5]

Treatments for cancer include chemotherapy, radiation, and surgery. Dr. Bernie Siegel's *Love, Medicine and Miracles* explains how a person's mental state and attitude can significantly influence the progression of the disease.[6]

DEMENTIA. Dementia is the loss of intellectual abilities (such as thinking, remembering, and reasoning) of sufficient severity to interfere with a person's daily functioning. The likelihood of developing the most common form of dementia, Alzheimer's disease, doubles about every five years after the age of 65. After age 85, the risk reaches nearly 50 percent. More than 50 diseases or conditions can cause dementia or symptoms similar to Alzheimer's disease. Currently, health care practitioners conduct a series of tests designed to rule out other potential causes of dementia. For more information on caring for people with cognitive impairment, see chapter 19.

INCONTINENCE. Incontinence is the loss of control over the elimination of urine, stool, or both. This loss of control can range from a slight leakage, such as stress incontinence triggered by a sneeze, to a total loss of bowel and bladder control. There are four main causes of the condition: urological (problems in the genitourinary tract), neurological (problems with the nervous system or brain), psychological (depression, nervousness), and pharmacological (adverse reactions to medication). Eighty percent of all incontinence is manageable; in extreme cases, surgery or catheterization may be necessary. The national organization that serves the needs of incontinent people is Help for Incontinent People (HIP).

Incontinence can be a very embarrassing condition, and the management must promptly deal with problems that arise. Take the time to find out the cause; often the problem is temporary and treatable. Many incontinence problems are caused by something as simple as a urinary tract infection, an adverse reaction to pain medication, or even lactose intolerance that develops unexpectedly. Explain this to the resident and urge him to seek a doctor's advice. Follow up with a call to the physician to determine the cause of the problem and to express your concern for the resident's well-being. Adult sanitary products, such as Attends or Depends, can allow residents considerable freedom to move about the community.

Teach your employees to look at an incontinence problem as an opportunity to learn more about this unpredictable condition and to be problem solvers. The housekeeping staff are usually the first to become aware of a potential problem and should be questioned routinely during weekly staff meetings to identify changes in a resident's status.

SUBSTANCE ABUSE. Too often we associate the problems of alcoholism and chemical dependency with youth, but these problems can occur in populations of any age or economic status. Alcohol dependency among elderly people living in senior living communities is a growing concern. According to the American Academy of Family Physicians about 6 percent of older adults are considered heavy users of alcohol.[7] The most consistent findings of cross-sectional and longitudinal studies are revealing:

- Alcoholic patients frequently require health care in many different settings, with the highest rates of care seen in emergency, hospital, psychiatric institution, and nursing facilities.
- Little change in alcohol consumption as people age.
- Stressful life events, such as bereavement or retirement can trigger late-onset drinking.
- Effects of alcohol at the cellular and organ levels are altered by changes in physiology related to aging. Absorption of alcohol from the gastrointestinal track is equally rapid among all age groups; however, the loss of lean body mass related to ag-

ing may reduce the volume of alcohol distribution, resulting in an increase peak in ethanol concentration with any given dose of alcohol.
- Alcohol interacts with numerous commonly prescribed drugs.
- Concomitant abuse of or dependence on other drugs, such as benzodiazepines occur in about 15 percent of older alcoholic patients.[8]

The body's tolerance for alcohol decreases significantly with age. This lower tolerance is attributed to a combination of factors, including a reduction in lean body mass and a decrease in the percentage of body water, which results in higher blood alcohol concentrations with the ingestion of a given amount of alcohol. In addition, the oxidation or metabolism of some medications and alcohol may be impaired by a decrease in blood flow and functioning of the liver. Alcohol affects some organ systems in the body preferentially. The nervous, cardiovascular, and gastrointestinal systems all have reduced functional reserves in elderly people, and consequently the elderly person who abuses alcohol may be at a higher risk of developing clinical illnesses of these organ systems.[9]

A strong correlation exists between alcohol abuse and depression in the elderly alcohol abuser. Alcohol induces depression by direct action on the central nervous system. The elderly person may self-medicate this depression with more alcohol. When alcohol abuse and depression coincide, the person is at greater risk for suicide.

In elderly people, alcohol abuse and dementia may be difficult to differentiate because frequently the symptom in both of these disorders is a slow, progressive loss of memory. Some common symptoms that may indicate alcohol abuse include a history of repeated falls, forgetfulness, depression, gastritis, confusion, hypertension, and malnutrition. Alcohol abuse can often be precipitated by stress, such as the death of a spouse or significant other; recent diagnosis of a significant illness; a significant downward economic shift; retirement; significant loss of memory, vision, or hearing; or social isolation.[10] Moreover, prescription and nonprescription medications can exacerbate the effects of alcohol abuse.

Many late-onset substance abusers can be helped. The treatment of alcohol abuse and chemical dependency goes through three stages: breaching of denial, detoxification, and rehabilitation. The breaching of denial is more easily accomplished in elderly people than in younger populations. Detoxification is also easier in elderly people, because they do not need to drink as much as young people to experience the same effects. Alcohol rehabilitation programs focus primarily on education, outreach to the family, group counseling aimed at improving day-to-day functioning, vocational training, and attendance at Alcoholics Anonymous (AA) meetings. A typical program is a two- to four-week inpatient or outpatient session, which is almost always followed by 6 to 12 months of continuing therapy at decreasing intensity. Interestingly, approximately one-third of all AA members are over age 50.

Health Resources for Older People

The National Institute on Aging publishes a *Resource Directory for Older People,* an excellent summary of the many active senior advocacy groups operating in the United States.[11] The directory lists the various resources in alphabetical order along with short descriptions of their services.

Emergency Planning and Advance Directives

As we age, we face an increased risk of life-threatening medical emergencies and the possibility that we may be unable to make our own decisions about medical treatment. All residents should be encouraged to plan for these contingencies, preferably in consultation with their families.

A simple but valuable precaution is an emergency information card for use by paramedics (see exhibit 6.4). This card, which can be attached to the resident's refrigerator, should include important medical information such as preexisting conditions, a list of current medications, any allergies, hospital and religious preferences, name and emergency telephone number of the resident's personal physician, medical insurance information (including Medicare number, if any), names of relatives to be contacted, the existence of advance directives, and other pertinent instructions and information. Copies of this emergency information should also be maintained at the concierge desk and in the resident's file and updated periodically. Computerized, state-of-the-art emergency call systems include a feature whereby individuals' emer-

gency information can be retrieved on the screen during an emergency. The information can be printed and sent with the paramedics to the hospital.

Every individual has the right to determine his or her own medical treatment, including the right to execute a health care proxy and advance directives on cardiopulmonary resuscitation and life support. A health care proxy is a legally recognized document that allows an individual to appoint someone as an agent to make medical treatment decisions on his or her behalf. Many people complete a health care proxy as a way of ensuring that health care providers respect their values and wishes regarding medical care if they lose the ability to decide for themselves. The document enables health care providers to rely on the proxy agent's decisions without fear of liability. Seniors who have Alzheimer's disease or another form of dementia should make known their preferences on these matters at first diagnosis, before they become impaired.

Patients who do not wish their lives to be prolonged by extraordinary medical interventions may also arrange with their physicians for a Do Not Resuscitate (DNR) order, a doctor's order directing that the individual not be resuscitated in the event of cardiac or respiratory arrest. The community may choose to assist in the storage and dissemination of DNR information, including positive identification of residents through photo documentation or bracelets. This practice allows emergency medical personnel arriving at the scene to determine the resident's wishes. The resident can wear the bracelet and keep the form available in her or his apartment. Some seniors load advance directives, a power of attorney, living will, and other emergency information onto a USB flash drive. Many of these drives come with a lanyard so that the drive can be placed around the person's neck before transport to a hospital. This way, the responsibility lies with the resident to communicate advance directives, rather than with management to sort out the information during an emergency.[12]

Honoring patient preferences is a critical element in providing quality end-of-life care. To help physicians and other health care providers discuss and convey a patient's wishes regarding cardiopulmonary resuscitation (CPR) and other life-sustaining treatment, the Department of Health has approved form DOH-5003, "Medical Orders for Life-Sustaining Treatment" (MOLST), which can be used statewide by health care

---

Exhibit 6.4   Emergency Face Sheet

Name: _____ Apt. no.: _____ Phone: _____

Date of birth: _____ Marital status: _____

Living will?   ❏ Yes   ❏ No

Known medical conditions (stroke, heart attack, diabetes, etc.): _____

_____

_____

Known allergies or reactions to medications: _____

_____

_____

Pacemaker? ❏ Yes ❏ No

Diet restrictions? (list) _____

_____

_____

In case of emergency, please notify:

Name: _____   Name: _____

Address: _____   Address: _____

City, State, Zip: _____   City, State, Zip: _____

Phone number: _____   Phone number: _____

Physician: _____   Office phone: _____

Address: _____   After-hours phone: _____

Hospital preference: _____

Copy of supplemental insurance cards   *Copy of Meicare card*

---

practitioners and facilities. MOLST is intended for patients with serious health conditions who:

- Want to avoid or receive any or all life-sustaining treatment;
- Reside in a long-term care facility or require long-term care services; and/or
- Might die within the next year.

Completion of the MOLST begins with a conversation or a series of conversations between the patient, the patient's health care agent or surrogate, and a qualified, trained health care professional that defines the patient's goals for care, reviews possible treatment options on the entire MOLST form, and ensures shared, informed medical decision-making. Although the

conversations about goals and treatment options may be initiated by any qualified and trained health care professional, a licensed physician, nurse practitioner, or physician assistant must always, at a minimum: (1) confer with the patient and/or the patient's health care agent or surrogate about the patient's diagnosis, prognosis, goals for care, treatment preferences, and consent by the appropriate decision-maker, and (2) sign the orders derived from that discussion.

The MOLST form is one way of documenting a patient's treatment preferences concerning life-sustaining treatment—providers may choose to use other forms. But under the laws in many states, the MOLST form is the only authorized form for documenting both nonhospital DNR and DNI orders. In addition, the form is beneficial to patients and providers as it provides specific medical orders and is recognized and used in a variety of health care settings.[13]

Some important guidelines for DNR orders can be found in exhibit 6.5.

Operators must decide whether it will be their policy to perform CPR routinely on residents or to first determine whether a physician-documented DNR order is on file. With the passage of the Patient Self-Determination Act of 1990, residents can arrange for advance directives that legally prohibit the use of life-sustaining care for the terminally ill. In most cases, however, the law protects employees from liability arising out of performing CPR on a resident against his or her wishes. In assisted living and skilled nursing communities, state regulations require resuscitation attempts unless it can be determined that the resident has been dead for some time. In most operations, policy should stipulate that CPR be initiated on any resident, staff member, or visitor who experiences an acute cessation of respiration, pulse, and consciousness. The facility staff should be trained to respond efficiently, safely, and calmly to such an incident and to enable an advanced life support team of paramedics to function efficiently within the facility.

When a resident, employee, or visitor is found unconscious and unresponsive, the staff member who finds the person should immediately alert the nearest supervisor or other person in charge. The supervisor should assess the person and begin CPR (if appropriate) according to the American Red Cross guidelines. The concierge or attending staff member should call 9-1-1 and ask for an advanced life support team. The concierge should also place a call to the resident's physician to notify her or him of the resident's condition and receive orders. The executive director or alternate should be notified as soon as possible.

The resident's legal right to privacy must be protected during transfer and discharge from the community. Often a resident who recovers consciousness will be embarrassed by all the attention and may want to refuse transport. When in doubt, transport, or allow the emergency services (EMS) personnel to make the decision. When the EMS staff arrives, they take over responsibility for the incident, and the staff should document the events in the resident's medical record or fill out an incident report, placing a copy in the resident's file. If a resident refuses medical attention or

transport to a hospital, he or she should be asked to sign the incident report, noting such refusal. If the resident is transported to the hospital, provide a copy of any living will on file. It is usually best to let the hospital handle the administration of the living will.

Medications

A significant problem for elderly people is the psychological and physical hazards associated with the array of medications they may be taking. The incidence of chronic health conditions increases with age. Many disease states are managed by one or more prescription or nonprescription medications and nondrug items. Residents may be routinely taking as many as eight nonprescription medications in addition to those prescribed by their physicians. Although most pharmacies screen multiple prescriptions for incompatibility, many do not, and doctors may be unaware of a patient's use of nonprescription drugs or drugs prescribed by another physician.[14] (See also the section on management of medications in chapter 18.) In one case, an elderly resident who was exhibiting inappropriate behavior in the community was ultimately found to be taking 44 different medications from three separate pharmacies! The following medications can be a red flag for current and future health complications:

Anticonvulsants (Clonopin, Depakene, Diamox, Dilantin, phenobarbital, Tegretol). These medications may be used to manage seizure disorders and are used as mood-stabilizing agents. Some of them are also sometimes prescribed to treat bipolar disorder. They may cause sedation. Dosage may need to be monitored by periodic blood tests. Noncompliance may trigger seizures, resulting in falls and other accidents.

Antidementia agents (Aricept, Exelon, Razadyne, Namenda). These agents are FDA-approved for the treatment of dementia. The primary effect of the first three agents is increased availability of a neurochemical, acetylcholine. Namenda, approved for more advanced dementia, appears to affect the NMDA receptors in the brain. There are newer drugs being developed on the horizon. There is even a 93 percent accurate blood test that can possibly predict people at risk for Alzheimer's disease up to 20 years in advance.[15]

Antidepressants for moderate depression (e.g., Celexa [citalopram], Cymbalta [duloxetine], Effexor [venlafaxine], Lexapro [escitalopram], Fluvoxamine [luvox], Paxil [paroxetine], Prozac [fluoxetine], Remeron [mirtazapine], Serzone [nefazodone], Wellbutrin [bupropion], Zoloft [sertraline]). These medications are typically used to treat moderate depression and may also relieve the anxiety that accompanies depressed states. These agents may modify serotonin, norepinephrine, and dopamine levels in the brain. It may be useful to determine the resident's behavior before he or she started taking the medication to anticipate behaviors that may become disruptive if the resident does not comply with the drug regimen.

Antidepressants—MAO inhibitors (Nardil, Parnate) **and tricyclic antidepressant agents** (imipramine, desipramine, amitryptyline, nortriptyline). These medications are typically used to treat severe depression when other agents have not been effective, and their use is more prevalent among "young elderly" people. Residents with severe depression may pose management challenges and have difficulty assimilating into the community. If not taken correctly and monitored carefully, MAO inhibitors can cause serious hypertension. They also interact with many foods: residents taking these drugs are likely to have many dietary restrictions, although a version of an MAO inhibitor is available with a skin-delivery system that avoids interactions with foods. Residents taking tricyclic antidepressant agents may require periodic cardiac monitoring and blood tests. Lithium carbonate is used to moderate bipolar states and requires blood tests to monitor dosage.

Antipsychotics—Typical (Haldol, Navane, Prolixin, loxitane, trilifon, Stelazine, Thorazine). These medications, often referred to as first-generation antipsychotic agents, are rarely used to treat psychoses and severe anxiety and for sedation. Behavior problems, such as confusion, delirium, short-term memory problems, and disorientation, may occur. Neuromuscular side effects, which can contribute to falls, are common in elderly patients.

Antipsychotics—Atypical (e.g., Abilify, Seroquel, Zyprexa, Risperdal, Geodon, Clozaril). These second-generation antipsychotic agents are used to treat psychosis, mania, and behavioral disturbance with dementia. These medications appear to have fewer side effects than older agents, but they require monitoring of blood and diet because they increase the risk of diabetes.

Barbiturates (Nembutal, phenobarbital, Seconal). These medications may be used to manage convulsive disorders. They are no longer widely used, but some doctors prescribe them to aid sleep. They may cause dependency and confusion, and continued use may lead to disruptive behavior. These medications require monitoring.

Hypnotics (Lunesta, Ambien, and others). These medications may be used to aid sleep. They are not recommended for long-term use but may have a role in the treatment of people with dementia who have disturbance of the sleep/wake cycle.

Spasmolytics (Daricon, Ditropan, Urispas). These medications are given to control urinary incontinence. The drugs decrease spasms in the bladder and increase its ability to hold urine. Side effects include severe memory impairment, blurred vision, and constipation. It may be important to determine if the resident is psychologically stable and independent in the use of other external control measures.

Tranquilizers—Minor (e.g., Ativan, Clonopin, Librium, Serax, Valium). These medications, often referred to as the benzodiazepine class, are given to treat moderate anxiety, including panic disorder. Prolonged use may cause dependency, confusion, and impaired attention.

This is by no means a complete list, but it does provide an effective illustration of the potential side effects of many medications that can be taken by older adults. In addition to the *Physician's Desk Reference,* there is an excellent reference book published by the Public Citizen Health Research Group titled *Worst Pills, Best Pills.* This book explains the risks and benefits of 287 of the drugs most commonly taken by older adults; it is intended to reduce drug-induced disorders and increase the likelihood of benefiting from appropriate drug therapy.[16] Online sources for understanding side effects for medications include webmd.com, epocrates.com, medscape.com, medlineplus.gov, and drugs.com.

With the advent of electronic medical record software, most assisted living communities use software right on their medication carts that can track medication administration using barcode scanners. This ensures the administration specifics are tracked by the nurse or medication aide, automatically documenting the actual date and time the medication is administered to the resident, while keeping a running inventory of each medication. This software can also be used to track refills and can be fully integrated with the resident's electronic chart. It can also provide real-time electronic communication between your clinical database and the primary pharmacy which is a giant leap in efficiency and accuracy.

Wellness Programs

A senior community should have a wellness clinic where residents can go on a weekly or bimonthly basis to have their vital signs and weight checked by a registered nurse or licensed practical nurse. These sessions allow a nurse to quickly identify potential health risks and provide counseling, and they may also help residents become more comfortable with the natural aging process. If a manager suspects that a resident may be developing a health problem, she can consult with the nurse and perhaps recommend an evaluation by the resident's personal physician.

Wellness programs should include an exercise component, such as walking programs or low-impact aerobics. Gerontologists agree that the people who generally live the longest are those who are physically, mentally, and emotionally active. Exercise combined with a healthy diet can significantly reduce or even eliminate the occurrence of cardiovascular disease. Seniors who regularly exercise generally feel better and remain stronger than their sedentary counterparts. Residents who are healthier are usually better balanced emotionally and easier to deal with. (See also chapter 17 for a complete system for managing functional trends and communicating with physicians and families.)

Managing Disruptive Health Problems

A resident whose health status is causing problems for the community and who is in denial or refuses to cooperate with an evaluation leaves the management with limited options. It is important to emphasize safety and outline to the resident and his family the risks involved in continued residency. The management may request that the family or physician attempt to influence the resident: physicians are usually trusted and respected by elderly people. Failing that, the management may request that the resident or family employ the services of a licensed home health agency, request that the resident transfer to a more appropriate level of care, or give the resident notice to vacate according to the conditions of the residency agreement. In extreme cases, the management may wish to notify the local or state department of adult protective services to report an inappropriate and dangerous condition. The Fair Housing Amendments Act of 1988 allows residents to remain in their apartments as long as they can afford to finance their additional care requirements. Most residents will agree to the management's recommendations if their options are made clear to them. For residents living in licensed communities, regulations are clear on the limits to the level of care that can be provided in each setting. Some residents may qualify for home health services provided under Medicare Part B.

Supportive Devices

Supportive devices, such as wheelchairs, walkers, and mobility scooters, are essential tools for some residents, but they may also carry negative perceptions and pose real hazards. Seniors do not like to be confronted with supportive devices because of their association with the stereotypical nursing-home resident. Help residents overcome this misperception by pointing out that the device does not define the person and that it is designed to allow independence, not promote dependence. The law clearly protects the rights of wheelchair users to be treated equally, and rightly so. The same principle applies to walkers. Explain to prospects that walkers are simply a supportive device to help people who may be experiencing mobility problems. When possible, the management should encourage residents to use supportive devices as rehabilitative tools, with the ultimate goal of abandoning the devices as they recover.

Managers should develop a clear policy on the use of motorized scooters or carts. Many of these carts are capable of speeds up to 12 miles per hour and may be driven by people who would not usually qualify for a driver's license. When used outdoors, they may tip over on slopes or uneven ground. Although the courts have not ruled specifically against the use of these carts in senior communities, they are sensitive to the hazards they may pose to residents. In addition, these carts can damage building fixtures and furnishings when operated using the typical "bump and go" method. Carts parked in the corridors can pose a significant obstruction to evacuation in case of an emergency. Operators who do allow the use of these carts in their communities are advised to impose speed limits, require the use of an audible device when carts are going around corners or backing up, and prohibit their use in elevators at busy periods, such as mealtimes.

NOTES

1. Quoted in R. L. Desatnick, *Managing to Keep the Customer* (San Francisco: Jossey-Bass, 1987).

2. Centers for Disease Control and Prevention, National Center for Health Statistics, US Life Expectancy at Birth, https://www.cdc.gov/nchs/fastats/life-expectancy.htm.

3. L. Hayflick, *How and Why We Age* (New York: Ballantine Books, 1994).

4. American Heart Association, https://www.heart.org/, 800-242-8721.

5. American Cancer Society, https://www.cancer.org.

6. B. S. Siegel, *Love, Medicine and Miracles: Lessons Learned about Self-Healing from a Surgeon's Experience with Exceptional Patients* (New York: HarperCollins, 1990).

7. "Alcoholism in the Elderly," *American Family Physician* 61, no. 6 (2000): 1710–1716. https://www.aafp.org/pubs/afp/issues/2000/0315/p1710.html.

8. "Alcoholism in the Elderly."

9. R. Jain and J. McGuiness, "Neuropsychiatric Aspects of Alcohol Abuse in the Elderly," *Geriatric Medicine Today* 9, no. 7 (July 1990): 60.

10. Jain and McGuiness, "Neuropsychiatric Aspects," 62.

11. National Institute on Aging, "Talking with your Doctor," https://www.nia.nih.gov/health/doctor-patient-communication/talking-with-your-doctor.

12. Free brochures are available from the Massachusetts Office of Emergency Medical Services, 617-753-7300 or https://www.mass.gov/orgs/office-of-emergency-medical-services (search for "comfort care" or "DNR order").

13. Medical Orders for Life Sustaining Treatment (MOLST), https://www.health.ny.gov/professionals/patients/patient_rights/molst/.

14. W. Simonson, *Medications and the Elderly: A Guide for Promoting Proper Use* (Rockville, MD: Aspen, 1984).

15. "Validation of Plasma Amyloid-B 42/40 for Detecting Alzheimer Disease Amyloid Plaques," https://n.neurology.org/content/98/7/e688.

16. S. M. Wolfe, L. Fugate, E. Hulstrand, et al., *Worst Pills, Best Pills* (Washington, DC: Public Citizen Health Research Group, January 4, 2005).

7

Transportation

The transportation department is the residents' conduit to the outside world. Those who can no longer drive rely heavily on bus and car transportation offered by the community to run errands, buy groceries, visit the physician, attend religious services, and take other routine trips. Occasionally, family members can augment this function, but operators should not count on them to do so.

In organizing a transportation department, the first step is to determine what transportation services will be included in the monthly service fee and what additional services will be billed to residents. Residents expect transportation for routine activities and occasional special trips. Much of this transportation can be handled in groups, using the community's bus or vans. Most communities post a specific schedule for their community van. A typical schedule might include a run to medical offices on Mondays, a visit downtown on Tuesday, an outing on Wednesday, a run to the grocery store on Thursday, routine servicing on Friday, and runs on weekends for lunch out and religious services. This information is best disseminated to the residents using a printed schedule that lists the normal transportation times and states policies and charges. It's best to start in a new community using a schedule, rather than making the van available to residents for errands and random appointments upon request. As the occupancy grows, catering to individual resident transportation needs becomes impossible, resulting in dissatisfied residents and families.

For scheduled trips, it may be best to designate specific times and places for drop-off and pick-up. This approach motivates the residents to be at the pick-up point at the appointed time (or risk having to take a cab back to the property), and it allows the driver to refuse special requests for alternative stops that are out of the way and may cause delays. In addition, a scheduled service allows the driver to return to the property between runs and perform other duties, such as delivering parcels to residents' apartments or doing routine maintenance on the vehicle. There is a good argument against the driver's remaining with the residents: under some circumstances, the community could be held responsible and perhaps liable for any mishap that might befall a resident in the driver's presence. It is better to leave the residents alone to do their business and let them exercise their independence.

EQUIPMENT

In determining the type of vehicle to purchase, the first concern should be the passengers' comfort. Larger van manufacturers can customize a van to meet the needs of a special population. Seats should be firm, with proper lumbar support. Armrests are unsuitable, as bags and parcels can catch on them. Larger 26-passenger vans that have three axles and adjustable air suspension give a smoother ride than two-axle vans. In addition, a larger van may accommodate luggage, groceries, and a wheelchair lift and storage area. Seniors are sensitive to temperature extremes, so the van should have adequate climate control and an engine big enough to power the system without overheating. Other considerations in the purchase of a new van include the intended uses and any potential limits on size. The distances traveled routinely to and from the community, terrain, street width, availability of parking, overhead clearance, and availability of service and parts are important factors in the decision.

The provisions of the Americans with Disabilities Act may require operators to provide a wheelchair lift. Although this may be an expensive option, it provides a great convenience—not just for transporting residents but also for moving heavy objects and supplies. For safety reasons, the driver should always accompany the resident on the lift as it is being raised or lowered: if an unaccompanied resident released the wheelchair brakes while on the lift, she or he could roll off the platform. Residents who use motorized carts should never sit on them in the van. Wheelchair tiedowns are not designed to handle the weight of these heavy carts, and they could break loose in an accident.

A wheelchair lift can be installed at the rear, the front, or the side. The rear-load location is convenient for the driver and allows ambulatory residents to use the other door while the driver assists wheelchair users at the back. The front- or side-load configuration has other advantages. Residents who use wheelchairs can sit up front and communicate with the driver and fellow passengers rather than feel like second-class citizens forced to the back of the bus. Also, when the front wheelchair areas are vacant, the tiedowns are usually recessed, and residents can store groceries and parcels in this location rather than wrestle them back to their seats.

In addition to passenger vans, larger communities often have a luxury sedan to provide more customized transportation needs. At the start of a new community's operations, it may be possible to structure the transportation program so that the sedan is used solely for transportation services that are billed to the residents. Not only does this arrangement generate additional revenue for the project, but it also discourages overbooking of the vehicle. For existing operations, it is best to set up a zone around the property, usually five to six miles, within which trips

are free. Trips beyond this zone can be charged by the trip or, preferably, by the hour. Drivers should be discouraged from waiting for the resident at an appointment; if it is necessary to wait, the resident should be charged for the wait time. Drivers must be directed to hold to the schedule and not get into the habit of accommodating special requests: one resident's request could result in another's inconvenience. There are few things that residents dislike more than being picked up late or missing an appointment, especially if the problem is caused by another resident. A simple solution for this is to drop off the resident and tell the reception staff at the medical office to call the concierge so that an Uber can be arranged for their return. This can easily be added as ancillary services to their monthly bill.

MANAGEMENT

When opening a new project, it is advisable to provide only limited automobile service. Otherwise the first residents to move in may become spoiled by having a car to themselves and will later resent sharing it with newcomers. Residents can be informed that, should more than one resident be going in the same direction or traveling at the same time, they may be asked to carpool.

Transportation should be scheduled through the concierge as far in advance as possible. Residents should give the date and time of their appointment; the destination, with a contact name and telephone number; and their own name and telephone number. The concierge relays the request to the driver, who then contacts the resident to confirm the arrangement. Residents should be made aware that leaving a transportation request with the concierge is not sufficient: it must be confirmed by the driver, preferably on the day it was submitted. To ensure fairness, transportation requests should not be accepted more than 30 days in advance. It is also advisable for residents to reconfirm appointments, especially medical appointments, the day before. Should their plans change, they should leave a message for the driver with the concierge. After the appointment, a resident should call the concierge and ask to be picked up by the driver. In some cases, residents may have to wait for a pick-up.

To avoid costly overtime, it is wise to establish a firm time by which the driver must return the vehicle to the community, such as 5:00 p.m. each day.

Residents who schedule a late appointment that will not allow them to return to the community by that time can request the concierge to arrange pick-up with a car service or nonemergency van.

It is rarely necessary to schedule transportation eight hours per day, seven days per week. Many communities limit transportation services to six days a week, with the seventh day reserved for servicing the vehicle. The amount of scheduled service depends on the community's size and budget. Abbreviated schedules can be offered during holidays and inclement weather.

All vehicles must be maintained in safe working order and have appropriate safety equipment on board, including distress signals, a fire extinguisher, a first-aid kit, and a cell phone. They should be managed as a fleet, with routine maintenance performed based on mileage and hours of service: a tickler system is a good way to maintain this schedule. Although major vehicle servicing may require the services of professionals, the lead driver should be responsible for routine maintenance in accordance with the vehicles' owner manuals. Services such as topping up fluid levels, changing the oil and wiper blades, checking tire pressure, doing paint touch-ups, and replacing burned-out lights and fuses can easily be scheduled and handled by the driver. Yet even with the best preventive maintenance program in place, community vehicles have a habit of breaking down at the most inconvenient times. I well remember being called at the corporate office in the Midwest by a resident on the cell phone of our stalled vehicle on the George Washington Bridge in New York City, during a summer heat wave, to be offered explicit advice on vehicle maintenance procedures.

As most community vehicles are conspicuously marked with the community's name and logo, they are a public reflection of the property's standards, and they should be cleaned and washed weekly. In addition, any scratches and scrapes, however minor, should be repaired immediately. A daily checklist, such as those used by car rental agencies to document deficiencies in appearance or performance, should be developed. Attractive van wraps turn the community van into a rolling billboard and are relatively inexpensive to install and remove.

All transportation employees' driving records and licenses should be verified at least annually in written form with the state, in accordance with Occupational Safety and Health Act rules, and a copy of each employee's license should be kept on file. All drivers should know how to handle an accident or emergency situation; these occur with surprising regularity. Proper reporting procedures should be kept with each vehicle at all times, along with insurance records and the vehicle's registration.

If a resident needs to be taken to the hospital, do not use the community's vehicle, regardless of the resident's entreaties. The driver cannot perform emergency care if it should become necessary. A subsequent inquiry could find the community negligent or guilty of exercising poor judgment in making the transfer decision, even if it was made at the resident's request. Personal staff vehicles should never be used to transport residents. The community's insurance may not provide coverage in the event of an accident, and there is no guarantee as to the mechanical soundness of the employee's vehicle.

Residents should always be assisted into and out of vehicles and helped with their parcels. When unloading the van, it should be residents only and then parcels. The likelihood of a resident becoming entangled with their shopping bags and falling is much higher when getting in and out of the van. Vehicles should be parked and locked when the driver is assisting residents into the doctor's office or other areas; I once had a sedan stolen (along with an entire trunkload of dining room linen returning from an outside laundry contractor) when the driver left the car at the curb with the keys in the ignition and the motor running.

If the driver has time available after the grocery and shopping runs, it can be used to deliver residents' packages to their rooms. In addition, during slow times the driver may undertake tasks for other departments, such as assisting the activity department in the set-up and take-down of events and special functions. Often drivers also double as security staff for the property; some even assist with building maintenance.

Staffing

The number of transportation staff needed depends on the resident population. To cover absences and to maximize flexibility, several employees should be licensed and trained to operate the vehicles, including the activity director and other management personnel. All potential drivers should be screened for driving his-

Table 7.1 Typical Transportation Schedule for 200-Unit Community

Days	Hours of service	Staff hours required per week
Monday–Friday	8:30 a.m.–5:00 p.m.	42.5
Friday nights	7:00 p.m.–11:00 p.m.	4
Saturday	10:00 a.m.–5:00 p.m.	7
Sunday	9:00 a.m.–5:00 p.m.	8
Total		**61.5 hours (1.54 FTE)**

tory, with a copy of their current driver's license on file with the insurance company providing automotive coverage. In addition, it is a good idea to have one or two on-call drivers on the payroll to fill in as needed. Often communities have a float person who is hired as a maintenance or activities assistant also qualified and trained to operate the van. Except for prearranged group trips, driver service should be available on a scheduled basis. Table 7.1 is an example of a transportation schedule for a 200-unit community that accommodates most residents' needs. This translates to about 18 driver minutes per week per resident.

The more active the population, the more transportation residents will require; however, properties that have a high proportion of assisted living residents may find it necessary to make more frequent runs to medical appointments. Once residents transfer to skilled nursing units, the services are mostly self-contained, and doctors visit them. A good rule is to schedule about 15 to 20 minutes of transportation time per week per unit, or more if there is a large number of shared units or a high percentage of frail residents who require frequent medical visits. Some economies of scale may be achieved in larger communities. For a 150-unit community, to provide minimum transportation service seven days a week will require 1.4 FTE (full-time employees), or 56 hours, which translates to about 22 minutes per unit per week. For a 225-unit project, the same transportation schedule translates to 15 minutes per unit per week, and such a program is still adequate for residents' needs. Supplemental transportation can be scheduled using the community sedan and charging users on a per-trip basis.

■■■■■■ OTHER TRANSPORTATION RESOURCES

Operators are increasingly turning to outsourcing the residents' transportation needs. Often residents

cannot secure a doctor's appointment, for example, during the scheduled run to medical offices in the community van. Options such as nonemergency community transport, Uber, Lyft, or family-owned companies dedicated to seniors, veterans, and disabled adults with disabilities can be tapped at the resident's expense. With GoGo Driver, seniors can order rides with their app or have something picked up such as groceries, prescription medications, meals, even schedule home chores and more. Onward Care's Onward app provides a comprehensive platform for those who need compassionate assistance for transportation, grocery, and prescription delivery. Drivers are highly vetted and trained to work with seniors and will happily assist at every stop. As with most services, discounts apply for seniors who ask for them. Many taxi services offer senior discounts. In larger cities, the local public transportation agency usually offers special or discounted bus services for seniors.

Financial resources may be available to nonprofit corporations. Section 5310 (formerly Section 16) of the Federal Transit Act (formerly known as the Urban Mass Transportation Act of 1964), as amended, declares that elderly people and people with disabilities have the same right as other people to use mass-transportation facilities and services and that special efforts should be made to ensure access for them. Section 5310(b) (formerly Section 16b) of the Federal Transit Act, as amended, authorizes grants to nonprofit corporations and associations specifically for providing transportation services that meet the special needs of elderly people and people with disabilities for whom mass-transportation services are unavailable, insufficient, or inappropriate.

Three categories of applicant are eligible for Section 5310 funds: (1) private nonprofit organizations, determined by the secretary of the treasury to be organizations described by 26 U.S.C. Section 501(c) as exempt from taxation, or that have been determined by state law to be nonprofit; (2) public bodies that certify to the state department of transportation that no nonprofit corporations or associations are readily available in the area to provide the service; and (3) public bodies approved by the state to coordinate services for elderly people and people with disabilities. Grant funds may be used to acquire vehicles for these purposes. But vehicles acquired by private nonprofit agencies may be leased to private for-profit entities where services could not otherwise be provided and where such arrangements result in more efficient and effective services for elderly or disabled people. For-profit organizations can, in fact, coordinate their transportation needs with those of nonprofit agencies receiving these grant monies; this possibility should be investigated in communities where transportation constraints have become an issue. Interested parties should contact their state department of transportation to obtain more details and the names of plan participants.

Activities and Enrichment

oday's senior communities are full of activity. Residents are attending classes, playing golf, traveling, and working in local service organizations. Variety and respect for individual preference are the keys to a successful recreational activities program, along with sensitivity to the emotional forces that motivate people in this age group. Activities must be designed to direct seniors' focus away from their limitations and toward positive, productive educational and social pursuits that will enhance their quality of life.

A quality life is a full life. We are constantly engaged with short-term and long-term memories, music, grooming, exercise, socialization, eye-hand coordination, and so forth, just in a normal day. When someone moves into an assisted living community, their day should not be reduced to care needs, food, and bingo. A well-designed multifaceted program can help residents maintain their independence and keep them as stimulated as they might have been before they moved into the community.

Many inquiries and subsequent admissions to senior living facilities are triggered by life-changing events, frequently losses: the loss of a spouse, of the ability to drive, or of the ability to care for themselves without help. It is human nature to mourn these losses and through this process to reevaluate our lives. We tend to compare actual accomplishments and position in life with the mental image of what we expected to be like at this stage. At forty, if

we come to the conclusion that life is not meeting our expectations, we feel we have ample time to adjust our priorities and get back on track. At eighty, the opportunities for change are more limited. John Barrymore once said, "A man is never old till regrets take the place of dreams." Research into the attitudes and behavior of seniors suggests that anxieties about future adverse health conditions are less important than fears about the loss of opportunities to be what they wanted to be.[1]

Old age is a time in life when we may perceive the physical world as continually shrinking. Seniors tend to focus on their limitations and the obstacles that aging presents. If the stress of this process is internalized, they may be vulnerable to depression. If left unchecked, depression in turn can inhibit activity and recovery from illness and lead to hopelessness and premature death. For example, depressed people tend to lack motivation to get up and move about. This inactivity makes them susceptible to urinary tract infections and pneumonia, which if not treated can lead to kidney failure and death. Residents who remain active are usually healthier and happier.

A community's life-enrichment or activity and recreation program thus offers more than entertainment: it helps maintain the well-being and satisfaction of residents. It should include activities that encourage intellectual and personal growth, physical activity and exercise, social contact, creative expression, and travel. In addition, the activity department may offer a bridge between the community and the neighborhood through intergenerational programs, fundraising, and the formation of residents' councils. The possibilities are numerous and may be individualized based on residents' preferences and the creativity of the program director.

The activity program should reflect the community's identity, catering to what residents like to do and to see, and representing values and pastimes important to them. This personality should be reflected in the appearance of the newsletter, the calendar, and even the holiday decorations in common areas. The same holds true in assisted living communities and nursing homes.

With the OBRA (Omnibus Budget Reconciliation Act) guidelines, CMS (Centers for Medicare and Medicaid Services), and in some cases JCAHO (Joint Commission on Accreditation of Healthcare Organizations) and CARF (Certification Administration for Rehabilitation Facilities), the activity programs of skilled nursing units are being scrutinized more closely than ever. This trend can be expected to proceed across the continuum of care as regulators look to assisted living communities as a more cost-effective setting in which to deliver care. The old standby of the "4 Bs"—birthdays, Bible, bridge, and bingo—as the basis for programming activities falls short. Many states now mandate weekly or monthly programming standards such as exercise, cognitive, reminiscence, recreational activities, and others. Regulations often mandate that the community will provide stimulation; promote or enhance physical, mental, and emotional health; and provide age-appropriate activities that are based upon input from the residents or family members. For this reason, the position of activity director must be filled by a qualified recreation professional who possesses the training and capability to recognize these complex needs and plan for them. There are good web-based programs available for activity ideas and scheduling. These include notjustbingo.com, which provides activity calendar ideas themed by month, and Illustratus .com, which provides online editing software for newsletters and calendars Pinterest.com has a large and varied section entitled Activities for Seniors and Crafty Dementia Activities. iCan is downloadable software in the nature of an interactive calendar add-on for mobile devices and PCs that enables users to access, down-

load, and deliver therapeutic, multifaceted interdisciplinary activities designed to stimulate, entertain, and engage people suffering from dementia and other cognitive disorders.[2]

■ STAFFING

It is best to hire an activity director who is a certified therapeutic recreation specialist (CTRS). This credential indicates not only that the individual has a bachelor's degree in recreation administration and activity programming for special populations but also that he or she is certified by the National Council for Therapeutic Recreation Certification. The CTRS is trained to perform activity assessments, programming, planning, documentation, evaluation, and supervision for elderly and special populations. This level of sophistication adds depth to an enrichment program while meeting the needs of both active, independent residents and frail residents who may need more care.

Communities with assisted living facilities and skilled nursing services may eliminate the need for outside activity consultants, at substantial savings. Regulations concerning activity consulting vary from state to state, and many states have specifically named therapeutic recreation specialists as qualified candidates for the position of activity director. In the CCRC setting, independent apartments are not currently regulated, but the skilled nursing component is. Operators should consider hiring a professional activity director with a clinical background and knowledge of the documentation required for therapeutic recreation programs and activity adaptations for people with impairments. The director should also have a high energy level and empathy for elderly people.

The director should be an active member of the local activity director association or, if he or she is a CTRS, of the local chapter of the American Therapeutic Recreation Association. These organizations provide continuing-education opportunities, programming information, networking resources, and updates on legislative standards for activity therapy in higher levels of care. Participation in these organizations will help the activity director avoid the isolation that leads to stagnation, which can be disastrous for the program.

Managing an activity program is demanding, both physically and emotionally. The activity director and staff are expected not only to keep the community decorated to reflect every season and holiday but also to rearrange furniture, arrange food service, set up functions, create signs and information boards, and physically assist with the residents' mobility and transfers. The activity staff must also give residents emotional support and encouragement. This constant giving requires great psychological strength. The management must recognize the strain involved in the job and encourage the activity staff to become involved in organizations in which they can share their frustrations and victories with peers. These organizations can provide a much-needed balance for the director and staff, allowing them to maintain their positive attitude, energy level, and creativity.

Activity assistants can be individuals with a high school diploma or graduates of a 36-hour activity therapy course who are interested in working with elderly people. Often caregivers will convert to the activity assistant position as they demonstrate an ability to energize and motivate residents to participate. This is also desirable as licensed caregivers can assist with resident care if call-outs result in short staffing. Mature individuals who may have aging parents are usually better at connecting with seniors. But people of any age with the right attitude, good communication skills, and a sincere desire to help older people can earn the trust and respect of the residents.

There are currently no industry guidelines for activity staffing ratios across all levels of care. Staffing for each community must be determined according to the residents' profiles and interests, the extent of programming offered in the service package, the number of volunteers, and the nature of the activities. External factors that may also affect staffing include regulatory requirements, the extent of programming offered by local competitors, the location of the community, the proximity to outside sources of entertainment, and the availability of transportation. For skilled nursing facilities, the staff-to-resident ratio should be no less than 1:50. Therefore, a 99-bed home should have one activity assistant and one activity director. The assistant may work Sunday to Thursday or Tuesday to Saturday or rotate weekends off to provide activity programming seven days a week. Coverage on the weekends is particularly important, as the activity level tends to fall off when the management is off-site. Additionally, families often visit their loved ones on the weekends and will evaluate the program

based on what they experience during their visits. A typical schedule also includes evening programs two nights a week.

In other types of senior housing, staffing requirements are lower: the recommended ratio of staff to residents is about 1:150 for independent living facilities and 1:100 for assisted living. The activity director may work alone or with one assistant, and a van driver may be available for community outings. Many smaller communities with staffing constraints have effectively used volunteers or entertainers, and they may offer courses and seminars to supplement evening and weekend programming.

The staff should be responsible for maintaining their own professional certification, and the activity director must keep records of all in-service training provided to activity assistants, aides, and nursing home staff members. Proof of all employees' credentials must be on file in personnel records or with the human resources director at the property for review by regulators. The community may choose to reimburse for some costs for continuing education and certification for activity program employees, particularly if the certification is a regulatory requirement.

VOLUNTEER PROGRAMS

Typically, the activity director also acts as the volunteer services coordinator. This double role is not always ideal, as the activity director's time may be at a premium. Recruiting a volunteer to act as the coordinator of volunteers is a good alternative; many residents have suitable leadership skills and management experience. Volunteers can run activity programs, teach courses, assist with large functions, and provide one-on-one activity support to residents in assisted living and skilled nursing facilities; some may even work in the business office or provide musical entertainment.

Recruitment of volunteers should start with the leisure interest survey given to residents when they move in (see exhibit 8.1). The survey may ask a resident if he or she is interested in working as a volunteer or has a talent to share with other residents. If the response is positive, the resident should be asked to fill out an application as an employee would; then, after receiving a thorough orientation, the volunteer can be matched with specific job descriptions provided by the activity director. In this way, the activity director and the

Exhibit 8.1   Recreation/Activity Program
Initial Assessment

Resident's name: _____

Admission no.: _____ Room no.: _____

PERSONAL DATA

Diagnosis: _____

Date of birth: _____ Age: _____ Date of admission: _____

Photo release: ☐ Yes   ☐ No   Special diet considerations: _____

Allergies/medical precautions: _____

SOCIAL HISTORY

Past occupation: _____ Education: _____

Marital status: M S W D   Name of spouse: _____

Children: _____ Family, friends, support systems: _____

Resident interested in church services: ☐ Yes   ☐ No   Describe: _____

INTEREST INVENTORY

(P) *Past interest*   (C) *Current interest*   (N) *No interest*

_____ News/current events   _____ Intergenerational programs

_____ Exercise   _____ Trivia/word games

_____ Arts and crafts   _____ Residents' council

_____ Spiritual services   _____ Task time

_____ Cooking club   _____ Gardening

_____ Special events/entertainment _____ Sing-along

_____ Community outing   _____ Audiobooks/magazines

_____ One-on-one visit   _____ Sensory stimulation

_____ Board games   _____ Music

_____ Bingo   _____ Movies/videos/slides

_____ Computer gaming   _____ Reading

_____ Pet therapy   _____ Other

LEISURE ACTIVITIES

Interview residents regarding lifestyle, attitudes, and interests (for example, "Describe a typical day at home"). Interview family, friends, or children for information:

_____
_____
_____
_____
_____
_____
_____
_____

COGNITION/COMMUNICATION

Orientation: Self: ❑ Yes ❑ No   Day/date: ❑ Yes ❑ No   Situation: ❑ Yes ❑ No

Attention: 0–5 Minutes ❑   5–15 Minutes ❑   15–30 Minutes ❑   1 Hour or more ❑

Communication system: _____   Dentures: ❑ Yes ❑ No

Comprehension/understanding: _____

Memory: _____

Safety awareness: _____

PHYSICAL

Vision: _____   Hearing: _____

Ambulation: _____   Bowel and bladder: _____

Sitting tolerance: _____   Transfers: _____

Right-handed ❑   Left-handed ❑

SOCIAL/EMOTIONAL

	Yes	No	Comments:
Aware of placement	❑	❑	_____
Responds to 1:1 conversation	❑	❑	_____
Initiates 1:1 conversation	❑	❑	_____
Aware of others in group setting	❑	❑	_____
Seeks social contacts in social situations	❑	❑	_____
Avoids social contacts/situations	❑	❑	_____
Expresses feelings/emotions appropriately	❑	❑	_____
Frustrates easily	❑	❑	_____
Touches others inappropriately	❑	❑	_____

Signature: _____   Date: _____

volunteer clearly establish their mutual expectations. The more structure provided to the volunteer, the better the outcome of the relationship and the less chance of misunderstanding regarding each other's roles.

Networking in the neighborhood is another way to recruit volunteers. Announcements can be directed to local houses of worship, high schools, and university recreation and leisure departments, gerontology and psychology departments, and schools of social service. Many academic programs require internships; the student intern is a wonderful asset for providing additional staffing at little cost. Students can be offered incentives such as a per diem allowance, a vacant apartment, meals for each day worked, or even a bus pass. Many communities hire temporary interns as entry-level employees after graduation, as they are already trained and familiar with the community's operations and residents. An activity director who is a certified therapeutic recreation specialist (CTRS) can act as a preceptor to university student interns in therapeutic recreation, gerontology, occupational therapy, and psychology. Larger counties often have an organized volunteer program designed to link willing volunteers with needy organizations in the community.

In addition to recruiting volunteers to help in the senior community, an activity program can help place seniors who want to serve as volunteers.

A well-organized community outreach program designed to promote volunteer activity within a community can help dispel the myths and fears among seniors about senior living. As volunteers become accustomed to the community and make friends there, they begin to realize its value and potential benefits to them. Clearly, the benefits of such activity programs may stretch beyond their intended value to the resident population.

MANAGEMENT

Organizing an efficient activity department begins with clearly written policies and procedures. Policy and procedure manuals are required by OBRA and CMS. Copies of the manual of the activity department must be on file in the executive director's office as well as in the activity office. Members of the activity staff should review and update the manual annually. It should be included in orientation for new employees to ensure that activity standards are consistent. The policy and procedure manual should include the following:

■ A philosophy or mission statement
■ Clearly stated objectives
■ A description of the organization of the department, including details on the responsibilities of all personnel
■ Human resource policies, including employee orientation, in-service training, job descriptions, staff meeting outlines, and descriptions of volunteer and student intern programs
■ Scheduling of activities, programs, and staffing
■ Documentation policies for activities, including skilled nursing facility initial assessments, the resident leisure interest survey, patient care plans, also known as individual care plans (ICP), such as the minimum data set (MDS), progress notes, and frequency and participation records
■ Descriptions of in-house activities, including program protocol information for each group, provided by the activity department
■ Policies for outings, including an emergency plan; programs involving residents who have dementia must have an escort policy for safety
■ Communication procedures, such as monthly calendars and newsletters, with the frequency of their distribution, along with guidelines concerning when and where to post and distribute them

■ A quality-assurance plan to evaluate participation in programs and the effectiveness of the activity department in meeting the needs of residents, including some criteria for resident satisfaction

BUDGET

Activity costs vary widely with a community's location, its demographics, and the interests of the residents. An activity program in a large city such as Chicago would likely include fine arts, entertainment, and spa activities, whereas a Utah community's program might include more arts and crafts programs and volunteer work. The former is likely to be more costly.

In addition to salaries and benefits, the activity budget may include categories for general operating services supplies, decorations, independent contractors, equipment rental, dues and subscriptions, educational programs, events, and refreshments. When budgeting, each category should be divided into subcategories such as arts and crafts, seasonal decorations, exercise videos, and movies. Include contracts for music therapists, entertainers, program calendar software, water aerobics, and equipment, to name just a few. Table 8.1 gives general guidelines for various program levels. Obviously the scope of the programs offered will depend to a large extent on what the community can afford, but a successful activity program need not require a large budget. Success depends largely on the creativity and energy of the activity director.

SUPPLIES

An activity program will need to purchase supplies such as arts and crafts materials, decorations, and computer software. Activity budgets are typically small, and the seasoned director becomes skilled at making every dollar count. Ordering supplies online may seem quicker and more convenient, but it is wise to establish accounts with local stores to take advantage of sales and specials. Also, with mail order, the

Table 8.1   Activity Budget Levels

Program level	Budget per resident per month ($)
Low	0–4
Moderate	5–8
High	9–11
Extensive	≥12

hidden cost of shipping may offset the convenience. The use of local vendors can also reduce receiving and administrative paperwork and foster good relations between local businesses and the property. Local accounts may include garden shops, stationery shops, and arts and crafts stores; even the company that delivers oxygen to the resident in unit 216 may be able to deliver a helium tank to inflate balloons for activities, marketing, special events, and to cheer ill residents. It never hurts to ask, and it can save considerable expense.

To contain costs, activity directors need to keep an organized inventory of all equipment, supplies, and decorations. How many times have executive directors heard that an iPad is missing or that "we can't find the Christmas decorations" when hundreds of dollars were spent on these items in previous years? Not only do lost items cost money to replace, but searching for them takes precious time. All materials should be kept in a designated storage area and checked out and signed back in by the staff. (A simple clipboard with a checklist for signing out items will suffice.) Seasonal supplies can be stored in large plastic tubs and labeled for each holiday.

In addition to an inventory of supplies and equipment, sales records, warranty information, and instruction manuals should be kept on file for all major purchases. It is a good practice to record the serial number inside the front cover of the instruction manual of expensive equipment to facilitate identification in the event that it is lost or stolen.

REFRESHMENTS

Most communities provide food and beverages for activities from the in-house kitchen. Given sufficient notice, most chefs can supply everything from birthday cakes to nonalcoholic beer. The activity budget should include a line item for food and beverage charges so that these are not included in the kitchen's meal-cost calculations for the resident population. A separate budget amount for this purpose will also create an atmosphere of cooperation with the chef. When planning an event, the activity director should fill out a special-function request form well in advance. Waiting until the last minute to request cookies or fruit plates may cause resentment among the kitchen staff. Depending on the community's accounting procedure, the kitchen or property accountant should notify the activity director of the food and beverage charges for the event. The activity director should keep a running tally of these charges against her own budget and earmark dollars for upcoming major events.

RESOURCES

Every activity department can benefit from maintaining a reference library of books and periodicals to provide new ideas. The activity director should also contact the editor of the local newspaper to receive lists of upcoming programs. The local chamber of commerce, to which most communities belong, is also an excellent resource, offering an important connection to the outside community and a source of programming ideas.

Local houses of worship may hold services or activity or study groups open to residents, or even initiated by residents. These events can be important resources for activity ideas. Schools are also excellent and inexpensive resources. Local elementary or middle schools may welcome residents as volunteers and may provide some valuable intergenerational interactions. In one community in Colorado, residents and high school drama students joined forces during the summer to produce a play that earned statewide recognition. Not only did it provide a creative outlet for interested residents, but it also served to bridge the generation gap. The press coverage in the local newspaper and on television made great progress toward dispelling the myth about a senior living community being an "old folks' home." Another successful school program involved a class project to document the history of the local community. Middle school students interviewed residents who had lived in the surrounding community most of their lives. The students asked the residents to share their impressions about how the town had changed over the years. The activity director and the schoolteacher had the completed reports edited and then archived them at the local library. In a skilled nursing home in Washington state, a lonely but highly educated resident, who was confined to her bed by rheumatoid arthritis, was recruited by the special-education director of a local elementary school to record audiobooks for developmentally challenged students. This activity gave the resident a new purpose in life and added significantly to the audio library of the school system. Residents can also attend community college courses or act as mentors or tutors of students in some circumstances. The opportunities are unlimited for someone with a bit of creativity.

RECREATIONAL ACTIVITIES

The rule for providing programs for independent residents is *listen, listen, listen.* The residents can be an excellent source of ideas; the activity department should incorporate residents' ideas into successful program offerings. Programs may be either sponsored by the community or offered on a shared-cost basis. Programs should include physical activity, music, social groups, spiritual and educational programs, community outings, special events, personal parties, arts and crafts, movies, and current events. Tables 8.2 and 8.3 offer some typical programming standards for independent and assisted living residents.

Educational Programs

Educational programs are of increasing interest in senior communities. Today's senior "is a member of the most information-driven segment of U.S. society," according to David Wolfe, an expert on the mature market. "They prefer news shows and documentaries to other TV viewing. They are big readers of newspapers and magazines. They travel to expand their horizons, rather than for the escapist reasons that widely motivate young people to travel. They are signing up at colleges and universities by the tens of thousands. They are creative about shaping their lives and are intellectually involved in life."[3] According to a Marriott study on seniors' attitudes, when asked if they were bored with their lives, most seniors (76.3%) said no. Asked what they would do differently with their lives, 68 percent said they would do more to help society, and 75 percent said they would get more education.[4]

Communities need to address this demand for stimulating, enriching programming. Classes should emphasize fun and personal growth and cover subjects of particular interest to seniors. These might include special studies in religion, literature, art, and social customs of different regions. Monthly book groups or literary reviews are always popular. Because seniors have rich and diverse life experiences, the classes should draw on the participants' own experiences and knowledge. Seniors have a continued thirst for information and love seminars. Creating a seminar series

Table 8.2	Sample Activity Programming Standards: Independent Living		
Program level	Intensive	Moderate	Low
Physical exercise			
Sitting exercise	3×/week	5×/week	3×/week
Regular	5×/week	3×/week	
Walking group	5×/week	2×/week	
Aquatic exercise	3×/week		
Dance	1×/week		
Social			
Bingo	2×/week	1×/week	1×/week
Birthdays	1×/month	1×/month	1×/month
Lunch out	1×/month	1×/month	
Shopping	3×/week	2×/week	2×/week
Doctor appointments	4×/week	3×/week	2×/week
Cards	2×/week	2×/week	2×/week
Happy hour	1×/week	2×/month	
Movies	1×/week	1×/week	1×/week
Men's activities	1×/week	2×/month	1×/month
Cultural			
Entertainment	4×/month	3×/month	6×/year
Trips—cultural	1×/month	6×/year	4×/year
Art classes	1×/week	2×/month	1×/month
Crafts	1×/week	1×/week	1×/week
Writing	1×/week	1×/month	6×/year
Acting (plays)	4×/year	2×/year	1×/year
Sing-along	3×/month	2×/month	1×/month
Intellectual			
Bridge	1×/week	1×/week	2×/month
Group discussion	1×/week	1×/week	2×/month
Current events	1×/month	2×/month	1×/month
Book review	1×/week	6×/year	4×/year
Spiritual			
Services in-house	2×/week	1×/week	1×/week
Services—external	2×/week	1×/week	
Study group	1×/week	1×/week	
Planning			
Resident council	1×/month	1×/month	1×/month
Activity steering committee	1×/month	1×/month	1×/month
Special			
Theme events	1×/week	2×/month	1×/month
Intergenerational	2×/month	1×/month	4×/year
Pets	4×/month	2×/month	1×/month
Plants	1×/month	4×/year	3×/year
Speakers—health	1×/month	6×/year	4×/year
Speakers—other	1×/month	6×/year	4×/year
Puzzles	1×/week	1×/week	1×/week

Table 8.3   Sample Activity Programming Standards: Assisted Living

Program type	Typical
Slow exercise	3×/week
Bingo	2×/week
Birthday party	1×/month
Cards	1×/week
Movies	1×/week
Entertainment	2×/month
Crafts	1×/week
Sing-along	2×/month
Group discussion	1×/week
Religious services	1×/week
Pets	2×/month
Puzzles	3×/month
Kids	2×/month
Plants	6×/year
Walks around building	5×/week
Change bulletin boards and decorations	1×/month
Newsletters (large print)	1×/month
Transportation	1×/week
One-on-one interaction with staff	7×/week

with outside speakers where families can also be invited can provide stimulation and free advice to enable them to recognize risks of aging and lifestyle changes as they manifest.

Seniors are also going back to school in increasing numbers. Local colleges and universities have expanded their curricula and programs to attract senior populations. Some schools are not just adding desks but developing elaborate university-linked senior living villages. The goal is to lure back alumni who want to live in a collegiate environment—auditing classes, picking up new skills for their postcareer career, or giving something back by mentoring younger students.

Clearly, educational opportunities and a rich activity program can enhance a community's marketing efforts. By making its classes available to the public, the community facilitates a better understanding of the concept of active retirement living. Potential residents can be invited to attend programs on subjects in which they have an interest, enabling them to get to know the community and its residents. A well-coordinated program can persuade prospects to move in sooner than they initially intended. Communities should also encourage residents to invite their friends to attend classes; this helps residents maintain strong relationships outside the community. Healthy interaction between residents and nonresidents helps spread the word about the positive attributes of senior living.

Attention to ethnicity and cultural origins can also highlight the community's diversity and provide a rich variety of activity programming: winter holiday celebrations might incorporate Hanukkah, Christmas, and Kwanzaa traditions. Often celebrating the differences and uniqueness of individuals enables a community to become unified and more accepting of others.

Outside the sphere of formal education, other shared-cost programs might include spa activities such as massage or fitness training. Another option is group travel. Travel agents may offer reduced group rates for cruises or package tours. One community conducted a series of classes on Mayan history and culture that culminated in a cruise and a tour of Mayan ruins in Mexico. (It should be made clear that all such travel by residents or any accompanying staff members is at their own risk.) Also popular are trips to a casino or theater. YouTube has wonderful travel videos that residents can enjoy without leaving the community. In addition, there are numerous searchable educational programs available on streaming services such as Amazon Prime, PBS, Discovery, Smithsonian, and the History Channel, which can be added to the activity calendar for those who do not wish to participate in group activities with the other residents, or who may be interested in a particular topic.

For frailer and less mobile residents, operators must make an effort to provide activities that meet their needs as represented by the MDS and the initial assessment. Each resident's needs are clearly defined on the patient care plan; efforts to accommodate their interests must be documented. For example, Mr. Cameron is admitted to a skilled nursing facility with a diagnosis of congestive heart failure and dementia. In his initial assessment, he states that he used to enjoy gardening and was an award-winning horticulturist after retiring from his law practice. The activity director writes into the care plan a specific goal: Mr. Cameron should participate in a horticultural group once a week. Staff interventions might include providing Mr. Cameron with a window garden in his room (if facility policy permits) or asking him to help select and care for plants in the common areas. Empowerment, choices, dignity, and respect must be represented clearly on the care plan.

Community Programs

When possible, an activity program should incorporate community-wide projects to which all residents can make a contribution. One outstanding example is a project that was coordinated in a care center in Phoenix, Arizona. This facility offered multiple levels of care, including dementia care. Seeking a way to enable residents at all levels to participate in a holiday bazaar fundraiser, the activity director created a long paper banner and taped it to a tabletop; she then provided brushes, sponges, paint, and glitter and let the residents wander in and out, decorating it as they pleased. After the paint dried, the paper was cut into smaller sections and given to bedbound residents to cut into small strips, then passed to residents on another floor to punch holes in one end. Next, the strips went into shoe boxes and were taken to another group of residents, who threaded red and green yarn through the holes and bundled the strips in bunches of 25 to be sold as gift tags at the bazaar. Thus residents of all functional levels helped to complete the project. Sales of the gift tags earned more than $300 for the residents' council fund. Each bundle bore a label stating that the cards were made by the residents of St. Joseph's Care Center, and both the program and the center received positive media exposure.

An ambitious project with a clear purpose has the potential to attract large numbers of participants, residents and staff alike. It provides both a sense of belonging and a sense of accomplishment. And if the activity director can devise creative programs that attract the interest of other staff members, it is amazing what can be accomplished.

Special social events may also be popular throughout the community and attract the attention of potential new residents, but they require planning. A theme dinner such as "An Evening in the Tropics" could be open to prospective residents as well as residents' guests and thus serve both a social and a marketing function. Planning a special event requires the coordinated efforts of the marketing, maintenance, housekeeping, resident relations, and food and beverage departments. Task sheets, an agenda for the evening, and a menu should all be prepared two to three months in advance, and all staff, including those at the reception desk, should be well briefed to respond to inquiries about the event.

COMMUNICATION

In evaluating the success of a program, feedback from the residents is just as important as the number of residents who attend. A morning exercise program may have 45 residents outside for a brisk walk each day, whereas the bridge club may have only four tables twice a week, but both activities may be valued highly by the participants.

Obviously, activities will be better attended and enjoyed if residents (and other potential participants) are made aware of them. Events requiring participants to sign up in advance should be publicized well ahead of time through community newsletters, bulletin boards, and other means; any fees or other costs should be clearly indicated. In skilled nursing facilities, the calendar of events should be posted by each resident's bed; given to residents; posted at desktops, in elevators, on bulletin boards, and at nursing stations; and given to all department heads. Additions or corrections should be posted and announced to keep everyone informed. Many communities post their activities and photos or even menus on television or computer monitors positioned throughout the building with scrolling screens that are easily updated.

The community newsletter can highlight ongoing programs by using residents' interviews or reviews, which often spark new interest. A well-produced and informative newsletter can also be used by the marketing department for mailings to potential residents and their families. Some communities produce two newsletters, one for the residents and staff and another for public relations and marketing. Both are effective in portraying the life of the community and generating interest in programs.

The best and most attractive method of communicating daily activities to the residents is in the elevators. A classic brushed brass or silver frame, open at the top and mounted on the wall of the elevator car, can announce daily activities with a one-page flyer. (But be sure to post the flyer where it will be visible to residents on the first floor as well.) I have even seen flyers posted on the back of the door of public bathroom stalls (called "TP Times") to encourage communication of important events.

Much of what it takes to get people involved is internal marketing. If a program looks and sounds attractive, people will come. Fortunately, today's computer software allows almost anyone to become proficient at developing attractive flyers, calendars, and newsletters. Most programs come with clip art, and vast numbers of additional images and decorative elements are available online at little or no cost.

BEST PRACTICES

A therapeutic, multifaceted interdisciplinary approach to activities, social and leisure programming provides specialized stimulation to create structure and support in meeting the physical, psychosocial, cognitive, and spiritual needs of each participant. This is especially important for people who are confined in a locked unit and unable to freely experience the outside world where most of the rest of us readily access a wide array of activities and stimulation during the course of our everyday lives. The best practices components listed below allow providers to focus on residents' wellness and their holistic needs, rather than the losses that aging causes. The following research-based programming should be scheduled to align therapeutic activities with common behaviors as they typically occur during the day. This provides stimulation within each resident's capabilities that is failure-free and success oriented, at specific times when they are most likely to respond favorably.

FAILURE-FREE. Activities that encourage participation at any functioning level, from low functioning to high functioning, while still building self-esteem of the participants. Participants are not at risk of being singled out or embarrassed in these activities. (Recommended frequency = Daily.)

EXERCISE. Seniors with dementia tend to be less careful ambulating than their non-demented counterparts who are constantly aware of and fear the consequences of a fall. Unfortunately, seniors suffering from dementia are at a significantly higher risk for falling than the general elderly population. Morning exercises and physical activities at least every two hours throughout the day keep joints limber and reduce the frequency of devastating falls. Elderly people need to support their own weight and/or walk at least every two hours. This helps them to maintain body strength and muscle mass while improving their coordination and circulation and avoiding pressure sores. Elderly residents can also experience dizziness when standing up. This is caused by blood pooling in their lower extremities (orthostatic hypotension). It is vital to let them stabilize on their feet for a minute after they have been sitting or lying for an extended period to prevent dizziness and a potential fall. (Recommended frequency = Daily.)

GROOMING. Residents who are well groomed feel better about appearing in public than those who do not dress appropriately and groom for their day. People with dementia who remain in their rooms in bedclothes without grooming are more at risk for isolation and vulnerable to depression. (Recommended frequency = Daily.)

CURRENT EVENTS. It is important to provide residents a window on the world and keep them informed regarding top stories in the news. This connects them to important events outside their senior living community and stimulates them to maintain cognition. (Recommended frequency = Daily.)

REMINISCENCE. This is the act or process of recollecting past experiences or events. Programs such as trivia, finish the phrase, memories that relate to holidays or the current month, or taking them back to "the good old days" can help to connect them to their past and ease the fears they experience daily in failing to remember people, places, and things. (Recommended frequency = Daily.)

LONG-TERM MEMORY. These are memories that many people hold on to until late in their disease progression. Activities that encourage working with familiar lifelong tasks of everyday living such as sorting laundry, setting a table, or winding yarn remind them what they did in their life, by cuing and using memory stations, and encouraging interaction with these familiar items. Programs that cue residents to access their long-term memories can highlight to them what they can still do, which builds self-esteem and confidence. (Recommended frequency = Daily.)

SHORT-TERM MEMORY. These are memories in the immediate past days or weeks. Loss of these is normally the first symptom noticed by families. Programs that offer structure, a calendar or written daily agenda, and note cards to refer to provide residents with a visual reference that anchor them to recent events. Using familiar photos, family albums, pictures of favorite foods or activities recently completed can help build confidence and reduce fear and anxiety. (Recommended frequency = Daily.)

COGNITIVE STIMULATION. This is an intervention that offers a range of enjoyable activities providing general stimulation for thinking, concentration, and memory, normally in a small social group setting. It is aimed at general enhancement of cognitive and social functioning. These activities include word games, puzzles, music, and practical activities like baking or indoor gardening. Improvements for participants following cognitive stimulation show a much higher functional status. (Recommended frequency = Daily.)

PSYCHOSOCIAL. Synaptic reserve, neuroplasticity, and perhaps other factors such as neurotransmission and neurogenesis may be impacted by lifetime intellectual achievement. The relationship of leisure activities or other forms of intellectual stimulation such as social interactions to diminished risk for dementia suggests several mechanisms are at play, including stress reduction and overall cognitive stimulation. Offering stimulation that reaches back to lifelong love and work for others helps to reflect on the past and validate the present. Creating activities surrounding lifetime accomplishments, travel destinations, and other bucket-list accomplishments gives a sense of life purpose to participants. (Recommended frequency = Weekly.)

EYE-HAND COORDINATION. Exercising the participant's creativity and fine motor skills can help build a sense of accomplishment. The more you build upon remaining abilities, the higher the quality of life they will enjoy. (Recommended frequency = Weekly.)

SOCIALIZATION. Humans are social creatures, but as people begin to lose their memory and become aware of their losses, they tend to seek isolation to avoid embarrassment and confrontation. Programs designed to be delivered in small groups will enable each participant to offer what they can without being singled out. Programs such as a group exercise activity (parachute) or finish the phrase or Wheel of For-

tune all offer a venue for socialization with other residents while allowing them to express themselves within their individual comfort zone. (Recommended frequency = Daily.)

ARTS AND CRAFTS. These activities can build self-confidence and offer a sense of accomplishment. Creating a door hanger or other artwork each month is fun and helps to communicate a sense of purpose and accomplishment of something meaningful. Higher functioning residents who help lower functioning residents with their art projects feel a sense of pride and contribution. Assisting others helps to overcome their own insecurities. Art therapy also helps to restore brain synapses through eye-hand coordination. (Recommended frequency = Weekly.)

MULTIMEDIA INTERACTION. Researchers surveyed people with dementia and reported that travel and engaging with nature and science were most important to them in terms of their quality of life. Surveying families can help identify lifelong interests such as travel, nature, sports, ancient history, oceans, cooking, or science. PBS or *Nature* series programs available to stream online are a great commercial-free way for people to access this. Programming exposure to these themes helps participants remain connected with their passions. (Recommended frequency = Daily.)

SING-ALONG. Many people with long-term memory remaining will respond well to sing- along programs and music therapy where they can participate at will and often surprise themselves with how well they remember popular songs of their younger days. Music bingo, holiday sing-alongs, and other singing games offer a great social and confidence building venue to residents to access past fond memories. (Recommended frequency = Weekly.)

SPIRITUAL AND RELIGIOUS. Remaining active spiritually is very important for elderly people, who tend to become more religious later in life. A balanced program that offers interdenominational services or even religion-specific services can help residents remain connected with their faith. At the heart of our being exists a core set of virtues—gifts that represent the essence of the human spirit and the content of our character. These gifts are universal, not defined or limited by gender, nation, race, or religion. They are inherent in the human experience. Research shows that seniors need to keep in touch with their spiritual self to live life fully.[5] (Recommended frequency = Weekly.)

LOW FUNCTIONING. Sensory stimulation to offer distraction and engagement is needed for even the lowest functioning participants. Programs that offer simple exposure to stimulate participant's senses of touch, taste, smell, sight, and hearing can provide engagement and reach into the spirit of someone who may be otherwise catatonic. In many cases it is impossible to tell if a participant is responding mentally to these stimuli, but research has shown that many people with advanced dementia are engaged by sensory stimulation even though they may be unable to physically respond to it. Bubble painting, name that smell, feels like, sounds like, tastes like, or edible art like "Hello with Jell-O" can all bring stimulation and quality to life. (Recommended frequency = Daily.)

SEQUENCING. Sequencing and muscle memory are among the last cognitive skills to erode for a dementia patient. Sorting silverware, folding napkins, word-find, or playing with musical instruments can restore confidence that participants can still access those skills and be successful in manipulating their form and function. (Recommended frequency = Weekly.)

NONVERBAL COMMUNICATION. Much of what we perceive about each other is not what is said but by how it is communicated. Activities designed to have fun with nonverbal cues can offer both verbal and nonverbal participants a fun and engaging experience. Introduce the topic by talking about body language. Define it for them if needed. Tell the residents that you are going to communicate nonverbally with your face and body and ask them to guess your mood. Use happy (smiling and joyful), sad (mouth turned down and sorrowful), afraid, amorous, hurt, and, yes, confused! Have fun with it and ask the residents to show you how they look for each of these emotions. (Recommended frequency = Daily.)

BEHAVIOR MODIFICATION. Many residents with dementia experience anxiety disorder. This is typically manifested in the afternoons and often referred to as "sundowning." Physicians normally treat this disorder with medications from the Benzodiazepine family. For many residents, these medications, while effective, can leave them depressed, dispirited, and even catatonic. There has been ample research that essential oils and auditory artifacts can moderate behaviors without chemical intervention. Aromatherapy is the art of using essential oils to benefit physical, spiritual, and psychological well-being. Aromatherapy can provide sensory stimulation or relaxation, increase self-esteem, and work against a sense of self-isolation. It can provide opportunities to communicate nonverbally and enhance reminiscence, memory retrieval, and mood stabilization. Binural beats or delta tones are very low-frequency auditory processing artifacts, or apparent sounds, the perception of which arises in the brain for specific physical stimuli. Delta tones have been used extensively with people who suffer from insomnia to induce relaxation, meditation, and creativity and to dissimulate the brain activity. Binural beats reportedly influence the brain in more subtle ways through the entertainment of brain waves and have been shown to reduce anxiety and provide other health benefits such as control over pain. (Recommended frequency = Daily.)

OTHER THERAPIES. Horticultural therapy is an interaction between people and plants. This process has a powerful benefit that gives someone receiving care the opportunity to become a caregiver themselves, as they nurture their plantings. The benefits to a dementia population are many—not only the physical benefits of utilizing fine and gross motor skills but also the emotional benefits of working with plants, sensory and mental stimulation, decreased anxiety, and improved orientation to reality with the stimulation of long-term memories. Pet therapy is another way seniors can stay connected to their past and is for many an opportunity to be the caregiver that is calming to both resident and pet alike. (Recommended frequency = Monthly.)

ENTERTAINMENT. Everyone loves to be entertained, whether it is live music, multimedia, or audio recordings. Having paid entertainers perform for the residents or staging an open-mic night can bring that musical stimulation many people crave and enjoy right into their community. Often school bands or dance groups can be engaged to come perform for the residents, which can offer the group experience of performing before a live audience. Regardless of the source or the reason, seniors love live performances. It stimulates so many emotions and offers a significant boost in their quality of life that is always enjoyed with eager anticipation. Where words fail, live music speaks—it is the sound of life. (Recommended frequency = Monthly.)

ACTIVITIES WITH CARE, NOT CARE WITH ACTIVITIES. Best practices enable staff to explore the use of different strategies to support coherence and quality of life in people. The aim is to support quality of life beyond building a secure and safe environment. It is important to look for habits and routines that seem to be of importance to people. One important task is to determine what the residents actually are able to do and what they want to do on their own. Since technology is contextual, it is also the case that technological artifacts at times will not play any role at all if they are not integrated into the user's daily routines or personal interests. On the other hand, when technology is integrated it also becomes invisible and hard to separate from the interlacing of activities and habits of which daily life is woven.

Best practices in assisted living and memory care activities ultimately offer the type of engagement critical in helping residents thrive. The industry standard is offering care with random activities. Best Practice operators are now reversing that paradigm to provide continuous therapeutic activities as their main focus, with the care that residents routinely need sandwiched into their day. This means offering *activities with care*, not *care with activities*. Quality of life goes on all day long at best practice communities. Quality of life is continuous, and people expect and need to be engaged in that quality of life so they can remain positive, focused, and enriched.

NOTES

1. D. B. Wolfe, *Serving the Ageless Market: Strategies for Selling to the Fifty-Plus Market* (New York: McGraw-Hill, 1990), 45–46.
2. iCan can be accessed at www.planetbenja.com by subscription and requires an iPhone or iPad to operate. It was designed based upon 20 years working with dementia populations to provide meaningful and therapeutic engagement.
3. Wolfe, *Serving the Ageless Market*, 46.
4. *Marriott Seniors' Attitudes Survey* (Washington, DC: ICR Survey Research Group, 1990).
5. Living virtues website (http://www.virtuesforlife.com /blog/) provides empowering strategies that inspire the practice of virtues in everyday life through simplicity which supports our residents to cultivate their virtues.

Food and Beverage Service

9

This chapter discusses the food service operation primarily as seen from the back of the house—the kitchen. Seniors' preferences are as different as they are, and residents are not shy about expressing their opinion on everything from how to make chicken soup to the amount of ice in a water glass.

CONCEPT AND DESIGN

The first step in planning the food service in a new community is to choose the menu plan and service style. This decision will depend on a number of factors. Everyone must clearly understand and accept decisions made at the project's inception. Once the service package is in place, it is very difficult to modify, and especially to scale back, without strong opposition from residents.

As with every other aspect of the service package, the financial objectives of the owner will dictate the overall assumptions and key criteria for food service. Another factor is the project's position in the market. If competing projects provide table service, for example, then you may also have to incorporate it into your offering. In addition, the labor costs and availability—for both high-level food service professionals and entry-level servers—may influence the decision. As the resident population ages in place, more labor may be required to provide essentially the same level of service.

In addition to deciding on operating hours, the food service director needs to decide on a style of meal service. There are basically three types of food preparation in congregate senior communities: the tray line or its more upscale derivative, the buffet; à la carte, or restaurant style; and seatings with table service, as on a cruise ship. Most communities incorporate two or three styles of service into their food program, depending on budget constraints, the level of care, and residents' preferences.

Buffet

Tray-line service and buffets were very popular in the early 1980s, but as the senior living industry expanded and the residents became more sophisticated, providers were forced to accept the added overhead of table service. Tray lines, with their clearly visible steam tables, turned into buffets where providers tried to give a more elegant appearance to the project while still saving on staffing.

A good buffet food service, like any other food product, must be based on a nutritionally sound menu consistently prepared and produced from the freshest ingredients available. Because it is truly a movable feast, however, it requires special attention to health and safety concerns. The buffet service must meet all local health and sanitation guidelines for mass self-service food distribution. Food stations must allow for resident and staff accessibility. No matter whether the setup is portable or permanent, the freshness, healthfulness, and sanitation of the presentation are the first priority, and any operation considering this type of food distribution system must be committed to training the food service staff diligently in this regard.

To contain costs and avoid waste, the layout of the buffet must guide diners to select appropriate portion sizes. The styling of individual servings, location along the line, and even the size of the serving utensils can all facilitate this process. Typically, buffets are arranged with inexpensive salads and side dishes first, leaving little plate room for the more expensive entrée or carving station at the end of the line. Offering a wide selection of salads and other dishes encourages the diner to try a little taste of each, in effect minimizing the food cost—as long as portions are kept small. The menu must also be carefully selected. Offering too many high-cost items at the same time can quickly absorb any potential savings inherent in buffet service. Convenience products (items that can be purchased partly or fully prepared) can be dramatic in appearance but inexpensive to produce. They include such elaborate entrées as chicken cordon bleu with a choice of two serving sizes.

Although buffet service can save on labor costs, it also imposes logistical demands: consider the possibility of several hundred residents lined up for a buffet meal. Food in a buffet presentation must be easily mass-produced and hold well. With the advent of COVID-19 many operators have discontinued or significantly modified resident self-serve options.

As residents age in place, the popularity of buffet service declines because of the physical difficulties: manipulating a buffet tray and a walker simultaneously, for example, may be too challenging for a resident. With a more active clientele, however, buffet-style service enhances socialization, giving the residents a chance to chat as they make their way around the food stations. As a community matures, operators may still want to offer buffet service at some meals.

Special buffets such as the Sunday brunch, a weekday theme dinner, a soup and salad bar lunch buffet, and a salad and appetizer bar at dinner can help control costs. These creative meals can also help sales counselors differentiate the community from the competition. Theme buffets can become the center of celebrations during holidays and events such as the Fourth of July and Mother's Day. Special meals can also provide an incentive for family members to visit the community and eat in the dining room, generating additional revenue.

À la Carte

Many congregate operations now offer à la carte dining with open seating, essentially the type of service available in a fine restaurant. This is the most expensive type of meal service. Food is prepared to order from raw ingredients. Residents must be committed to leisurely dining: that is, they must be willing to wait as each course is prepared to their specifications. In a busy congregate dining room with à la carte service, a resident could spend more than ninety minutes over dinner.

Menus for à la carte dining can be sophisticated, with dramatic presentations. Besides incorporating sound nutrition, variety, color, and texture, they must also employ a variety of cooking techniques.[1] This distributes work more evenly among the cooks so that no station in the kitchen becomes overwhelmed. Cooks working an à la carte line are considerably more skilled than the typical kitchen prep cook: they must make independent decisions about degree of doneness and temperature continuously each meal.

Dish-up to Order

With dish-up-to-order food service, meals are served to residents at specific seating times. When many diners must be accommodated in a relatively short period and their numbers can be anticipated, this style of service benefits the diner and the management alike. It has become increasingly popular in senior communities as former hoteliers have entered the business. Seatings create a restaurant-style dining experience that allows residents to order from a menu and be served multiple courses while also making meal preparation easier for the kitchen staff.

The kitchen is essentially geared toward banquet preparation for all courses; some entrées are cooked to order but in multiples rather than individually. Although the food is plated and garnished to give the appearance of individual preparation and presentation, it is actually mass-produced. The plating guidelines in exhibit 9.1 can help ensure a good-quality presentation.

This style of service has a number of benefits, discussed above. To run smoothly, however, it demands planning, preparation, careful menu design, and a specialized kitchen layout and equipment. Kitchens

1. The main portion of the entrée is placed at the bottom (six o'clock) of the plate.
2. The plate should provide a contrast of colors, shapes, and textures.
3. Sauces and food must always be wiped from the rim of the plate.
4. Cooking juice must always be drained prior to plating the item (unless the juice is a vital part of the dish, as in a bouillabaisse).
5. Sauces must never be allowed to blend together on the plate (unless an artistic painting of sauces is intended).
6. Simplicity is often better than an overly ornate presentation.

Table 9.1   Dish-Up Times, per Serving

Activity	STYLE		
	Banquet (seconds)	Dish-up-to-order (seconds)	À la minute (seconds)
Read ticket	0	5	5
Set up plates	5	5	5
Garnish	3	4	4
Meat	5	7	420
Sauce	3	3	3
Vegetables	5	5	5
Starch	3	3	3
Wipe rim	3	3	3
Check and cover	3	5	5
Total	**30**	**40**	**453**
Meals per minute	2	1.5	0.1
Minutes per four-top	2	2.7	30.2

planned for this style of service need large areas devoted to the preparation and holding of food, as well as more walk-in refrigeration and more cook-and-hold equipment than à la carte kitchens. Because diners enter together and expect quick service, staging areas in the kitchen and service pantry become essential for loading trays efficiently while maximizing space and minimizing steps for the service staff. Menu design requires special attention to recipe preparation time, a product's holding capacity, and whether recipes can be prepared in phases to allow customization for individual diners.

In determining staffing needs and expectations, a simple study of the length of time the average order takes to be filled or the number of meals dished up per minute illustrates the demands made on the kitchen. A cook should not be expected to dish up more than 1.5 meals per minute if orders are to be filled accurately and attractively. Table 9.1 shows average dish-up times by style of service. When too many orders hit the line at once, they cause a bottleneck. Establishing two seating times can considerably relieve this pressure.

Clearly, the more customization requested by the diner, the longer the dish-up time. Residents should be advised that cooked-to-order (à la minute) selections involve longer plate-up times than do standard menu selections. If residents know that their special order may delay the dinners of their dining companions, they may opt for the standard selection.

The key to smooth operation of a dish-up-to-order service is a plan that controls the amount of food prepared and reduces the risk of running out of food. Sloppy production methods and inappropriate shortcuts should never compensate for poor planning.

Finally, communication between the front of the house (service) and the kitchen is essential to eliminate runs on any of the menu items. Seatings are very fast and can sometimes overwhelm the kitchen, but when managed properly they save considerably on labor at the front of the house.

MANAGEMENT AND STAFFING

The most efficient and cost-effective food service kitchens are staffed with generalists rather than specialists, people who are cross-trained and competent in all aspects of food production. This trend is evident not only in senior housing but throughout the entire hospitality industry. Today's executive chef must not only have experience in preparation and production, nutrition, sanitation, and administration but also be adept at managing and motivating a staff in a harsh work environment. Chefs are now being called on to manage the entire food service, from concept and design to financial accountability and even working on the line. As this function is highly specialized, its advisable to have all chef candidates for employment screened with a pre-employment exam to determine technical skill levels.

The menus in senior communities require careful attention to nutrition. The position of dietary manager, a fairly recent innovation, bridges the gap between dietitian and food and beverage manager. In certain regulatory environments, the dietitian will need to ensure proper preparation and planning for therapeutic diets; however, other than ensuring that items low in sugar, fat, and sodium are available, accommodations for residents with these special needs are not usually made in residential living environments.

Line staffing depends not only on the style of the service but also on the physical layout of the kitchen, the number of meals served, and the waiting time acceptable to the diners. Kitchen staffing needs should be calculated for peak dish-up hours. In most communities where many diners come to eat at once, it is advisable to preplate salads, salad dressings, and desserts.

The number of cooks needed depends on the total output desired in the time available. In the dish-up-to-order cook staffing example in table 9.2, with a kitchen serving 135 meals, at 1.5 meals per minute (see the breakdown in table 9.1), all meals can comfortably be dished up to order in 30 minutes using three cooks, with each cook dishing up 45 meals. For fewer meals, consider implementing two seatings: this practice reduces the number of orders placed at a given time and so can reduce peak staffing needs. For longer meal periods or food service with additional courses, fewer line cooks may be required for the same number of meals. If the management is willing to extend the average dish-up time, then the staffing can be reduced. For example, if all meals are targeted for dish-up in 45 minutes rather than 30, the number of cooks can be reduced from three to two (plus a backup if required). Catering to special requests may require an additional backup cook for finishing or for preparing à la carte orders.

Table 9.2   Cook Staffing

	Dish-up-to-order style (peak hours)	
Desired dish-up time (minutes)	30	45
Total number of meals	135	135
Total dish-up time (meals per minute)	4.5	3
Average production per cook (meals per minute)	1.5	1.5
Meals per cook during dish-up time	45	68
Number of cooks	3	2
Plus backup (if needed)	1	1
Total cooks	**4**	**3**

Economizing on effort and resources is the key to productivity in the kitchen. The line staff should aim to work at a consistent pace with minimal wasted movement. Work is usually organized through the use of a production plan, discussed below. Such a plan requires a precise job description for each position on the kitchen line staff and discussion with all team members to ensure that they understand their roles.

The utility staff in the kitchen are responsible for cleaning and ware washing. They should also be responsible for maintaining the cleanliness of not only all food storage areas and coolers, but also other back-of-house areas, including hallways and delivery areas. (The housekeeping staff should concentrate on front-of-house common areas and residents' apartments.) The number of staff members required to perform this function will vary according to the number of meals served, kitchen size and configuration, dishwasher capacity, and the precise job duties for the position. As a rule, a 100-unit community that serves one meal per day will require utility workers approximately 8 to 12 hours per day (1.4–2.1 full-time employees [FTE]); for two meals, 12 to 16 hours per day (2.1–2.4 FTE); and for three meals, 16 to 24 hours per day (2.4–4.2 FTE). Another way to budget for utility staff is to allow one FTE for each 100 meals served. For continuing care communities that operate two kitchens, additional staffing may be necessary to comply with nursing home regulations.

■■■■■ LAYOUT OF THE KITCHEN

In designing a new kitchen or remodeling an old one, the main considerations are traffic flow and the holding of food. Too many people going to the same location at one time or crossing paths in the kitchen during busy times cause congestion, inefficiency, and potential hazards. Planning ahead will enable the chef to establish work areas and traffic flow so that different functions complement rather than interfere with each other.

To save time and avoid exposure to theft, the storerooms and loading dock should be as close as possible to each other. The storerooms should be kept locked at all times and be within sight of the chef's office.

The dining room should have dual access, permitting one-way traffic. One door is used to take food out of the kitchen, while the other is used to return the dirty dishes. This system helps the staff avoid accidents and keeps the serving and clearing functions separate. Although satellite dining rooms can be popular among residents and add variety to the dining experience, the time needed to set up and service these areas adds costs to the operation.

The kitchen has to be sized to hold food for the largest projected number of meals to be served so that employees can be positioned at self-contained stations. Ideally, the kitchen and all its components (purchasing and receiving, dry storage, ware washing and utility, and dining room access) should be set up like the spokes of a wheel whose hub is the production and cooking line.

The equipment selected for the kitchen must be appropriate to the style of food service and to regional preferences. For buffet or tray-line service, the kitchen must have steam tables and additional radiant and Alto-Shaam ovens—in short, more holding and slow-cooking capacity than capacity for immediate cooking. This style of cooking also requires more holding space in the coolers or walk-in refrigerators. Allow about 18 feet for the cooking line and about 14 feet for the tray line. This type of kitchen also requires more pantry space to accommodate larger quantities of the same type of food coming in regularly. This is in sharp contrast to a typical restaurant setup. A restaurant may produce 250 meals per night, but they may be served to the clientele over three or four hours, so food goes through the kitchen and into the dining room a little at a time.

An à la carte setup will require a standard restaurant line. A kitchen serving 250 à la carte meals will require two convection ovens, a grill, a six-burner range and oven combination, a steamer, and a 50-gallon jacketed steam kettle or tilt skillet. A fryolator is also useful if residents like deep-fried food. The front of the line would include two cook's reach-in refrigerators, a sandwich station, and a five-compartment steam table.

A dish-up-to-order meal service requires a banquet-style food preparation area with additional refrigeration. It is also advisable to set up the kitchen with an à la carte line. This combination allows the staff to plate up most meals banquet-style and finish-cook special orders when necessary. This format lends itself to almost any style of operation in a fraction of the space required for a banquet setup.

This style of operation also requires a much larger ware-washing area than a traditional restaurant does. The meals will all go out within 30 minutes, and the dirty dishes will come back all at once. Therefore, the area should be large enough for rapid turnaround, including space for setting down trays of dishes, scraping, sorting, and loading and unloading dishwasher racks, with access to rolling-stock storage areas that does not cross the path of the servers carrying food to the dining room.

Ware Washing and Utility

To minimize breakage and maximize the dishwasher's efficiency, servers should break down their own bused trays and sort the dishes and glassware into racks for the dishwasher. Servers usually have time to do this if the dining operation is properly staffed and managed. They must be reminded to wash their hands after breaking down a tray to avoid contaminating fresh food.

A high-capacity commercial dishwasher must be operated with care and regularly serviced according to the manufacturer's recommendations. It should be run at temperatures high enough to sanitize the serviceware but not high enough to damage it (the recommended temperature for the final, hottest rinse is 180°–190°F). Chemical baths are just as effective at sanitizing, but hot water does a better job of cleaning soiled dishes and removing greasy stains. Booster heaters may be needed to raise water to the correct temperatures.

Flatware, whether silver plate or stainless steel, needs special attention to prevent corrosion or staining. Soaking soiled flatware as soon as possible loosens food, thus reducing the tarnishing and corrosion that result from contact with certain types of food, such as egg. Special presoak solutions for flatware are available. Silver-plated flatware can be detarnished during soaking by placing the flatware in an aluminum pan or placing a strip of aluminum foil in the bottom of the presoak pan. Stainless flatware, by contrast, must never come into contact with aluminum, or pitting can result. Therefore, it should not be soaked with other kitchen utensils. Flatware should not be allowed to dry between presoaking and washing. It should be washed with the handles down and stored with the handles up.

Serviceware is most efficiently stored in plastic dishwasher racks on castered carts, commonly referred to as rolling stock. This storage method minimizes handling and breakage and allows the carts to be easily moved around the kitchen and dining areas. In addition, racked serviceware is easy to count for inventory purposes.

Other cleaning duties include cleaning the floors, hood filters in cooking areas, and refrigerators and freezers. Typically only spills and paper or litter are cleaned up from floors immediately, and the main cleaning is left until the end of the day. Hard-surface floors should be stripped of all mats, which can be steam-cleaned behind the service entry. The floors should then be swept and wet-mopped. Some kitchens also use a pressure washer to clean their floors, but the management should be certain that the floor has been sealed before using this method. Pressure washing or steam cleaning can take longer than mopping, as any standing water needs to be removed and the floor allowed to dry before mats are replaced (although they can always be replaced by the morning staff).

The hood filters should be cleaned daily, especially if the fryer or broiler is used. Dirty filters can be a fire hazard. They are easily cleaned by running them through the dishwasher.

Reach-in and walk-in refrigerators should be thoroughly cleaned at least weekly. The inside doors of the coolers should be wiped down and the floors mopped daily. A critical element that is often overlooked is the fan coil unit. This unit can accumulate mold, which the fan then disperses to contaminate the entire contents of the cooler. Temperatures inside the coolers should be monitored during cleaning. Occasionally the entire contents of the cooler may need to be removed to defrost or clean the shelves. In this case, the food must be kept chilled and not returned to the cooler until the temperature has returned to 40°F or below.

HEALTH AND NUTRITION

Planning an appealing and nutritionally adequate menu for seniors can be challenging. As people age, their caloric requirements decrease, while the requirements for many vitamins and minerals remain the same or increase. Some nutrients become less available to older people because of gastrointestinal changes: many seniors, for example, cannot efficiently absorb vitamin B_{12}, commonly found in animal foods, and may require fortified foods or dietary supplements. By contrast, many older adults need to restrict their intake of certain substances, such as salt, sugar, and fat. Allowances have to be made for individual health, pharmacology, poor dentition, decreased activity, loneliness or other emotional factors, past eating habits, and decreases in the ability to taste and smell. It is imperative to provide a wide selection of nutrient-rich food choices while allowing for smaller appetites.

The operator and food service director must make every effort to provide a menu plan that meets the nutritional needs of this population. Technically, operators of independent living communities without any continuing care components are required to provide a healthy menu plan but are not required to provide therapeutic diets for residents. Diet is the responsibility of the resident, though the food service staff should educate the new resident in the options provided by the community's menu plan. Although federal guidelines do not mandate the services of a consulting dietitian, the operators of independent living communities without a dietary manager on staff should nevertheless consider regular menu reviews by a nutrition professional.

Seniors benefit from four to five smaller meals per day and a high-quality evening snack. The USDA 2015–2020 *Dietary Guidelines for Americans,* in conjunction with the MyPyramid eating plan, provides guidelines for health-promoting, balanced diets for people with differing caloric needs. The guidelines specifically encourage eating fewer calories and promote activity. The *Dietary Reference Intakes for Older Adults* recommends a diet consisting of 45 to 65 percent carbohydrates, 10 to 35 percent protein, and no more than 35 percent fat.[2]

The Tufts University *Food Guide Pyramid for Older Adults* provides a guide for people 50 or older and is specifically designed for seniors over 70 years.[3]

Recommended daily food choices from the Tufts food pyramid are as follows:

■ **Fish, poultry, lean meat, and eggs.** Two or more servings to provide protein, iron, and zinc. Dry beans and nuts are also good sources of protein and fiber.

■ **Low-fat and nonfat dairy products.** Three or more servings to provide high-quality protein, calcium, and vitamin D for strong bones.

- **Brightly colored vegetables.** Three or more servings of dark green, red, orange, or yellow vegetables. Fresh, frozen, or canned vegetables are acceptable. These are rich sources of potassium, magnesium, vitamin A, vitamin C, folic acid, and fiber.
- **Deeply colored fruit.** Two or more servings of fresh, frozen, dried, or canned fruit packed in juice. Juices fortified with calcium provide a nondairy source of calcium. Fruits provide extra fiber not found in juice and are good sources of vitamin A, vitamin C, and folic acid.
- **Grains and cereals.** Six or more servings of wholegrain enriched and fortified cereals and grains to provide folic acid, B vitamins, iron, and fiber.

One of the main recommendations of the Tufts pyramid is that older adults consume at least eight servings of fluids per day. Low-fat milk, beverages such as fruit or vegetable juice, reduced-sodium soups, and decaffeinated tea or coffee are counted as fluid. Adequate fiber and fluid intake can help prevent constipation.

Soft drinks typically are unpopular among seniors. A limited selection should be available on request. At least three flavors of fruit juice should be available for all meals. Orange and grapefruit juice should at least be the frozen concentrated type. Clear juices such as cranberry and apple juice are good for the urinary tract and are popular with seniors. For diabetic diets, servings of fruit juice should be no larger than four ounces. Sugar-free soft drinks should be available.

Catering to Taste and Smell Deprivation

The taste and smell of food greatly influence food intake and nutritional habits. As the aging process affects the body's sensory and biochemical responses to food, seniors do not enjoy their food as much or absorb it as well, and as a result they can become vulnerable to malnutrition, which in turn can aggravate other health problems.[4] They may try to compensate for sensory loss by using too much salt at the table or by eating too much dessert because they can still enjoy a sweet taste. Such habits may lead to nutritional imbalances and could be in direct conflict with prescribed therapeutic diets. Adapting menus to compensate for sensory losses and make food more enjoyable is a challenge for food service planners in senior communities.

Seniors almost unanimously identify meals as the single most important aspect of daily life in a senior community. Mealtime brings residents together for socialization and companionship, and for many it is the only time they can share their frustrations about aging with others who can understand. This is particularly true for new residents or those with serious medical conditions. Residents who skip meals because they do not feel hungry or do not enjoy their food are therefore likely to miss out on an important source of stimulation and emotional support.

When the body smells, tastes, or simply sees appetizing food, a number of biochemical responses are set in motion. Saliva builds up in the mouth, gastrointestinal juices are released into the stomach, and insulin is released into the bloodstream. All these responses aid the absorption of food and promote overall nutrition. Conversely, impaired sensory response to food also impairs digestion.

Loss or alteration of taste and smell arise not only from the normal aging process but also from certain disease states, pharmacological and surgical interventions, radiation treatment, and exposure to environmental toxins. Most people have experienced the metallic taste of orange juice after brushing their teeth; the chemical in toothpaste responsible for this effect is sodium lauryl sulfate, which is also used to help fat-soluble drugs dissolve. Most elderly people take their medications with their meals to offset the potentially harmful effects of the drugs on the stomach lining, which in turn affects their ability to taste and smell their food. Their senses are inhibited by these drugs, as is their digestive system, and this effect can at times induce a negative reaction and in severe cases lead to malnutrition.

Many medications commonly taken by elderly people are prescribed to be taken with food. Typically, residents in a senior community take their medications in their rooms before coming to the dining room. By the time their meals arrive at the table, 30 minutes or more could have passed, giving the medication time to adversely affect the ability to taste and smell food. Simply advising residents (when appropriate) to take their medications after they eat rather than before can have a profound effect on their overall dining satisfaction. In fact, at one community, after the residents were educated about this concept, resident satisfaction with food and beverage service increased by 10 percent over the previous survey, while perceptions of all other conditions remained constant.

Measurements of taste and smell dysfunction in older adults reveal a progressive decline with age. Those losses tend to begin around 60 years of age and become more severe in people over 70. In most senior living communities, the chef and cooking staff have an ability to taste and smell that is more than twice as acute as that of the people for whom they are cooking.[5] Therefore, even the best-qualified chefs working with the freshest natural ingredients are working at a considerable disadvantage, and they may feel frustrated at being unable to please their diners.

Studies suggest that the enhancement of foods and beverages with naturally derived flavoring agents can increase satisfaction as well as nutritional intake and absorption in elderly people with known chemosensory losses. Flavor-amplified foods not only are preferred from a sensory standpoint but also can stimulate the body's biochemical responses to food, promoting better absorption and, as a result, improving the health of elderly people. In a study by Schiffman and Warwick, elderly people were offered regular food for three weeks, then flavor-enhanced versions of the same food. Blood samples taken before and after the use of the flavor enhancement showed an increase in lymphocytes, crucial components of the immune system.[6] This research suggests that the use of flavor enhancements improves health and increases resident satisfaction. And if their use is explained to residents, they are likely to feel appreciative that the management is concerned about their well-being and enjoyment.

In addition, residents feel better about their dining experience, and opioid (endorphin) levels increase as their ability to sense their food improves. It has been proved that residents become physically stronger as well. With flavor enhancement, residents are less interested in fatty foods and in adding salt to their entrées, and thus are better able to adhere to their prescribed dietary guidelines.

PLANNING MEALS

Meal plans and budget should be determined in the early stages of planning a new community. Planning should address the number of meals a resident will receive per day as part of the service package, any à la carte meals not included in the monthly fee, the question of whether these meals are full-course or abbreviated meals, and the choice between full-course hot breakfasts versus continental breakfasts. At the planning stage, it is tempting to build many different meals and mini-events into the plan as a means of impressing prospects and guests. But in addition to the direct cost of the food, a more significant expense is the labor associated with serving it. Once the number of meals per day has been determined and the budget for each of those meals established, creativity and technical skill take over.

Breakfast

Breakfast is a great time in any senior community. There is always plenty of activity and much conversation among residents discussing their plans for the day. When breakfast is included in the monthly service fee, residents will come. Additionally, in areas where people go out less at colder times of the year, the dining room becomes a congregating point for residents and breakfast an event. Many communities use a combination of different breakfast offerings: for example, a basic continental breakfast of fruit juice, breakfast pastry, and a hot beverage is offered, along with some à la carte hot breakfast selections. This allows the property to offer some variety at little additional cost.

Deciding on a type of breakfast service involves tradeoffs. À la carte breakfasts alone usually do not attract enough residents to justify their cost, and they offer little marketing advantage. The costs of pastries for continental breakfasts, however, far exceed those associated with some hot breakfast items. Although a self-service breakfast saves on serving staff, the opportunity for residents to take a little something extra for a mid-morning snack can also increase costs if the breakfast is not properly supervised. Whether the property offers a simple continental breakfast, an enlarged continental breakfast, or a hot breakfast, the most important issue is not the food cost but the cost of labor and dining room maintenance.

Continental breakfasts are a popular alternative to the à la carte breakfast. A continental breakfast can be offered "light" (coffee, juice, and muffins) or "heavy" (including hot cereals and a selection of fruit and breakfast meats). Many congregate communities offer a light to medium continental breakfast to their residents and include the cost in the monthly service fee. A nice buffet-style continental breakfast with an assortment of juices, pastries, fruits, hot cereal, and a chef's daily special can usually be produced for less than $2 per person. A true continental breakfast should not require the presence of a cook. The fruit can be sliced the day before and left covered in the walk-in cooler, and the server who opens the dining room can easily be instructed in the making of hot cereals.

Different types of coffee, milk, and juice should be clearly labeled. Cold cereals can be purchased in bulk and stored in self-serve containers; this option is more economical than offering single-serving cereal boxes, which can be removed from the dining room. Self-service juices and milk can be poured into one-liter plastic carafes and kept cold in an iced bin. Toasted items do not hold well but can be prepared ahead in small quantities for serving in a heated tray. Servers should avoid taking specialized toasting orders, as these can create delays in the kitchen.

A continental breakfast buffet can be set up conveniently close to the kitchen entrance doors on skirted banquet tables or, preferably, on a built-in breakfast bar. It is a good idea to provide some type of floor protection or to install special slip-resistant tile in the breakfast bar area.

Lunch

Some communities offer lunch as the main meal of the day, with a soup and salad bar setup at dinner. Many residents prefer this arrangement, finding that it promotes better digestion during the day and better sleep at night. Operators may also find that it alleviates crowding at dinner and enables them to staff full-time positions with employees from breakfast through lunch, rather than the typical short shifts in the evenings. In tight labor markets, breakfast and lunch shifts are easier to fill than evening shifts, when workers would rather be home with their families. Employees who are willing to work a part-time evening shift after another full-time job are usually more stable.

Always a favorite of the community's marketers, lunch provides residents a chance to entertain friends, family, and associates. It is an excellent time to add revenue with a limited à la carte menu. Menus should offer dishes on the small side, feature chef's specials, change frequently, and be priced consistent with the going rate for lunch at nearby restaurants.

Another lunch option is the shared-menu concept, which allows residents the opportunity to have their main meal either earlier in the day or in the evening. Older, less active populations find this an attractive option, and it simplifies production in the kitchen.

Dinner

Dinner is usually the critical meal of the day; in many facilities it accounts for as much as 75 percent of the total food cost. Developing a menu for senior dining is different from the process in other venues in that the clientele is a largely captive audience. Overcoming boredom by providing variety is the greatest challenge.

One way to vary the menu is with the rotation system, by which a selection of dishes is offered over a number of days and then repeated. Menu rotations must take into account the number of total menu days, number of courses per day, and number of selections per course; the availability, color, texture, and variety of foods; the schedules and skill level of the staff; the style of service; and the merits of cooking from scratch versus the use of convenience products. No two entrée choices should come off the same position on the cooking line: if they do (e.g., two grilled items or two sautéed items), timing complications can ensue. Good results can be achieved with a two-, three-, or four-item entrée selection. Fewer selections make achieving the necessary variety more difficult and may require implementing a number of standing menu items. A four-item entrée selection that includes braised, roasted, sautéed, and grilled items creates diverse selections for residents, especially if multiple accompaniments and sauces are provided. This pattern of organization also maximizes the distribution of the workload throughout all the cooking positions in the kitchen.

The standard dinner menu should feature a choice of soup or salad, a choice of at least two entrée items (to include meat, fish, poultry, or the chef's special), and the chef's selected dessert or ice cream. All primary meals should be served with fresh rolls and butter, as well as a selection of hot and cold beverages. Residents should be permitted to have seconds or to order a smaller portion. A chicken or fish alternative should be available, cooked to order. Some communities offer premium alternatives—such as shrimp, filet mignon, or prime rib—for an additional cost, charged to the resident's bill through a check or chit system. Some communities have generated as much as $15,000 per year in additional revenue from their premium foods. Once the entrées have been selected, other courses can be chosen so that they complement the entrée.

The Menu

A well-written menu is the key to a cohesive food service operation. Not only does it satisfy residents and boost the community's reputation, but it also it helps control costs. Menu writing is constrained by residents' preferences and dietary requirements, the budget, and the availability of ingredients. The chef must understand the nutritional needs of elderly people and be sensitive to the problem of diminished senses of taste and smell. In the absence of such experience, the management may choose to employ the services of a qualified consultant to develop menu plans. Generally speaking, it is better to survey the residents to determine their likes and dislikes, and then to design the menu around their preferences, than for an outside consultant to second-guess them.

The availability and cost of the menu items selected are particularly important, especially if a menu rotation is used. Selections should take advantage of seasonal availability in the wholesale food market to minimize food cost. Each individual entrée item should also be put out to bid and negotiated to obtain the lowest price possible. Companies that operate several communities can take advantage of group purchasing strength by developing corporate menus, with each entrée specified by price and vendor code number for ordering. For example, the corporate food and beverage director can negotiate the use of broken shrimp for seafood casserole at $5.40 per pound rather than buy whole shrimp at $7.10 per pound. Savings such as these add up over several repetitions of a four-week menu rotation.

Careful consideration must be given to the color and texture of menu components to avoid combining food products that are too similar in appearance; for example, too many light-colored soups, sauces, poultry, vegetables, and starches. Another pitfall in menu planning is offering too many dishes prepared in the same way. For example, the stuffing menu—stuffed tomato salad, baked stuffed pork chops, stuffing for the starch, and baked apples stuffed with a dried fruit mélange—can become very repetitive. Although these selections may sound slightly far-fetched, writing a five-week menu cycle with two soups, two salads, one appetizer, four entrées, two vegetables, two starches, and two desserts offered per day for 35 days is a task that might strain anyone's creativity. Although some repetition is acceptable, the sheer number of items in each of the categories can make it difficult to avoid some unappealing combinations. The menu plan is further complicated by the addition of garnishes and sauces.

Another factor in menu planning is the skill of the kitchen staff, who must be able to produce each item consistently and well. A menu that is too labor-intensive or that requires special expertise to prepare will cause delays, criticism, and waste. Although some creativity should be encouraged, simple, well-prepared, "home-style" food consistently presented is what most people are used to eating, and it is usually far better received than a half-hearted attempt at competing with the latest culinary trend. Consistency is paramount in any food service, especially where the clientele returns to the same location to dine daily. Standardizing recipes and training all cooks to prepare them correctly and consistently will help ensure good results.

Equally important—because it is directly associated with the amount of labor required in the kitchen—is the choice between scratch cooking and the use of convenience products (see below). In weighing these options, it is necessary to evaluate the trade-off between direct cost differences and time saved. The kitchen staff do more than just cook during their shift: on most days they must receive and store food deliveries and deal with sanitation, deep cleaning, in-service training, and administrative tasks.

Purchasing

Once the menu has been designed, the next step is to develop a cohesive purchasing plan. There are different ways to purchase: contract buying, triple-bid purchasing, use of specified product directives, or a combination of all three. No matter which method is used, however, sufficient funds must be allocated to purchase the appropriate foods. It is a good idea to check on the cost and availability of products when the menu plan is created.

Before any purchasing, specifications for the primary food categories and their planned use should be prepared. For example, what grade of meat will the property serve: commercial/select, choice, or prime? Will you use fresh, frozen, or canned vegetables? Any of these is acceptable as long as it is appropriate to the community's target market and meets budget criteria.

A recent study found that a dollar spent buying directly from a farmer has about twice the impact on the local economy as spending a dollar on food that goes through a middleman. Many seniors frequent local farmers markets to buy their food fresh, and a community that advertises itself as a farm-to-table operation will certainly be more attractive to families. Community supported agriculture (CSA) has become a popular way for consumers to buy local, seasonal food directly from a farmer while also investing in their agricultural community. Here are the basics: a farmer offers a certain number of shares to the public. Typically the share consists of a box of vegetables, but other farm products may be included. Interested consumers purchase a share (also called a membership or a subscription) and in return receive a box (bag, basket) of seasonal produce each week throughout the farming season. This can be a great way for the community to purchase ultra-fresh food, get exposed to new vegetables, make a field trip to the farm at least once a season to develop a relationship with the farmer who grows their food and learn more about how the food is grown.

Using less expensive cuts of meat can still yield high quality. Cooked by the appropriate method, cheaper or tougher cuts of meat can produce very appetizing meals. Alto-Shaam ovens that use moist heat can produce a very tender product with minimal shrinkage. Alto-Shaams are also useful for holding food from one meal period or seating to the next without drying it out.

Using a bid process with several different purveyors can help stretch the food budget. The chef should use at least four meat, fish, and poultry purveyors and two produce purveyors. Case prices on produce can result in savings of $0.30 to $8.00 for the same items. Purveyors also feature weekly specials that can allow the chef to adjust menus to lower costs. Menus featuring popular local dishes and ingredients can take advantage of regional price breaks and vendor specials, savings that a corporate menu plan often fails to realize.

Convenience products can save both time and money. These are labor-saving products, such as ready-cut produce and portion-sized meat, fish, and poultry, not necessarily precooked. In no way do these products compromise the quality of a community's offerings. Rather, their use enhances the production power of the kitchen by freeing chefs and cooks to do what they were trained to do—cook, not break down vegetables and butcher meat, fish, or poultry. Their use can also save money. In addition to reducing waste from raw product preparation and helping to control labor costs, these items give your food service a consistency that is sometimes lacking owing to absences and labor shortages. The convenience-product industry has made tremendous strides and now offers many products that meet the standards demanded in fine restaurants. Even so, residents' response to these products, as to everything else, is mixed, and so they should be limited to no more than 20 percent of the menu.

Convenience items are worth using only when the pricing is comparable with or less expensive than the cost of the raw product plus labor costs. Using convenience items really does not enable an operation to save on labor. Generally the labor is scheduled based upon coverage regardless of the menu.

Other cost-saving strategies include better use of leftovers. For example, one can freeze leftover fish to use in Newburg dishes, stir-fries, and stews. Leftover chicken and steak can be offered to top salads on the à la carte menu the following day to create additional variety and avoid waste.

When and how often to purchase food is contingent on the available storage space and the depth of the menu. There must be sufficient lead time between the purchasing and the proposed date of use to allow for receiving, storage, and preparation of the products. One simple rule is that the entire inventory should be turned over every five to seven days. Budget dollars used to purchase food that is not readily used and will remain in inventory for more than seven days are not well spent. Excessive inventory resulting from poor planning is usually the main cause of cost overruns. Inventory in dry storage and coolers should not exceed 12 percent of the monthly food budget: a well-devised purchasing plan will help keep this level in check. All deliveries should be made to the community during nonproduction times, allowing the order to be verified against the purchase order and properly checked in.

All purchasing arrangements should be made in writing. The chef should prepare weekly vendor bid sheets and purchasing logs that list all items purchased, along with vendor name, accepted price, amount of product, date ordered, and delivery date. At no time should there be a question about the status or location of the food products to be used. All senior living communities should maintain an inventory of three days perishable and seven days nonperishable food on hand at all times. Food rotation priority is: perishable first, freezer second, canned/boxed third. During infectious disease outbreaks, deliveries may become delayed, so some operators stockpile heat-and-serve emergency entrées in the freezer. Exhibit 9.2 itemizes additional cost-saving strategies.

▪▪▪▪ PLANNING PRODUCTION

A smoothly running food service operation requires a cohesive production plan. None of us can remember everything we are told. The food service manager must plan the day's production and communicate to the entire staff the tasks to be accomplished and the parties responsible for each. Kitchens and dining rooms are exceptionally busy places, and in the rush of activity much can happen to distract individuals from their primary tasks.

The planning and responsibility for food preparation fall to the executive chef. The cooks, prep staff, and utility staff follow and rely on the chef's lead. They expect to be provided with the tools, information, and supplies they need to produce the food on time.

A thorough production plan creates the basis for many of the daily functions of the food service department. The production plan not only specifies the quantity of each item to prepare but also documents the actual consumption. This information aids the chef in the difficult but essential task of predicting the amount of each entrée that diners will order. Historical data on residents' preferences and volumes ordered are also useful for managers creating new menus and purchasing, scheduling, and reviewing the staffing needs of the operation. Menu planning based on historical *production* plans can also help with budget management and resident satisfaction. For example, chefs can put a high-cost entrée on the menu with a very popular lower-cost item to

minimize the number of high-cost orders. They can also include a popular item on the menu on the same night that they try out a new creation or a new convenience product. Careful menu and production planning is the hallmark of an experienced chef.

In food service—whether in a restaurant, a hotel, or a senior community—timing truly is everything.

Exhibit 9.2	**Cost-Saving Tips for the Kitchen**

Establish low-labor emergency menus in case you lose an employee for a day or more.

Plan for staff vacations. Prepare and freeze items such as breaded foods, quiche, and pesto ahead of time.

Always prepare food one day in advance.

Plan menus with labor balance. If you have high-labor entrées, use low-labor vegetables and salads.

Buy foods competitively. Use three or four purveyors for fish and meat, and two sources for produce and grocery products.

Take advantage of purveyors' insights into fluctuating markets. Consider using Community Supported Agriculture (CSA) to avoid the middleman.

Adjust preplanned 30-day menus to eliminate overpriced items. When raspberries are $42 and strawberries are $10, switch to strawberries.

Minimize the number of entrées. More entrées mean more inventory and more expense.

Forecast menu items so that you do not prepare too much product.

Minimize food inventory in the walk-ins and dry-food storage areas. Inventory should not exceed 10 to 12 percent of the monthly food budget and should be turned over completely every five to seven days.

Use leftovers in attractive lunch specials, employee meals, or soups.

Slow-roast expensive meats to increase yield and tenderness.

Install soap dispensers in dishwasher and pot sinks to minimize soap waste.

Train all personnel to properly care for all equipment and utensils to maximize life.

Keep the kitchen and food storage areas locked at night.

If production planning in the back of the house has not gone well, all the dining room ambiance and clever, diplomatic conversation by servers and managers will not disguise the fact that the food is not ready or the orders are backed up. Most residents are understanding of an occasional bad or chaotic meal, provided it is the exception rather than the rule, because anyone who has ever cooked for themselves has known disaster. But they will always complain when they begin to see consistently negative trends, because they have a vested interest in the quality of food service: they have to live with it every day. In addition, because most residents pay for meals in advance, they pay for a meal whether they like it or not. No one can guarantee perfection, but good production planning can minimize mistakes.

As important as the cooking of orders is the dish-up. Every movement of the line staff, whether they are cooking à la minute or dishing up to order, should be analyzed to maximize efficiency. A well-designed steam table, with like foods grouped together, promotes a logical dish-up progression and facilitates quick and smooth filling of orders. Every item necessary to fill menu orders must be prepared and available before each meal period.

▬▬▬ INVENTORY SYSTEMS AND COST CONTROLS

The industry commonly uses several methods to calculate food costs. Some companies calculate their costs very simply at the end of each month using the direct method, while others track their daily food cost by splitting their inventory into direct and indirect items and using a storeroom requisition system. There are advantages to each system.

Under the monthly system, the month's expenditures are totaled on a receiving report or collected from weekly vendor invoices. As these items are delivered and stored, the cases and individual items are marked with their corresponding cost. This can be found on the extended vendor invoice and should include shipping charges.

It is also essential to keep a count of all meals that leave the kitchen, including guest meals, marketing meals, and employee meals. At the end of each day, week, and month, the meals are totaled. The calculated cost per meal is only as accurate as the meal counts: too low a meal count (which is common), results in an artificially inflated cost per meal.

An inventory is taken on the last day of each month, priced, and extended. The increase or decrease is calculated based on the inventory of the preceding month. Decreases are added to the total food costs from the receiving invoices, and increases are subtracted. Usually the chef subtracts the raw food costs incurred for banquets and parties, which are charged to the budgets of other departments, such as activities. The adjusted total is then divided by the total number of meals served to yield a cost per meal.

The monthly system has the advantage of minimizing paperwork and the inevitable errors associated with it. All food purchased and used each month is considered a direct charge to the food cost. The daily system is considerably more complicated, but it can produce an estimate of daily food costs that enables chefs to monitor the food cost and budget throughout the month rather than wait until the month's end to discover that they have missed the target.

Under the daily system, all food items received are classified as either direct or indirect. Direct foods are generally perishables that will be used during the month in which they are delivered. Direct foods can include fresh meat and deli meat; frozen convenience entrées; frozen meat; fish and poultry; all fresh produce; all dairy products; dispenser juice and coffee; ice cream, sherbets, and yogurts; fresh herbs; and fresh breads and rolls. Direct purchases are not requisitioned as they are used; rather, they are accounted directly to the food cost for the month in which they are received from the vendor. Indirect products are those that generally have a longer shelf life and are requisitioned from the storerooms. Indirect foods can include any product in the dry storeroom and all frozen desserts, frozen vegetables, and frozen breads and muffins.

Under the daily system, a running or perpetual inventory is kept for the indirect food items. When the chef removes indirect items from storage, they are itemized on a requisition form. The daily inventory is calculated by using the closing inventory from the previous month, plus inventory purchases that are put into storage each day, less requisitions, to yield the closing inventory. The difference gives the daily total food cost. In other words, the gross daily food costs are equal to the daily direct purchases plus inventory requisitions. This figure will fluctuate on days when deliveries occur, but it tends to balance out as the month progresses. Total daily costs are divided by the daily meal counts in the same manner as the monthly system to yield the daily cost per meal. A full inventory of all indirect foods is performed on the last day of each month to calculate an ending inventory and make any adjustments to the monthly food cost. Goods in production (items already requisitioned that day) and direct issues (perishables) are not included in the inventory.

The main advantage to the daily system is control, but with control comes complexity. The system can easily break down if food is improperly classified, if the chef fails to requisition the issues from indirect storage, or if storage areas are accessible to other staff members. The daily system is useful for communities in the fill-up stage, in which the costs to feed the growing population are constantly changing. Once the community has stabilized, however, this system becomes more trouble than it is worth. It is difficult to teach to new employees, and it can be a source of frustration to the accounting department, which usually performs the daily calculations.

Another method of calculating food cost is by recipe cost. This is done by multiplying the recipe cost per portion by the number of portions served. This method is useful in calculating the cost of an individual entrée or menu, and it is often used to estimate the cost of a banquet, special function, or catered meal. Under this system, portion control is vital: too much variation in the portion size will render the estimate inaccurate.

Recipe costs can be calculated with computer-generated recipe cards, taking care to ensure that the ingredient costs are current. Portions served are determined by noting the number of attendees at the meal and by keeping accurate meal abstracts (records of portions of each dish consumed). The cost per portion multiplied by the number of portions served and then divided by the total number of diners served will yield the average cost of that meal.

The cost per meal is often confused with the daily food cost. Depending on use, a continental breakfast costing approximately $2.50 per person to produce, combined with a dinner that may run as high as $6.50, can yield a combined daily food cost of $9.00, but the average cost per meal is only $4.50. When comparing food costs from different communities, one must be sure that the data compare similar items: food service

packages and methods of counting meals vary. For example, many communities include the cost of kitchen labor in their calculations, which can add $3.00 to $3.50 per meal to the cost. Food cost ranges depend on the number of meals offered per day and can be based on costs of dinner and breakfast or lunch and dinner. Finally, some chefs subtract guest and employee meal revenues from their food cost to yield a lower cost per meal. In a typical breakdown of daily food costs, the main meal (either dinner or lunch) accounts for half the daily cost; breakfast accounts for one-third of the remainder, and the other meal for two-thirds. For example, a food cost per meal of $3.00 translates to $9.00 per day; dividing by two sets the main meal cost at $4.50. Dividing the other $4.50 by three sets the cost of breakfast at $1.50, and the remaining $3.00 is the approximate cost of lunch. The actual costs may vary slightly in proportion, depending on the menu selections at each meal.

■■■■■ SANITATION AND FOOD SAFETY

The importance of a well-designed, well-managed, and well-implemented sanitation and food safety program outweighs all other facets of a food service operation. Operators must set clear policies that meet or exceed federal and local standards and provide appropriate employee training. All food handling employees should receive instruction in safe food handling practices. The National Restaurant Association has online training resources such as ServSafe that has training packages for managers, handlers, alcohol, allergens, and COVID-19 precautions.[7]

Additionally, most states have certification programs for food handlers, and some of these are mandatory. A certified food service supervisor should be available during all operating shifts in both the front and the back of the house. Therefore the chef, sous-chef, food service director, dietary manager, and dining room managers should have local certification.

A food handling and safety training program is intended to safeguard the health of residents and employees alike. Food must be undamaged, clean, free from adulteration and contamination, and completely suitable for human consumption. Residents expect to be served safe, appetizing food that has been prepared and handled in a sanitary manner in a clean environment. The food service supervisors and managers are responsible for knowing, understanding, and enforcing the standards and practices called for by the program.

Although it is difficult to run a top-quality operation, supervisors must be aware of their employees' practices, the condition of the equipment, and the ability of the food service staff to adhere to the policies and regulations at all times. A good food service team looks for ways to set standards, and careless attitudes should not be tolerated. Should any food safety problem arise, it is generally the responsibility of the food service supervisor to contact the local authorities and take any immediate action necessary to protect the health of the community.

All employees should receive training within their first week of employment to eliminate the possibility of acquiring any inappropriate food handling and safety habits on the job. Thereafter, employees should receive ongoing and review training. This can be provided, and safety awareness reinforced, through in-service meetings, video demonstrations of correct procedures, display of work-area posters depicting proper sanitation and food handling techniques, and individualized methods, such as completing daily sanitation side-work sheets. The cost of these efforts is minimal compared with that of transmitting a food-borne illness, which could endanger the lives of diners, devastate the community's hard-earned reputation, and significantly hamper marketing efforts. Safe handling and preparation of food are learned behaviors that should become second nature to employees. Supervisors are ultimately responsible for food safety in the community.

Good food safety standards and practices include the following:

Employees should not be allowed to work with food when they are sick.

All cuts and abrasions should be cleaned with soap and disinfectant and covered with a bandage or waterproof protector.

Gloves should be worn at all times when handling food.

Personal protective equipment should be worn by staff during any communicable disease outbreak.

Employees should not be allowed to work if they have a wound that may be infected.

Employees should bathe daily.

Employees should wear freshly cleaned outer clothing or uniforms daily.

Employees must restrain or cover their hair at all times.

Employees may not smoke, chew gum, or eat in food work areas.

Employees must sanitize or wash their hands with warm water (110°–115°F) and soap

when entering the kitchen
after using the restrooms
before and after any food, coffee, or cigarette breaks
after handling garbage
after handling any soiled equipment
after handling raw food products, such as meat and poultry, and cooked foods
after coughing or sneezing
after handling hair, facial hair, soiled uniforms, or any skin

Hand sinks must be used only for washing hands, not for working with food.

All equipment must be sanitized after each use. All food contact surfaces must be sanitized frequently.

Food contact surfaces must not be wiped with kitchen rags.

Sanitizing solution must be available at each work station.

The proper color-coded cutting boards must be used for different foods.

All food products coming into the facility should be checked immediately to ensure that they meet the community's quality and freshness standards and be returned to the appropriate vendor if they are in any way questionable. All stock must be rotated so that the oldest products are used first. Table 9.3 lists the shelf life for common fruits and vegetables. Dry foods should be stored out of their original packaging. Raw foods should never be stored above cooked products. Spoiled, damaged, or otherwise unwholesome food should be held in separate storage areas before disposal. Ice for human consumption must not be used for any other purpose. Food requiring refrigeration must be cooled to an internal temperature of 40°F or lower. Cooling time for cooked food should never exceed four hours. Frozen food should be stored and maintained at 0°F or lower.

Table 9.3   Shelf Life for Common Fruits and Vegetables

Apples, fresh   Store in fruit or vegetable box 3 weeks to a month. Inspect daily and remove any rotten fruit so that the balance will not be contaminated. Watch for blue mold or black rot.

Apricots   Easily stored for 1 to 2 weeks.

Asparagus   May be kept in refrigerator 1 week after ripening.

Bananas   May be kept at 50° to 60°F and used within 2 to 3 days after ripening. Do not store in the cooler at any time.

Berries   May be kept for a week to 10 days. However, should be used as quickly as possible for best flavor.

Broccoli   Can be stored for 8 to 10 days.

Cabbage   Early variety will keep about 2 weeks. Late variety is much sturdier and will last about 2 months.

Cantaloupe   If unripe, store at room temperature and inspect daily for ripeness. When ripe, may be held in the cooler for 1 week.

Carrots   If in good condition, may be kept in the storeroom for a few days. Under refrigeration, will last 3 months.

Cauliflower   May be kept for 2 weeks if the leaves are not cut away. After the leaves are removed, will deteriorate rapidly.

Celery   Should not be kept longer than a few days. If it is wilted, placing in cold water will freshen it.

Corn   Should be used within 24 hours.

Cranberries   May be stored under refrigeration for up to 2 months.

Cucumbers   Should be used within 1 week.

Eggplant   Should be used within 1 week.

Garlic   Can be kept for about 2 months at temperatures from 55° to 66°F. In vegetable cooler at 32° to 36°F, will last 4 months.

Grapefruit   May be stored for 6 weeks at 32° to 36°F.

Grapes   White seedless or red Tokay grapes will keep for 4 weeks. Red Emperor, obtainable in fall, will keep for 2 months.

Kale   May be stored at 32° to 36°F for up to 3 weeks.

Lemons   May be kept from 1 to 2 months at 50° to 60°F.

Lettuce, iceberg   If in good condition and inspected regularly, whole heads may be kept for 4 weeks. However, should be used as soon as possible after arrival.

Limes   May be stored for a maximum of 2 weeks.

Melons   May be stored for a maximum of 3 weeks. However, it is recommended that they be used as soon as the proper degree of softness is achieved.

Mushrooms, fresh   Sliced, will keep for 1 or 2 days. Whole, will last 4 to 7 days.

Onions, green   If kept under refrigeration, will last a week to 10 days.

Onions, yellow   If stored in a cool, dry place, unrefrigerated, will last 3 months.

Oranges   Should be used within a week if possible. If necessary, may be held in a reasonably good condition for a month to 6 weeks.

Parsley   Will last for a week if well iced.

Parsnips   Can be stored for 2 to 3 months at 32° to 36°F.

Peaches   Most varieties will last about a week; the yellow cling variety will last about 2 weeks. Must be inspected and sorted each day.

Pears   Summer or Bartlett variety: before ripening, may be kept 3 weeks at 65° to 75°F; after ripening, must be refrigerated and used within a few days. These require gentle handling to prevent bruising and must be sorted every 5 days. Bosc or Comice variety may be kept 6 weeks before ripening if sorted weekly.

Tomatoes   Should not be kept more than a week after ripening. Must be inspected and sorted daily for ripeness.

Turnips   Will keep 10 days to 2 weeks without refrigeration. Under light refrigeration, will last 3 months.

Watermelon   May be held for a week to 10 days.

A pest-control program must be implemented immediately on operation of the food service. Chemicals must always be stored separate from food.

Once a basic food safety procedure is in place, a facility can consider voluntarily implementing a preventive food safety management system. The FDA provides a model, HACCP (Hazard Analysis and Critical Control Point), that emphasizes the prevention of food-borne illness through proper food handling, monitoring of procedures, and record keeping.[8]

NOTES

1. The National Association of Nutrition and Aging Services Programs (NANASP) publishes national standards for congregate and home-delivered food services and programs as well as a newsletter titled *Many Hats*, which includes tips for site managers and has activity updates. The association also sponsors regional and state training seminars on senior nutrition and programming. It can be contacted at 1612 K Street, NW, Suite 400, Washington, DC 20006, phone

202-682-6899, fax 202-223-2099, https://www.nanasp .org.

2. US Department of Health and Human Services and US Department of Agriculture, *2015–2020 Dietary Guidelines for Americans*, https://www.dietaryguidelines.gov /resources/2020-2025-dietary-guidelines-online -materials.

3. Tufts Food Guide for Older Adults, http://globalag.igc .org/health/us/2007/guidelines.pdf.

4. C. Lucas, B. W. Pearce, and S. S. Schiffman, "Reactivating Appetite," *Contemporary Long Term Care* 17, no. 12 (December 1994): 55.

5. S. S. Schiffman, "Taste and Smell in Disease," *New England Journal of Medicine* 308 (1983): 1275–79, 1337, 1343.

6. S. S. Schiffman and Z. S. Warwick, "Effect of Flavor Enhancement of Foods for the Elderly on Nutritional Status: Food Intake, Biochemical Indices, and Anthropometric Measures," *Physiology and Behavior* 53 (1992): 395–402.

7. ServSafe National Restaurant Association training courses, https://www.servsafe.com.

8. U.S. Food and Drug Administration, Center for Food Safety and Applied Nutrition, www.cfsan.fda.gov.

10

Dining Services

As chapter 9 shows, running a successful food service in a senior community requires meticulous attention to menu planning, budget, equipment, supplies, staffing, and food safety in the kitchen, or the back of the house. These efforts must be complemented by equal attention to the front of the house, or the dining room: the appearance and cleanliness of the room and tables, the scheduling of meals, the presentation and serving of food, and the residents' overall satisfaction. Dining is the most important experience in the daily lives of some residents, and the one which attracts more attention and comment than any other aspect of the community's service package.

SERVICE PACKAGE

The style, interior design, and even architecture of the property establish certain expectations about the services offered. If the property is lavish in appearance, the residents and guests will expect top-quality food service, and if the food does not live up to these expectations, residents and guests will be critical. On the other hand, if the food quality and service meet or exceed the expectations created by the physical property, they will say so.

Each community tailors its food service package to the local market, the needs of its current and target resident population, and its budget. Some communities provide food services à la carte, whereas others include food in the monthly service fee.

In addition to the usual daily food service, most communities sponsor special events, such as a weekly afternoon tea or cocktail hour. These events encourage residents to mingle and socialize and welcome new residents. They are generally staged in one of the common rooms. Teatime features finger sandwiches, cookies, and pastries and residents are served tea, coffee, or punch. During weekly cocktail hours, residents provide their own liquor, and the community provides mixers, limited garnishes, ice, glassware, and dry snacks. A resident volunteer or activity director generally tends the bar.

Whether the community can offer residents alcoholic beverages depends on state and local licensing laws. Most states and municipalities require that a community possess a liquor license to sell alcoholic beverages to residents. If the community is located near a school or library, this activity may be prohibited. Residents can, of course, consume their own spirits in their own apartments or in the common areas. Many residents enjoy a predinner cocktail or wine with their meal. Residents can pour their own wine or have an employee who is of age do so.

Liquor sales in larger communities can be a significant source of income to the property. One 340-unit congregate community in Chicago had a bar service that yielded $1,000 per month in additional revenue to the project without any additional labor costs. They were able to attract 20 percent of their residents to the lounge daily, with each visitor consuming an average of 2.5 drinks. Residents generally pay for their drinks by signing a chit that is charged to their monthly accounts. Good security and portion control of the liquor are essential to running a successful bar.

STYLES OF SERVICE

The number and type of meals offered will vary with the type of community. Assisted living communities generally offer three meals a day, whereas congregate or continuing care retirement communities offer an allotment of meals, typically 30 a month. For most communities, a light breakfast and a dinner with a choice of two or three entrées is sufficient. A cost-benefit analysis should be done before giving any consideration to adding lunch, which can effectively double labor costs by converting the four-hour breakfast shifts into full eight-hour shifts. Unless this additional cost can be recovered from the residents through à la carte billings or a rent increase, offering lunch will effectively decrease the operating margin of the community.

One fundamental decision about meal service is dining room hours. The dining room can be open continuously, open for a specified dining period within which all residents can be served, or opened and closed for shorter periods using prearranged seating times. Generally speaking, the longer the dining room is open to the residents, the higher the labor cost for both the front and the back of the house; longer dining hours, however, provide maximum flexibility for the residents and lessen the institutional feel of a community. Residents who were used to eating whenever they wanted before moving into the community typically have some difficulty adjusting to predetermined dining times.

The problem with open seating times in the dining room is that even though it must be operated like a restaurant, offering flexible seating and preparing meals for residents as they arrive, most people come down to eat at roughly the same time. Restaurants are inefficient in feeding large numbers of people quickly. They count on the fact that their customers will arrive to eat at different times over several hours. If all of their customers were to arrive in a two-hour period, seating, service, and production capacity would quickly be overwhelmed. When the restau-rant reaches capacity, it simply turns people away or asks them to wait. This can never happen in a senior living community, where residents have already paid for their meals through their monthly service fees.

Multiple seatings offer a way to give top-quality service within a limited time and with limited staff. This concept can be applied to one or all meals. The dining room is closed for 30 minutes between seatings to allow the food service staff to reset the room and the cooking staff to prepare the next set of entrées and vegetables. The advantages of the two-seating arrangement include the following:

Operating costs are lower. Staffing costs are lower because only one-half to two-thirds of the population needs to be served at one time. Usually 60 percent of the population will choose the first seating when offered a choice.

Food is plated and served more quickly. Far fewer orders are placed at one time, eliminating the bottleneck that usually occurs in the kitchen when the majority of residents come to the dining room and place their orders within a one-hour period. Moreover, the kitchen can anticipate the number of diners at each seating and save effort by preparing multiple servings of each dish.

Food is fresher. The kitchen can prepare the food in two batches, which reduces the tendency for certain dishes, especially vegetables, to become overcooked when held in the steam table. In addition, if the kitchen runs low on one entrée, alternatives can be prepared between seatings to avoid running out of food.

Residents do not have to wait to be seated. The dining room is set and ready for the residents at the beginning of each seating. They do not have to wait for a dirty table to be bused and reset. The dining room can be completely cleaned, bused, and reset between seatings using all service staff, the utility staff, and any available personal care aides. Diners at the second seating receive the same quality of food and service as those at the first seating.

Seatings can accommodate different resident profiles. Most communities serve both active and frailer residents. Often the two profiles do not mix well, particularly at mealtimes; assigning them to different seatings can alleviate the problem. The typical senior community also has two types of diner: those who are lined up outside the dining room 15 minutes before opening, and the leisurely diners who may start the evening off with a cocktail. The early diners are generally interested in *eating*; the late diners are generally interested in *dining*. Whereas the early diners will usually eat and leave the dining room within an hour, the late diners will usually relax with coffee and dessert, taking up to 90 minutes to complete their meal. Separate seatings can accommodate both dining styles: one starts at 4:45 p.m. and ends at 6:00 p.m., and the other starts at 6:30 p.m. and ends at 8:00 p.m. The dining room is closed from 6:00 to 6:30 p.m. to bus and reset the tables.

Increased resident satisfaction. Residents perceive staffing and food quality as improved when they are seated and served in two smaller groups than in one large one. The system maximizes the efficiency of the kitchen, while providing the residents with the service and promptness that they expect and deserve.

LAYOUT OF THE DINING ROOM

The design and layout of a dining room should maximize flexibility and efficiency of service. Architects should remember that most residents eat two to three meals per day in the dining room seven days per week. Variety in design can significantly contribute to the diner's satisfaction. Dining rooms that are divided into smaller dining areas, or communities with country kitchens or cafés in addition to the main dining areas, give residents some choices, although they can also increase the work of the serving and cleaning staff. These areas can also be used for theme dinners and special occasions.

The layout of all dining areas should take into account traffic flow and afford a clear and unobstructed path to and from the kitchen. Designers should examine the kitchen layout and service path to determine the best locations for the servers' stations, keeping in mind that the farther the service staff have to walk, the longer it will take them to fill each order. To promote social distancing, many operators have designated separate eating areas or seating times to obtain appropriate distances between diners during communicable disease outbreaks. During uncontrolled and spreading outbreaks, often resident's meals are delivered directly to their rooms to prevent cross-contamination.

The dining areas should be easily accessible. Booths and bench seating are unsuitable for residents with limited mobility. Room dividers and planters can obstruct efficient service and may collect trash.

The dining room should be big enough to accommodate at least 75 percent of the residents at one time, plus an allowance of 10 percent for residents' and marketing guests (see chapter 20 for dining room design specifications).

Larger or remote dining rooms should be equipped with side stations to improve efficiency and quality of service. These are areas that can accommodate a coffee warmer, soup kettle, chafing dishes, dessert tray, condiment storage, and a small busing area. Remote storage areas for linens, paper goods, silver, and glassware are also helpful.

A storage area for walkers and wheelchairs should be located adjacent to dining areas to minimize obstructions in the dining room.

EQUIPMENT

For many businesses, packaging is everything, and packaging in food service involves the presentation of the meal. How residents perceive this package conditions their response to the product itself. Therefore, the quality of the tabletop setting must be consistent with or better than that of the food that will be plated onto it.

When determining the type of equipment to use in the setup of the dining room, the owner or operator should consider the initial cost, the availability of replacements, durability, and ease of cleaning and storage. Some operations use customized china, silverware, and glassware, which may lend a touch of class to the dining room and discourage theft. Yet these customized items are almost always more expensive, and replacements must be kept in inventory by the community instead of by the supplier. Some suppliers offer to customize china with the community's logo for a small additional charge, which enables them to do special runs for larger orders that they do not have to keep in stock.

An inventory of china, glass, silverware, and linen should be performed quarterly. The house stock (items in inventory at the community but not in service) should be counted and kept in a secure location. As the working stock of items in service becomes depleted, the dining room manager can check out inventory from the house stock piece by piece and deduct the amounts from inventory. In this way, it is never necessary to count the entire inventory but only the working stock, to which is added the house stock, less any removals. Operational losses for all equipment should not exceed 25 percent annually. Loss expectations for different categories of serviceware are noted below.

China

China is usually the single most expensive investment of the dining operation, both at the initial purchase and for ongoing replacement. The cost per place setting for china can run anywhere from $25 for café china to $100 for Lenox. The choice of china must be based on what the primary market can afford, because every dollar of capital expenditure (or savings) will affect the residents' monthly service fee.

China has a shorter life than silverware but a longer life than glassware. Annual china losses should be less than 10 percent for operations with a good grade of china and well-designed warewashing and storage areas. A well-trained dish crew following proper guidelines for loading, unloading, sorting, and stacking, as well as incentives for reducing breakage and loss, is essential.

Functional considerations include durability; chemical composition; thickness and weight; engineering and construction; shatter resistance and resilience to shock; resistance to warping, scratching, and fading; porosity; washability; thermal characteristics; and heat resistance for microwave and broiler use. Good restaurant china is resistant to breakage, chipping, and scratching. In fact, some manufacturers guarantee certain china against chipping and replace at no cost any products that become chipped.

China is usually broken by hitting other china. Seventy-five to 80 percent of all breakage occurs in the soiled dish area and may be traced to careless servers or utility staff. In many cases, china is broken accidentally by staff because the warewashing area was not designed with a spot to place a tray full of dirty dishes, forcing the busser (or server) to empty trays on top of other soiled dishes or in a sink. A critical component of kitchen and dining staff orientation is training on how to properly handle dirty dishes and load the dishwasher trays.

In some cases in which it would appear at first to be cheaper to switch from existing china to another more durable, less expensive, and manufacturer-stocked item, it is a good idea to use some of the china on a trial basis for a number of months before the initial purchase. Heavy or thick plates are not necessarily more durable or resistant to breakage, though they tend to hold heat longer than thin plates.

Plates with raised rims are better for sight-impaired residents, have a tendency to frame the food on the plate, and make small portions appear more plentiful. Colored or metallic borders should be avoided, as they deteriorate with repeated exposure to the 180°F final rinse cycle of a commercial dishwasher. Also, elaborate plate designs may be confusing to residents with cognitive impairment or dementia.

Glassware

The considerations for china also apply to glassware. Glassware, especially stemware, is generally less durable than china. For senior communities, a place setting consisting of a 10.5-ounce goblet for water, a multipurpose wine glass, and a 5-ounce juice glass works well for most applications. (Residents prefer goblets for water and wine. They are lighter than a highball glass and more easily handled by residents with arthritic hands.) In addition, a sherbet cup for desserts, an octagonal salad plate, and a matching cereal bowl provide the most versatility and require the least storage space and expense. These items should all be microwave-safe, and the undersides should not hold water when inverted in the dishwasher. Stackable glassware is much easier to store and handle.

Most restaurant operators purchase glassware that is mass produced (or pressed) and consequently less expensive than either hand- or machine-blown or custom-made crystal. Mass-produced glassware is usually thicker than blown glass and much more durable. Glasses should have sturdy stems, weighted bottoms, and rolled rims: these are the points where most breakage occurs. Costs for good-quality, durable glassware run from $1.00 to $6.00 per stem. Some operators use the same glassware for all beverages. Although this may save on storage and inventory costs, it tends to increase food costs because the larger water goblets are also used for juice or wine.

Some manufacturers guarantee their stemware against chipping and loss of serviceability for more than 50 washings. As with china, most glass breakages occur in the soiled-dish area. Designing the warewashing area to include a shelf for glassware racks allows servers to rack their own dirty glasses rather than push them at random onto the dirty-dish counter.

Loss rates for tabletop items—which include salt and pepper shakers, creamers, sugar caddies, bud vases, and cruet sets—are in the range of 5 percent. Salt and pepper shakers should be of the tower variety, with smooth surfaces that do not collect food particles. Sugar caddies need to be large enough to hold regular sugar as well as other sweeteners (e.g., NutraSweet, Equal, Splenda, Sweet'n Low, stevia). Bud vases should be short and weighted on the bottom so that smaller (and less expensive) flowers and greens can be used to decorate the table without blocking the residents' view of one another. Cut glass with a simple design works best for the tabletop items because they are easier for elderly people to grip. They are, however, harder to keep clean.

Silverware or Flatware

The feel of the flatware and its appearance on the table can either enhance or detract from the message of quality. The selection of flatware, however, is much easier than that of glassware.

Most restaurants use silver-plated flatware, which is considerably less expensive than sterling but still substantially more costly than stainless steel. Silver-plated flatware tends to tarnish and peel over time. Good-quality stainless is a wiser investment. The quality of stainless is measured by its relative chrome and nickel content. Lower-quality stainless steel flatware contains roughly 13 percent chrome, while high-quality contains 18 percent chrome and 8 percent nickel. The best-quality stainless is 18/10 flatware, with an even higher nickel content, which is harder and resists scratching and corrosion.

When selecting a pattern, the operator should consider the weight of the utensil, its pattern, and its functionality for seniors with limited grip strength. In general, the larger and the lighter, the better. Larger knives with rounded handles work well, for example, when they are hollow and not too heavy. Salad and dessert forks are often too small to handle easily and can be replaced with larger dinner forks. As the size of the flatware increases, it becomes easier to grip but heavier to hold. This is especially true of 18/10 flatware; the 2 percent increase in nickel content makes it only slightly heavier than the 18/8, but it *feels* more substantial. Complex patterns with too many ridges are harder to clean and have a tendency to pit.

Losses in flatware tend to be greatest and can be as high as 30 percent annually. For a 90-unit community, replacement can cost as much as $2,500 per year. Flatware is easy for employees to steal, is often left in residents' apartments from tray service, and is often inadvertently thrown out by servers scraping food waste into the garbage. Some operators have controlled losses by asking residents to use their own flatware for room service, providing incentives to staff to control losses, or periodically dumping the trash barrel and sorting through the food waste from the night's meal service.

Table Linens

Many high-end senior communities use tablecloths and cloth napkins at some or all meals. Historically, white tablecloths have symbolized fine dining. White is still preferred for formal service, but with the advent of dyes colorfast enough to withstand repeated commercial laundering, many restaurants have begun to use colored tablecloths and napkins to match their decor.

The two primary natural fibers for use in tablecloths and napkins are cotton and linen. Mercerized cotton is relatively inexpensive, has a good sheen, starches well, and has a long life because it holds up well to soap, bleach, and detergent. Yet 100 percent cotton fabrics wrinkle or crease easily unless the fabric is treated to be wrinkle free. Linen is relatively expensive and does not have as long a life as cotton. It has a moderate sheen and crisp texture (it wrinkles and creases more easily than cotton), but it absorbs moisture well, sheds dirt easily, and is lint free. Polyester fibers (such as Dacron) are usually combined with cotton (in 50:50 or 60:40 blends) for greater serviceability. This fabric resists wrinkling, but it may produce excessive lint. Because of Dacron's no-press, no-iron characteristics, some communities purchase wash-and-wear tablecloths and launder them in-house. The higher the percentage of cotton, the better the item holds starch; this means fewer wrinkles and more possibilities for creative napkin folding. Napkins made of polyester blends are not as absorbent, however, as those of 100 percent cotton or linen, and they tend to spread water or spills around rather than absorb them. Service cloths or side towels should be absorbent, lint-free, and capable of withstanding frequent bleaching. They are usually made of cotton, linen, rayon, or combinations of these fibers.

Most tablecloths need to be replaced after each seating. Some can simply be reversed and used for the next seating. Another option is to use a tablecloth covered by a Lexan or plexiglas tabletop, which can be wiped clean. Residents will accept the use of cloth placemats and paper napkins for breakfast and lunch provided the tabletop itself is attractive. Paper placemats are used in some communities and can be purchased in a variety of attractive and classic colors and seasonal designs. The use of paper communicates an informal or diner atmosphere, however, and should be carefully considered only for breakfast or lunch in the overall packaging of the meal.

All linen should be counted and sorted nightly. If linen is given to an outside laundry service, it should be inventoried before it is sent out. All deliveries should then be counted to verify the delivery receipt. This step alone can save the operation several hundred dollars per year: rarely are linen delivery counts accurate.

Chairs

Chairs with sturdy frames, arms, and high backs with casters on the *front legs only* are best for residents with disabilities. Chairs with casters can be hazardous on some floor surfaces if they roll too easily, as residents may use them to steady themselves. Purchase chairs that are designed with casters, as the addition of casters to existing chairs can affect the structural integrity of the chair and void the manufacturer's warranty. Select chairs without piping, cushions, or pockets in which food scraps can accumulate. The upholstery should be washable or protected fabric with a *firm* cushion. Wooden chairs seem to work best because they are easily repaired, re-covered, and refinished. Chairs must be light enough to allow residents to draw themselves to the table, yet sturdy enough to last for many years of hard use. Cross-bracing of the legs can add significantly to their durability and safety. Composite chairs have been introduced into the marketplace that are extremely durable and maintain their finish indefinitely.

Stackable chairs are a must for large events and parties. Good-quality stacking chairs are designed to be stacked without becoming marred. The chairs should be made in one piece, without mechanical or folding devices that eventually wear out and fail.

Chairs to be used by seniors should have arms and be lightweight and durable. It is helpful if stacks of chairs can be moved using a furniture dolly or chair cart. Ease of storage is another important consideration: when not in use, these chairs can make the common areas look cluttered.

Tables

Many residents prefer tables for two (30×36 inches), especially when they first move in and have not yet found regular dining companions. The other tables should seat four (42×42, 36×36, or 30×42 inches) or be convertible from square to round to accommodate additional diners. Round tables should be large enough for six diners (54 inches in diameter). Standard table height is 29 inches; it is useful to have several adjustable tables that can be raised to 31 inches to accommodate wheelchairs. Several banquet tables and half- or quarter-rounds should be available for theme parties and events.

When selecting dining room furniture, choose tabletops that look attractive when left uncovered. Such tables can be set with or without a cloth and can be used for other purposes, such as games, crafts, and cards.

In the dining room, there should be a minimum of 2 feet of aisle space between the backs of two adjacent chairs plus 18 inches for each chair. Therefore, the total distance from the edge of one table to the next should be 5 feet (18 inches + 18 inches + 2 feet).

Folding tables for continental breakfast, theme meals, parties, and special events are essential. This way food can be conveniently served in other locations within the community. These tables can be purchased in a variety of sizes, eight feet being the most popular. Wishbone-style folding legs (as opposed to pedestal or straight legs) maximize seating possibilities. Knockdown cabaret tables with pedestal tops (center-column) and bases offer considerable flexibility, but they are not as sturdy when set end to end for heavy items such as ice sculptures. These tables can be covered with standard square tablecloths from the dining room and skirted with matching cloth. Skirts are best attached to the tables using plastic Velcro clips.

Equipment for Functions and Banquets

Buffet and display equipment, such as serving platters and trays, can enhance the appearance and marketability of food even more than the china, silver, and glassware. This equipment must be highly functional and durable. It is generally cumbersome to store, and it tends to receive rough treatment. Chafing dishes and soup tureens can be purchased in silver plate, chrome, stainless steel, or crockery and are priced according to the design and the material. A large silver chafing dish with stand, insert, and lid may cost more than $1,000. Stainless steel is much less expensive, and silver-plated equipment can be replated for a fraction of the cost of new equipment. Chafing dishes can be heated with canned gels, liquid fuel, denatured alcohol, bottled gas, or electricity; most use canned gels.

Other equipment—such as mirrored or glass gourmet display trays, beverage housings and ice trays, ice carving pedestals, drip collectors, cake tiers, cubes and columns, various baskets, large shell bowls, serving stones, and rainbow glows—can add elegance and professionalism to any buffet. When garnished with fresh greens and edible flowers, the entire display becomes enticing.

■ DINING ROOM MANAGEMENT AND STAFFING

The management of the dining room operation can range from a lead server in small operations to a dining room manager and hosts in large communities. Any operation serving more than 70 meals at a time (communities with open seating that are 70 units or larger or communities with two seatings that are 140 units or larger) needs a dining room manager to help seat residents and manage the staff. Once the residents have been seated, the dining room manager can assist with beverages, ensure proper communication with the kitchen, and monitor resident satisfaction. During staff shortages, the dining room manager should be prepared to take on serving duties.

Between meals, the dining room manager is responsible for scheduling; selection and training of employees; ordering supplies; managing linens; inventorying china, silver, and glassware; planning functions; setting up events; sanitation in the dining room; and side work. As with the executive chef, the dining room manager is a working manager.

Dining rooms in congregate or continuing care retirement communities require server-to-resident ratios of approximately 1:30 for a continental breakfast and 1:16 for all other table service. These ratios provide each server with four tables, which, with the proper side work and a dish-up-to-order style of service, should permit efficient service. Assisted living communities require a higher ratio (1:12) because some residents require assistance with meals. Communities with residents who have dementia require ratios of 1:5 or 1:7 servers or care managers to residents. More may be required if residents need to be fed or if the food texture needs to be altered, such as by pureeing or chopping (see table 10.1).

These staffing ratios will produce good-quality service for most resident populations, provided the necessary side work and premeal setup are done. Salads and desserts can be preplated and stored on sheet pans on a covered rolling rack in the walk-in cooler. Salad dressings can be poured into small plastic ramekins and kept on a shelf in the server's reach-in cooler. Soups can be dished up in the kitchen at the

Table 10.1   Staffing Model for a Three-Meal Dining Room, 112 Residents

Meals per month	$112 \times 3 \times 30.5$	= 10,248	Breakfast	7:30–8:15	or	8:30–9:15
Guest meals per month	2×30	60	Lunch	11:00–12:00	or	12:30–1:30
Total		10,308	Dinner	4:15–5:15	or	5:30–6:30
Daily		344				

	Number of meals served (total daily meals / 3)	Meals per served seating (2 seatings)	Server to diner ratio	Servers needed (1 server per 12 diners, rounded)
	114.42	57.21	1:12	5

Shift	Number of servers	Serving hours	Nonserving hours	Total hours	Staff hours/day	Staff hours/week	FTE
7:00–2:30	5	2	5	7	35	245	6.13
3:45–7:00	5	3	0.50	3.5	17.5	122.5	3.06
Total		**25**	**27.5**		**52.5**	**367.5**	**9.19**

server's station or in the dining room from an electric soup tureen at a side or busing station. The entire operation must be organized to minimize servers' trips to the kitchen and maximize time with residents at their stations. Servers should be assigned to specific residents or a specific workstation, in much the same way as the personal care aides are assigned. This approach allows servers to learn residents' individual food preferences and thus builds resident satisfaction in the food service operation and confidence in the management.

For operations with open seating serving 300 or more diners per night, the staffing required is staggering. Some large congregate or continuing care retirement communities use busing staff or assistant servers. These people can perform beverage service, remove plates, and clean and reset tables. Assistant servers can be hired at a lower rate (these can be regarded as trainee positions) and expedite the delivery of the food. The disadvantage to having assistant servers is that the senior servers may slack off and not bus their own tables, sometimes even making an empty-handed trip to the kitchen to direct a busser to their station.

Labor cost and overtime can significantly affect the total delivered food cost and ultimately the bottom line. Nonserving hours should be used efficiently for side work, delivering trays, sanitation, dishwashing, inventory, and special functions. In addition, servers who have the flexibility to work short or split shifts can save the operation thousands of dollars annually.

Dining Room Service Plan

The dining room manager should develop a service plan that details the entire operation. It should describe each meal and state whether it is buffet or table service; specify how the dining room will be divided among the servers; and list numbered stations and serving assignments. It should also include a complete description of the setups for each side station in the dining room and in the kitchen (including approximate numbers of each needed item to be stocked). The plan should include policies and procedures, such as job duties during nonserving times, the guest meal policy, the reservation policy, telephone etiquette, kitchen rules, sanitation practices, minimum training standards, standards of professionalism, the procedure for a quality audit, resident preferences and dietary restrictions (by station if known), and dress code or uniform guidelines. When the dining room manager is absent or policy questions arise, the service plan can be used as a resource.

The plan should reflect the opinions and ideas of the servers. Thus premeal and sanitation side-work schedules and assignments can be agreed on with the staff and documented in the plan. Staff are more likely to support and follow the plan if they play a part in its development.

The chef or lead cook should hold premeal meetings with the dining room staff before each meal, explaining any important information about the meal before the servers offer it to the residents. The meeting should detail each item on the menu, from the soup and salad to the entrées, alternates, and dessert options. It should list the main ingredients, note anything special about the preparation or taste of the dishes, list the sauces available and explain how they were made, describe the portion sizes available, and specify any alternative items and how long they will take to prepare if requested. The servers should also be made aware of menu items with reduced fat, sodium, cholesterol, or sugar. Some chefs will even plate up a sample of each entrée and allow the servers to taste each one, with sauces, so that they can describe the meal to the residents. All resident plates should be prepared by gloved staff to promote infection control. By spending a few minutes with the servers before each meal, the chef will establish a partnership with the people who will be representing her creations to the residents, and the servers can help ensure that the residents receive what they expect and are satisfied with their dining experience.

Side Work

Side work refers to tasks related to setting up the dining room, service areas, and busing stations to ensure the smooth serving of meals, and these tasks are typically performed by servers before and after the meal service. They include vacuuming; wiping down and sanitizing furniture; cleaning side stands, counters, and cabinets; removing dishes and serving equipment; resetting all tables; restocking all tabletop equipment; and restocking side stations for the next shift. Exhibit 10.1 gives a manager's checklist of side-work tasks that a gloved kitchen or dining room staff can perform.

The supervisor should distribute side-work task sheets to each person during scheduled shifts. Estimated completion times should be given for each task, and the manager or shift supervisor should check each employee's work before the end of the shift. The manager and the employee should then sign off for the work completed each day. The dining room manager should also walk through the dining room before and after each meal period to correct any deficiencies.

Well-placed and fully stocked service stations are necessary to maximize the servers' efficiency. The cold station in the kitchen should be stocked with all food and equipment necessary for an entire meal service. This includes all preplated salads, cold appetizers, and condiments such as salad dressings, cottage cheese, sauces, mustard, and ketchup. Dessert items ready for dinner should be placed on trays on rolling racks in the walk-in coolers. The server's station should be located in the kitchen as close as possible to the walk-in cooler. The area should accommodate a stainless-steel work table for setting out trays of plated cold food as well as several rolling racks of plated cold food. Any underliners, such as those for bread and butter plates, utensils such as salad forks or spoons, doilies, creamers, teapots and teabags, and the like should also be stored here. During service, a line cook or utility person (but not a server) should continue to refresh and restock the area as needed. This station should be totally set approximately 15 to 30 minutes before the opening of each meal service.

Service stations in the dining room should adhere to the following guidelines:

Each station should be set up for the use of two or three servers.

Each station should be equipped with serviceware and linen to handle the appropriate number of meals for a second seating.

Each station should be supplied with a complete line of condiments, cracker baskets, lemon slices, and other adjuncts.

At least two soup stations inside the kitchen must be maintained and equipped for easy server access, with adequate serviceware and flatware for each seating as well as serving utensils.

A little preparation can ensure that during the evening's service all equipment is immediately available at the server stations, so that the server need not

Exhibit 10.1   Side-Work Checklist for Managers

- ❑ Replenish all the flatware on assigned stations.
- ❑ Replenish all glassware on assigned stations.
- ❑ Refill all cracker baskets and sugar caddies.
- ❑ Restock coffee cups, saucers, and bread plates.
- ❑ Clean the coffee and juice machines, service station refrigerator, and milk machine.
- ❑ Collect and inventory all teapots and stainless creamers and wash them by hand.
- ❑ Wipe down chairs and tables on assigned stations.
- ❑ Clean all kitchen countertops.
- ❑ Clean the microwave and the salad station.
- ❑ Collect all the flower vases from each table and store them in the reach-in refrigerator.
- ❑ Organize all trays and breadbaskets.
- ❑ Empty the garbage can in the dining room.
- ❑ Polish all the flatware used for the shift.
- ❑ Replenish all the flatware on every station for breakfast setup.
- ❑ Replenish all the linens and napkins in the dining room, including every station.
- ❑ Replenish condiments in the kitchen, including soup station.
- ❑ Maintain the bread warmer. See that there are enough rolls and bread for the shift.
- ❑ Refill and wipe down all salt and pepper shakers individually. Ensure that salt and pepper shakers are emptied and washed at least once a week.
- ❑ Set up flatware, glasses, china, and tabletop on every table.
- ❑ Wipe down and refill oil and vinegar sets every night.
- ❑ Organize all specialty beverages, juices, sodas, and milk inside the service refrigerator.
- ❑ Wipe down all the menu holders or update menu board.

leave the dining room to replenish supplies. Closing side work must include completely restocking these service stations.

■ TRAINING THE SERVERS

All food service operations require courteous service. Good training can help staff respond appropriately to difficult or demanding customers without becoming frustrated or angry. In addition, making servers aware of the special needs of an elderly population can provide them with the insight they need to avoid a potentially embarrassing or confrontational situation. A few comments in several categories may be helpful. In general, it is easier in the long run to accommodate residents whenever possible than to argue with them.

Seniors tend to know what they want and how they want it. They are value-conscious, and they may be well-off financially but still frugal; and they are not easily persuaded. The staff may perceive their behavior as demanding. Assigning servers to specific residents promotes awareness of individual needs. As habits and preferences are recognized, communication improves, and the chances that residents' requests will be misunderstood or neglected are minimized. Servers can even be in a position to alert the management when a resident's habits change, or they note signs of diminished appetite or illness.

To cater better to seniors, menus should be printed in large, easily legible typefaces, with significant contrast between the type and the background paper, and should not have a surface that produces glare. Many communities use a menu board at the entrance or post their menus on a video monitor in the lobby that residents can see during the day to plan their choices.

A resident who is taken ill at a meal should be offered any assistance necessary for comfort. The person should not be moved. The lead server should summon professional assistance quietly, and servers should try not to embarrass the person or arouse commotion in the immediate area. Any accidents should be quickly cleaned up to avoid ruining the appetite of other residents. Servers should be properly trained to recognize and respond to choking emergencies. All diners should be encouraged to sanitize their hands at a sanitizer station prior to entering the dining room.

Residents who are visually impaired should be treated with as little extra fanfare as possible. If unescorted, they should be led to their seats by the host or their server. Most visually impaired people follow by grasping the leader's elbow. A visually impaired resident may ask to have the menu read and should be spoken to when being served. The server should assist as necessary, and it may be necessary to cut or portion larger items for the visually impaired resident.

Should a hearing-impaired resident ask for a menu explanation, the server should explain the menu while directly facing the resident. Many hearing-impaired people can read lips, but they need to see the speaker's mouth. A gentle nudge or a visible approach to the table should be used so that the hearing-impaired resi-

dent realizes that he or she is going to be served. Some hearing-impaired residents may be able to speak (sometimes in monotone), and others may need to point to specific menu items to place an order.

Many elderly people experience uncontrollable shaking or palsy in their hands. Therefore, beverage glasses and cups should be filled only to within two or three inches of the rim.

Residents with short-term memory deficit may forget what they ordered or see a different entrée ordered by their tablemate and request the same. Any refused food should be promptly returned to the kitchen; the server should never try to offer an unwanted meal to another resident. Residents may also be confused about which meal they are eating. Some will order breakfast items at dinner. These requests should be accommodated when possible. Well-fed residents, even those who have eaten pancakes for dinner, are generally healthier and happier than those who leave the table hungry or dissatisfied.

Residents who arrive near closing time deserve the same courteous service as residents arriving at the opening, and management should plan for late-arriving customers. The residents may be served in a separate dining area or in their rooms so as not to be disturbed by staff cleaning or resetting the main dining room. If a resident arrives near closing time, the host or server may do a couple of things: (1) politely inform the resident that the dining room is closing, but she will make every effort to serve him; or (2) politely inform the resident that she must check with the manager or the chef to see if he can be seated. This sets the stage for politely asking the resident to leave as soon as he has finished eating.

Do not seat an inebriated resident if this can be avoided without giving offense. The other residents in the dining room deserve a quiet meal, and a drunken, disruptive resident can ruin their evening as well as yours.

All noteworthy incidents should be documented daily in the food service log book or computerized tracking system. A record should be kept to note residents' complaints and staff reactions, returned meals, residents' preferences, comments made by residents or changes in their behavior, training needs, and daily meal counts and the number of residents' guests. This information enables the supervisor to track resident eating patterns, complaint patterns, and workload and to follow up on resident questions and incidents

Visiting children require additional or special service. Their ages will dictate how much special attention they require, but children generally enjoy being treated as adults. The server should not ignore a child or use baby talk. A highchair or booster chair should be offered if required. A child's portion of a popular dish should be recommended—spaghetti, hamburger, chicken fingers, or a peanut butter and jelly sandwich—and brought to the table as quickly as possible. If a child is irritable, food may quiet her. The server should never reprimand a child for misbehavior.

International guests or residents may not speak or understand the language. The guidelines for visually impaired or hearing-impaired residents can be applied to international residents as well.

VIPs deserve special service, but this should not be observed by other residents in the dining room lest they feel like second-class citizens. VIPs should be served in private dining rooms to the extent possible, or in areas of the dining room that are not readily visible to other residents. VIP guests should be given the best available server and certainly never an inexperienced one.

The efficient performance of a dining room operation cannot be left to chance: good training is essential. Although an employee's attitude, friendliness, smile, and willingness to serve are uniquely her own, proper service can be taught. The dining room manager therefore must hire for attitude and train for skill. A quiz like exhibit 10.2 can be helpful in assessing servers' skills.

■■■■■■ PERFORMANCE STANDARDS

Adherence to defined performance guidelines will provide the kind of service that enhances residents' community-living experience and makes for long-term success (see exhibit 10.3). The keys to this service are alertness, attention to detail, and follow-through. Exhibit 10.4 lists the characteristics of *poor* service. Exhibit 10.5 lists tips for safety and accident prevention, and exhibit 10.6 offers a list of questions dining room managers can use for monitoring performance.

■■■■■ Service Protocol

A spirit of partnership and communication between the servers and the kitchen is essential to successful food service. How the food is served and presented affects overall perceived quality as much as its ingredients and preparation. Any breakdown in communication between the front (dining room) and back (kitchen) of the house is quickly detected by residents and can negatively affect their opinion of the food.

Once the food leaves the kitchen, the chef can do little to influence its reception by the residents. When residents complain about the food, the servers must accept responsibility for correcting it, not blame the kitchen. When serving begins, it is the server's responsibility to make sure that the food plated by the cook is exactly what the resident ordered. Every plate cover must be lifted and checked against the order to ensure accuracy. If it is incorrect, the server should refuse the meal. The servers do not work for the chef or cook: during serving times, the cook works for them. Some communities utilize dietary preference cards for each resident. These can be kept in the kitchen and identify preferences such as portion size, beverage of choice, special dietary restrictions, mechanical issues, or allergies. This customization shows attention to detail in customer service, and avoids food-related mistakes in service. Dietary cards should be reviewed by the nursing staff to ensure that any physician orders or allergies are accurately depicted.

Most senior living communities offer American-style plate service: food is dished onto plates in the kitchen, not at the table from a silver tray (Russian service) or a serving cart (French service). Trays should be used to carry food to the tables. This is advantageous for many reasons: many items can be carried at one time, thus saving trips to and from the kitchen; entrée plates can be covered and stacked, thus keeping food warmer; carrying a tray requires less skill than professionally carrying three or more entrée plates with side dishes; and a tray is then available to bring dirty dishes back to the kitchen.

All trays brought from the kitchen should be covered with an open napkin so that if the tray is damaged or stained, it remains sanitary and fresh looking. When extra flatware is brought to the table, it should be placed on a cloth napkin on a side plate. Flatware should never be taken from one table and given to another.

Coffee cups should always rest on a saucer unless mugs are being used. Hot tea should be served with

Exhibit 10.2 Skills Training for Dining Room Servers

Site: _____

Dining room manager: _____

Server: _____

Date: _____

1. What type of service is available at this retirement community? (choose one)
   ___ a) American plate service
   ___ b) French service
   ___ c) Cart service

2. When approaching a table, what do we ask the guests first?
   ___ a) What are your names?
   ___ b) Would you like a beverage?
   ___ c) Do you have any food allergies?

3. When do we begin to take the residents' orders?
   ___ a) After they ask what the soup is
   ___ b) When they stop talking to one another
   ___ c) After we return with their beverages

4. How do you learn about the day's menu?
   ___ a) By asking other servers
   ___ b) By reading the menu before the service
   ___ c) By attending the premeal meeting and asking questions

5. When taking an order, whose order is taken first?
   ___ a) The person closest to you
   ___ b) The person facing the kitchen door
   ___ c) Ladies' orders are always taken first

6. Beverages are always served from which side?
   ___ a) The side closest to you
   ___ b) Either side of the resident
   ___ c) From the right side of the resident

7. Food is always served from which side?
   ___ a) Either side of the resident
   ___ b) Always reach across the resident
   ___ c) From the left side of the resident

8. When extra silver is required at the table:
   ___ a) We take it from another table
   ___ b) We hand it to the resident
   ___ c) We bring it on a linen napkin

9. When a meal is not up to the resident's liking, we:
   ___ a) Tell them everyone else liked it
   ___ b) Say it's too bad and walk away
   ___ c) Apologize and offer to replace it immediately

10. When assembling a tray, we always try to:
    ___ a) Make it pretty
    ___ b) Have everything appropriate to the order on it at one time
    ___ c) Keep the order small

11. When carrying a tray, we always try to:
    ___ a) Show how good we are at balancing
    ___ b) Keep the tray at shoulder height
    ___ c) Carry it with the other hand

12. When you are busing a table, always remember to:
    ___ a) Scrape the dishes in the dining room to help the dishwashing staff
    ___ b) Leave the dishes until everyone in the room is finished
    ___ c) Bus dishes to a tray and remove them to the kitchen immediately

13. When serving coffee, what condiments are always served?
    ___ a) None
    ___ b) Cream and sugar
    ___ c) Condiments requested by the resident

14. When should the correct condiments be served with menu items?
    ___ a) Only after people ask
    ___ b) When the items are served
    ___ c) We don't serve condiments

15. Should a server know the daily desserts?
    ___ a) No, that's why we have a printed menu
    ___ b) The dining room manager should tell the residents
    ___ c) Servers should know all the daily desserts

16. When or by whom is the side work in the dining room done?
    ___ a) By the last person serving
    ___ b) By the dining room manager
    ___ c) Preceding the opening and after the closing of the dining room

17. Table settings are considered complete when:
    ___ a) Every place setting is complete as well as the table center
    ___ b) You have set them with whatever is available
    ___ c) They all have about the same thing

18. How often is a tablecloth changed in the dining room?
    ___ a) Each time the table is used
    ___ b) When the spots are noticeable
    ___ c) Once a week

19. Is your name tag considered part of your uniform?
    ___ a) Only when you are waiting on someone you don't know
    ___ b) Yes, always
    ___ c) Only when there are big parties

20. When writing the ticket for food, how important is it to write clearly?
    ___ a) It's not important; you can always tell the chef
    ___ b) It is important to write legibly
    ___ c) It's not important; only the server has to read the ticket

Total Score: _____ /20 × 100 = _____ %

hot water in a cup on an underliner. A lemon wedge should be placed on the underliner. The server should offer a selection of three teas, including regular tea, when delivering the tea water. Milk (not cream) should be offered with tea because it is the traditional accompaniment to English tea. Tomato juice and V-8 juice should always be served with a fresh lemon wedge, and all lemon wedges should be at least 1/6 count.

Even in the finest restaurants (or your mother's kitchen), an entrée occasionally turns out badly. Residents do not expect perfection, but they do expect a generally consistent quality of food and service. They will become upset only if they perceive that the food or the service is consistently bad and that their opinions are not respected. The kitchen staff should make every effort to forestall complaints by recognizing and intercepting a substandard meal before it gets to

---

Exhibit 10.3   Service Guidelines

- Always be courteous.
- Never stand around. If you are waiting, always look for something to do for the residents and be available to them.
- Always greet your residents, by name if possible. Introduce yourself, make eye contact with guests, and smile.
- If another resident is waiting, smile and say that you will be right with them.
- Answer any questions a resident may have. If you do not know the answer, apologize and inform the resident how to obtain the answer. Any resident who appears to need assistance should receive it immediately from any nearby employee.
- If a resident appears confused or in need of assistance, cheerfully inquire as to how you may be of service.
- Never argue with anyone, especially a resident.
- Do not complain about food to kitchen personnel; tell your supervisor.
- Do not blame the kitchen for slow service. Accept responsibility for the entire food service operation.
- Never hurry residents.
- Never make negative remarks about the property, fellow employees, management, or residents in the presence of a resident.
- Inform management of any problem that may disturb resident satisfaction, or any resident problems you may have dealt with. Try to prevent problems or solve them yourself whenever possible.
- Avoid talking to other employees, especially in the presence of residents.
- Always maintain a pleasant tone of voice. Do not shout or give loud orders in the dining room or kitchen.
- Walk briskly, but never run. Move more slowly when leading residents to their seats.
- Maintain good posture. Do not lean on chairs or put your foot on a chair rung. Stand erect or bend from the waist to hear. Do not crouch down or bend at the knees.
- Never use profanity.
- Do not eat, drink, smoke, or chew gum or tobacco in an area where you may encounter residents. This includes the concierge area and lobby, other public spaces, and the dining room. Never eat during service or in the kitchen.
- Do not point in the dining room or gesture at a table.
- Do not lean on walls or side stations. Do not rest anything on the resident's table. Do not perform any functions on the resident's table, such as stacking dishes, placing soiled silverware on plates, or writing the residents' orders.
- Do not put your hands in your pockets or on your hips.
- Do not cross your arms in front of your chest. Grasp your hands in front or behind you.
- Do not mop your face with the side towel. Never carry a side towel under your arm or on your shoulder.
- Replace your towel when it becomes crumpled or soiled.
- Use a clean, sanitary towel to polish silver or glassware only before opening the restaurant or when out of residents' view.
- If the resident spills something or you spill something on a resident, apologize, clean it up, and advise the dining room manager or supervisor.
- If a resident drops a napkin or piece of silverware, replace it with a clean one. Do not take replacements from adjacent tables!
- Do not carry pencils, books, or other items where they are visible, for example, in pockets, in your hair, or behind your ear.
- Carry menus in your hands, not under your arms or tucked into pockets or clothing.

Exhibit 10.4	Seven Sins of Poor Service

1. Apathy   5. Robotism
2. Brushoff   6. Quoting the rules
3. Coldness   7. Runaround
4. Condescension

Exhibit 10.5	Safety and Accident Prevention

- Be alert for tripping hazards, such as chairs pulled away from tables, briefcases or purses near tables, and unexpected motions of diners. Be especially aware of residents pushing chairs back from the table as you walk by.
- Always make sure residents are aware of your presence before you begin serving.
- Clean as you go: wipe up spilled food, drink, and ice immediately. Use a service towel to wipe up spills from tables and chairs. Use a rag to clean the floor.
- Always hold glasses by the base. If you hold water glasses between your fingers so that the rims touch, the glasses may slip from your hands.
- Always close drawers and cabinets that you have opened. Someone may hit an open drawer or door while passing by, resulting in injury.
- Hold hot plates with a clean, dry side towel to avoid burns. Warn the residents when plates are hot.
- Clean up any broken items immediately. If items are broken near food, warn others. If breakages occur in or near the ice bin, cover it with a tray immediately. New ice should then be brought in an ice pail to use until the bin is cleaned out and refilled. Never pick up broken items with your hands: always use a towel or dustpan and broom.
- Use a metal ice scoop to fill glasses with ice. *Never* scoop up ice with the glass: if a glass breaks in the ice bin, the whole bin must be emptied.
- If you discover broken or chipped glassware, or ragged or bent silverware, take it out of circulation and give it to your supervisor.
- Avoid overfilling containers with food and liquids, especially those that are hot and may cause burns.
- Bend at the knees when picking up heavy items. This will give you more support and guard against back injury.
- Always return items to their proper place.
- Be familiar with the fire prevention and evacuation procedure.
- Know the location and contents of the first aid kit.

the dining room. The server should check with the resident soon after the entrée is served to ensure that everything is satisfactory. The dining room manager should also greet all residents at least once during their meal.

If a resident rejects a dish, a substitute should be offered and served immediately, and the dining room manager should be notified. Under no circumstances should kitchen personnel seek to dismiss the resident's complaint or argue with food service personnel about the incident. The food should not be thrown away before inspection by a manager or supervisor.

If a server spills food or beverages on a resident's clothing, the dining room manager or server should apologize and offer the resident a signed, dated cleaning ticket (if appropriate). If the resident cannot remove the stain with normal cleaning, he or she should be asked to bring the clothing to the dining room manager with the cleaning ticket so that the clothing can be professionally cleaned at the facility's expense. All spills should be recorded in the dining room daily log book, noting the server's name, so that any patterns can be traced. Excessive spillage is often a result of poor training.

Many residents will want to take food from the dining room back to their rooms, especially if they are on a limited meal program or have a pet or a guest. The community should make it clear that "doggie bags" are not permitted: residents may eat as much as they wish at the table but may not take food to their apartments. The removal of food from the dining room can cost an operation thousands of dollars over the course of a year. Moreover, although the community should encourage residents to eat as much as they need to stay healthy, the risk of food-borne illnesses increases when food leaves the supervision of the food service department, and the community may still be held liable for contamination, as the food effectively remains on community premises. Often residents take food from the dining room for a snack if they are unable to purchase food outside the property. A trip to the local grocery store or arrangements for groceries to be delivered can provide residents the opportunity to stock their own kitchens.

Exhibit 10.6   Questions to Ensure Great Service

- Are salads properly chilled?
- Are water glasses promptly refilled?
- Are hot food and beverages served on hot plates or in hot cups?
- Is hot food served hot and cold food served cold?
- Is apartment delivery service timely?
- Are telephone callers put on hold for less than 30 seconds?
- Are apartment delivery trays picked up in less than three hours?
- Is all equipment retrieved?
- Does the food service director or host inspect all stations and tabletops before opening?
- Are dishes and glasses free of chips?
- Is the flatware on tables polished and free of spots?
- Are the glasses free of spots or streaks? Hold them up to the light to check.
- Are chairs and booths free of dirt, stains, and crumbs?
- Is there enough china, flatware, and glassware?
- Is the flatware set straight on tables?
- Are sugar bowls clean inside? Take the sugar packets out and look.
- Are the salt and pepper shakers full and free of grease? Touch them. Are the ketchup bottles clean and full?
- Can you be sure that you will not run out of any items?
- Are the residents recognized by a smile, a hello, or eye contact when they arrive at the door of the dining room?
- Are residents acknowledged within one minute of being seated?
- Does each resident get a menu that is clean, dry, and presentable?
- Are the bread and rolls fresh?
- Are meals presented attractively and creatively?
- Is the food picked up and served without sitting in the window too long?
- When orders arrive, are they complete? Do the servers know who gets what without asking?
- Do the service personnel have pleasant attitudes?
- Is proper service etiquette observed?
- Does meal service start on time?
- Are debris, bits of paper, and spilled food *immediately* picked up from the carpets or floors in the dining room?
- Do residents get the best possible value for money?
- Does the resident get exactly what the menu describes?
- Does the food service director or host speak with residents at each table during a meal?
- At breakfast, are residents served coffee immediately on being seated?
- Does the food service director personally inspect the continental breakfast at least once a week?
- Is the coffee steaming hot?
- Are the continental breakfasts or specialty buffets replenished quickly?
- Are the coffee cups free of stains?
- Are the tables and chairs solid and stable?
- Are clean, fresh towels, not paper napkins, used to wipe down tables?
- Do servers clean as they go?
- Are uniforms clean and attractive?
- Do all employees wear name tags?
- Do all employees abide by grooming standards?
- Are special requests for food items honored when possible?
- Are servers familiar with the menu items they serve?
- Is there consistency in glassware and china?
- Do servers assist residents when necessary?
- Are crumbs removed from tables after the entrée?
- Are all sauces and dressings presented in a ramekin on the side?
- Is extra flatware presented on a cloth napkin and underliner?
- Are napkins refolded when residents leave the table during a meal?
- Does everyone know the table numbers in the dining room?
- Is glassware always handled by the stem or at the base?
- When not picking up a food order, are servers attending to other tasks?
- Are the servers responsive to residents' requests?
- Are residents' expectations well managed?

Order of Service

1. The dining room manager or host greets residents at the door, seating them at the appropriate table. She assists residents with their chairs, placing the first resident in the seat facing the door.

2. A clean, fresh-looking menu is set before each diner.

3. The server acknowledges the table within one minute.

4. The server approaches the table with a friendly greeting within three minutes, pours cold water, and presents a breadbasket and butter. He explains the daily menu and offers beverages and margarine.

5. The server returns with beverages and asks if there are any questions about the menu.

6. The server returns to the table after two minutes to take orders, moving clockwise around the table. The order is taken on a captain's order pad, with person number 1 (chair with back toward the front door) at the top of the list. Each order includes appetizer or soup, salad, and entrée. All questions must be addressed in a patient, friendly manner. Substitutions are possible when ingredients are available.

7. The first course (soup, salad, or appetizer) is served, from the right with the right hand. Salad dressing is served on the side in a separate ramekin. Extra sauce for an appetizer should be placed at the left of the setting.

8. Freshly ground pepper is offered.

9. The server should return during the first course to check the water and beverages.

10. The first course is cleared only when everyone at the table has finished, not as the residents individually finish. Plates are cleared from the right with the right hand.

11. Before the entrée is served, the server should check whether any fresh flatware is needed.

12. The entrée is served, with any sauces placed at the left of the entrée plate, in a ramekin on an underliner. The plate should be set down with the main (meat) item closest to the resident and served from the left with the left hand.

13. If the order was correctly recorded using the seat-number method, there should be no question regarding who gets what.

14. After serving the entrée, the server should offer to replenish the breadbasket as well as the beverages.

15. Residents should not be rushed, regardless of how busy the dining room is. This meal may be the residents' primary social event of the day, and the experience must never be compromised.

16. Residents should never leave a primary meal hungry. Thus, if a resident wants another little taste of something, it should be provided, served on a salad plate.

17. The entrée should be cleared once all residents have stopped eating. Everything that is not needed for dessert should be removed: entrée plate, bread and butter plate, breadbasket, side dishes, and salt and pepper shakers. The server should never stack dishes or scrape plates in front of a resident.

18. The server should wipe crumbs away from each place setting.

19. The server describes the dessert presentation, mentioning other items, such as ice cream, that may be available; some communities may present a dessert tray. Coffee and decaffeinated coffee should be offered. Decaffeinated coffee must always be freshly brewed for each order. Because many residents drink only decaffeinated coffee for medical reasons, it is essential that regular coffee never be mixed or confused with decaffeinated.

20. If a guest is present, a guest meal ticket must be given to the resident for signature. Once dessert has been served, the server should bring the check to the resident in a check presenter or face down on a salad plate. All guest checks must be filled out correctly with the resident's name, apartment number, number of guests, price, and totals.

How to Set a Table

All tabletops should be set according to a sketch provided by the food service manager. All tables should be covered with a clean tablecloth, falling evenly, with the seam side down. Each table should be equipped with a clean, full set of salt and pepper shakers and a clean sugar bowl with white sugar, raw (coffee) sugar, and artificial sweeteners. Figure 10.1 shows a properly arranged place setting. Of course, all silverware, china, and glassware should be clean and polished, and linens should be spotlessly clean and pressed. The type

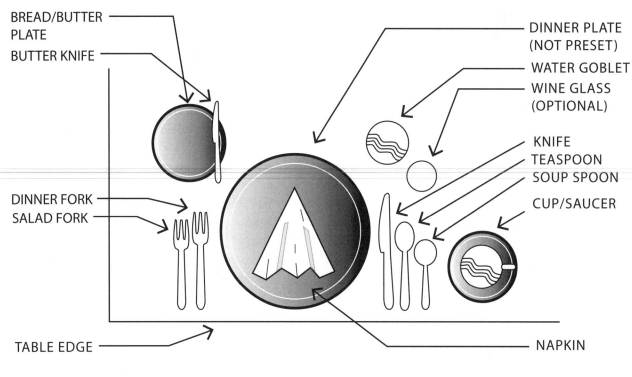

BREAD/BUTTER PLATE
BUTTER KNIFE
DINNER PLATE (NOT PRESET)
WATER GOBLET
WINE GLASS (OPTIONAL)
KNIFE
TEASPOON
SOUP SPOON
CUP/SAUCER
DINNER FORK
SALAD FORK
TABLE EDGE
NAPKIN

Figure 10.1   Place Setting

of napkin fold should be changed periodically to add variety to the place setting.

How to Bus and Reset a Table

1. All tables are bused onto trays, which are placed on tray jacks, and never into bus tubs. Trays should never be placed on tables or chairs.
2. All soiled items should be removed from the table. Glassware should be placed in the middle of the tray for stability, flatware around the edge, and the soiled tablecloth on top.
3. The tabletop, salt and pepper shakers, sugar caddy, and candleholder or vase should be thoroughly wiped.

4. Chairs should be wiped and litter and debris removed from around the table.
5. Trays can be heavy; bus staff should squat and lift the tray with the leg muscles. The tray should be placed in a predefined location in the dishwashing area.
6. Condiment bottles and linen napkins should be removed from the tray and cleaned.
7. The table should be reset according to the guidelines above.

Housekeeping

n planning a community, the management needs to decide on various aspects of housekeeping and maintenance services: the frequency of housekeeping visits to the apartments, tasks performed at each visit, annual deep cleaning, linen and laundry service, cleaning of common areas, pest control, maintenance of air conditioning filters, and scheduling.

It is much easier to keep a clean facility clean than it is to clean up a dirty one. If the management allows the community to become dirty over time, it is difficult to raise the bar or improve cleanliness with existing staff members, because they feel as though they are being asked to work harder for the same pay. Unfortunately, dirt gets noticed by residents and visitors; cleanliness generally does not.

INFECTION CONTROL

As the coronavirus continues to spread across the globe, scientists are learning more about its effects on people. Not all patients with COVID-19 will require medical supportive care. According to recent findings, the CDC reports that 80 percent of people who become infected with the virus will only experience mild to moderately ill effects and can safely be treated as you would treat the flu—staying at home, getting plenty of rest, and pushing fluids. Approximately 15 percent will become severely ill and while still able to remain isolated at home may experience more significant symptoms such as shortage of breath while the virus runs its course. The remaining 5 percent of the victims can become critically ill and will require hospitalization; they may develop pneumonia in both lungs, experience multiorgan failure, and in some cases die. Clinical management for hospitalized patients with COVID-19 is focused on supportive care of complications, including advanced organ support for respiratory failure, septic shock, and multiorgan failure. While most people recover from this virus, the fatality rate is now estimated at between 2.8–3.4 percent for the overall population but rises to 8 percent in patients between the ages of 70–79 and 14.8 percent in patients over 80.

From the data that is available for COVID-19 infected patients, and for data from related coronaviruses such as SARS-CoV and MERS-CoV, it is now clear that older adults, and persons who have underlying chronic medical conditions, such as immunocompromising conditions, are at significant risk for more severe outcomes.

Given the highly transmissible nature of the coronavirus and the limited treatment options available in severe cases, prevention will be the senior living community's first line of defense. Planning for a potential emerging infectious disease pandemic, like COVID-19, is critical to protecting the health and welfare of residents who are most vulnerable to the effects it can cause. A comprehensive communicable disease response plan should be designed with the involvement of public health officials, the community medical director, and nursing clinicians to apply educational, clinical, operational, and preventive measures to assure the safety of the residents and the staff who serve them to the highest clinical certainty possible. Exhibit 11.1 is a sample infection prevention and control plan (IPCP) adapted from HHS Pandemic Influenza Planning resources, recommendations of the Centers for Disease Control and Prevention for health care facilities, and the Assistant Secretary for Preparedness and Response (ASPR).

Covid-19 and other communicable diseases have changed the face of senior living communities where its population is much more vulnerable due to multiple comorbidities already weakening the body's natural immune response. Following proper infection control procedures can significantly reduce potential exposure to residents and staff. All staff and visitors should be screened for temperature and complete a brief exposure summary before granted entry.

■ COMMUNICATION AND RESIDENT RELATIONS

An organization is only as good as its frontline staff. Often housekeepers are treated as invisible, when to the residents they are the company's main representatives. No company understands this better than the Disney Corporation. At Disneyland theme parks, the management knows that the cleanliness of the park is of paramount importance to a good-quality experience. It also knows that the cleaning staff, who are constantly visible at their work, will handle more guest inquiries than any other employees. The management gives these employees extensive training in guest relations to equip them to enhance the guests' experience. They are among the most thoroughly trained employees at the parks, second only to those portraying Disney characters in costume.

In a similar way, the housekeeping department of a senior living community plays a vital role not only in keeping the property clean but also in maintaining relationships with the residents. Often the housekeeper is one of a resident's few regular visitors, and the resident may look forward to cleaning day for the company it provides. Strong friendships can develop between the resident and the housekeeper, who may be the main conduit of information between the management and the resident. After all, the housekeeper is spending more one-on-one time with the resident than any other staff member.

It is therefore critical that the housekeeping staff be trained to represent the community well. They should be trained to give appropriate, consistent answers to common questions from residents and families. Often, residents or their families ask the same questions of different individuals to test how the responses may vary. Conversely, the management can learn a lot from what the residents tell the housekeeping staff: residents typically test out rumors on their housekeeper and pass on the response to other residents. Weekly discussions with the staff at the beginning or end of the shift can be a valuable tool to monitor and manage resident satisfaction and expectations.

Resident referrals are a vital (and inexpensive) source of leads for the marketing staff. All community personnel should understand the importance of these referrals and what each can do to promote them. Managers will want to be certain that the message being delivered by the sales staff reflects reality in the operations and is consistent with the views of the housekeeping staff in particular. Consistency equals credibility. The more consistent all staff members are in communicating the features and benefits of the community, the more credibility the entire operation will demonstrate to the residents.

The housekeeping staff should also be asked to note and communicate to the management any change in the health of the residents they visit each week. Often this obligation can test the employees' loyalties, as residents may attempt to hide problems from their families or the management for fear of being asked to transfer out of their apartment to a higher level of care. This phenomenon is common in communities with independent apartments, assisted living facilities, and even life-care communities, where a resident's greatest fear is placement in a nursing home. The housekeeping staff must understand the importance of early detection and reporting of a change in health. It is in the resident's best interest to receive the treatment he needs if his health deteriorates. This proactive approach usually leads to more comfort and independence for the resident, not less.

Any change in a resident's health should be reported to the housekeeping supervisor, who should inform the appropriate management staff. In extreme cases,

Exhibit 11.1   Sample Infection Prevention and Control Plan

IPCP Task

Determine incident management activation/configuration based upon local impact as well as incident action plan cycle and development process.

Determine methods for resident/family information provisions. Designate a point of contact for family/resident information or questions.

Identify subject matter experts (SMEs) and information sources to determine extent and spread of contagion and risk profiles. (CDC and public health websites as well as medical director.)

Determine staff communication mechanisms and information management process.

Determine strategies to maintain services for at-risk residents during outbreak period unrelated to contagion. Hospice, PT, HH, medical director, care conferences may access residents electronically with voice or video conferencing.

Determine likely resource shortages and identify relevant vendor, cache, and options for managing shortages. Allocate secure storage for sanitized products. Contact vendor to determine their emergency plans for inventory acquisition, substitutes, and delivery.

Pharmacy services: Follow federal guidelines for notifying the community regarding nonavailability. If medication is unavailable, staff to contact resident's personal care physician (PCP) for alternate.

Food services: Food labeled for will-call at distribution center or dropped outside kitchen with notice. Stockpile heat-and-serve emergency entrées in freezer. Order take-out boxes for employee take-home meals.

Food rotation: Perishable first, freezer second, canned/boxed third.

Maintenance/housekeeping: Over-order toilet paper, paper towels, cleaning supplies, laundry products, bleach for disinfecting. Recommend purchasing three-month supplies of each.

Nursing: Over-order gloves, face masks (N95), isolation gowns, face shields, hand sanitizers with refills, and incontinence products. Masks can be used routinely by staff and reused unless soiled or contaminated. Gloves must be changed between residents. For any quarantined, or contagion positive resident, staff-to-resident contact will require a gown and full PPE and will be disposed of after each use.

Develop service restriction plans in case of staff shortages or increased demand (e.g., physical therapy, hospice, home health, activities, offsite appointments, and van transportation).

Evaluate plan for providing just-in-time staff education via electronic and other non-classroom means, including information about contagion, transmission, infection prevention measures, usual clinical symptoms and course, risk factors, and complications.

Update communicable disease policy and procedures to include the potential for triage decision-making (who, process, communication, considerations) and staff management (how staff expertise will be maximally utilized versus adding additional training for some staff).

Develop indicators and possible triggers for implementing alternate care sites in conjunction with public health and emergency management, including what support may be required from the health care system and it's availability to your residents.

Develop a plan for implementing facility security/controlled access plan (which may be phased) particularly during peak outbreak weeks to assure controlled facility ingress and egress and monitoring.

Provide residents and staff with information about stress responses, resilience, and available professional mental health resources. Develop monitoring for those exposed to high levels of cumulative stress or specific severe stressors (e.g., possible death of a resident or family member). Medical director and director of nursing to update families on resident conditions.

Consider ways to maintain staff resilience and morale when congregate gatherings and close physical contact are discouraged. This may need to include memorial service attendance for staff members

(continued)

Exhibit 11.1 Sample Infection Prevention and Control Plan *(continued)*

for a deceased resident. Employee appreciation demonstrated by appreciating and encouraging staff every day; providing delivered meals and treats. Keeping employees informed of updates regarding the contagion risks and spread.

Provide daily reminders for all staff regarding isolating themselves while at home to keep their families and the residents safe. Provide a daily meal at work and take-home meals to limit their need to go out into the community to secure food. Temperature screen and log temps upon entering building to report for their shift. Masks and gloves to be worn all day.

If there is an active contagious presence in the community or in the event of a contagion related death in the community, and any resident goes out of the building to an off-site appointment, the destination site staff must be made aware of the presence.

Define the differences between isolation and quarantine and how this will impact visitors. Determine how visitors will be informed and provide alternate methods for families and visitors to communicate with their loved ones (phone, webcam, FaceTime, Zoom, etc.). Isolation = Separation from others of people currently ill to prevent exposure to an infectious disease. Quarantine = Separation of people who have been exposed and have higher risk of developing disease.

Anticipate the possibility of public health officials closing schools and what impact this will have on staff scheduling. Source childcare resources and consider sheltering staff children within the facility during staff shifts. Evaluate the possibility of hiring and orienting employee applicants without family obligations and hiring on a per diem basis. Staff members who bring children into the building will remain in vacant apartments or secured area with a babysitter. Meals and limited entertainment will be provided.

Develop resources and supplies to establish rooms for quarantine stays similar to respite and guest suites.

Develop procedures for notifying the state agency for health care administration of licensed bed availability/capacity change as a result of conta-

gious disease outbreaks. All communication and updates should also be reported through the State Regulatory agencies.

Develop a plan for reporting resident/staff who are symptomatic to public health officials, physicians, and the hospital. Designate a point of contact for health officials. Physicians are mandated reporters of these diseases to public health officials; coordinate with them and/or community medical advisor. Any staff who has been without symptoms for 3 days without medication **AND** has been out for 10 days without symptoms may be able to return to work—in accordance with CDC guidelines.

Acquire test kits for contagion and training on their use in the event the pandemic reaches the community.

Develop infection control/isolation plan for ill suspect or confirmed cases. Isolation plans should be documented and submitted to the state or county health officials.

Emphasize hand and respiratory hygiene and other infection prevention techniques through education, policies, signage, and easy availability of supplies. Require all staff to view YouTube infection control video, https://www.youtube.com/watch?v=t_KT6dPIMwI.

New move-ins: Determine with medical director and/or nursing director changes in thresholds for admittance of community residents directly into the facility. Screening all new admissions or readmissions for signs/symptoms of current contagion and known exposure to anyone with symptoms over the past 14 days. Also requiring a note from the referring/discharging physician that to his/her knowledge the patient has not displayed these symptoms and had these exposure risks. Conduct extensive screening on potential new residents; if they or their loved ones have traveled recently or show symptoms, quarantine them for 7 days before moving them in, and isolate them for 7 days after moving in.

Restricting move-ins: Restrict new admissions to your communities temporarily yet remain available as a resource to public health officials. This is done to prevent any possible contamination from entering the community that may originate from an environment without the protections that this plan has implemented.

Readmittance from hospital: Isolate patients transferred back from the hospital. A safe assumption at this point is that anyone entering the emergency department is exposed to the contagion. Quarantine those returning from the hospital 14 days, plus negative test result.

Resident isolation: Isolate residents in apartments with delivered meals in disposable products and discontinue communal dining when recommended by health officials. Restructure activities to engage residents while in isolation. All active staff wear gloves and masks at all times.

Process for screening patients who need further assessment. Any patient of concern should be discussed with the medical director, director of nursing or the residents' PCP.

Evaluate potential staffing and responsibility changes and how less-trained staff and families could contribute to operations. Develop a process for rapid credentialing and training of non-facility supplemental health care staff. Work with a staffing agency who already has screened employees (criminal, references, etc.).

Develop cleaning plan and disinfecting strategies and frequencies in accordance with CDC guidelines. Utilize only EPA registered cleaning agents.

Create a tracking spreadsheet (confidential lists) of the residents and employees with disease symptoms, which is maintained and used to track and monitor the course of the disease and the outcome of the individual. These lists are not to be shared with anyone, except for the department of health and the wellness team to maintain infectious disease records confidentially.

All door handles, keypads, and wheelchair accessible pads wiped down with (EPA registration number 777-66) Lysol All Purpose Cleaner. All visitors sign in and then utilize sanitation station prior to entering resident areas. Cleaning checklist task sheet implemented. See https://www.epa.gov/pesticide-registration/list-n-disinfectants-use-against-sars-cov-2.

Ask all staff and visitors if they (personally) or anybody they have come into contact with have had any symptoms within past 14 days. All persons requesting entry to the community must sign a form attesting to this: Symptoms personally or symptoms on anyone else they have been in contact with. Common symptoms include: fever, cough, shortness of breath, body aches, temperature greater than 100.4. Maintain all records.

All people entering the building will be screened with an infrared digital or forehead thermometer. Temperature logs to be kept. Any results that exceed 100.4 will not be allowed to enter resident areas. Only one visitor per day; all visitors must be adults. Items for residents may be dropped off. The doors are to be locked when not attended by a concierge. Maintain all records.

As part of our assessment process, all move-ins need to be screened for flu symptoms. If they have symptoms, then wait 14 days to move in. All move-ins must be approved by the medical director. All furniture for residents moving in/out will be handled by facility personnel and staged in the parking area.

All vendors and contractors must show their own communicable disease response plan or be prohibited from entry.

All nonessential vendors and contractors prohibited entry.

All events and activities that include outside entertainers/presenters and family groups (such as happy hour, communion) may be canceled or held virtually.

All family care conferences and collaborative care dashboard updates will be accomplished remotely by phone, webcam, Skype, Zoom, or FaceTime. All morning stand-up meetings with staff conducted via conference line.

All nonessential visitors are restricted from entering the facility. Any hospice visits by nursing personnel

(continued)

Exhibit 11.1 Sample Infection Prevention and Control Plan *(continued)*

will be encased in full isolation PPE and only admitted every 14 days as required to maintain eligibility. Letter sent to families and vendors from the medical director justifying this measure.

Establish viewing windows for residents to see families and talk to them by phone. Communities equipped with iPads for families to connect to residents via Facetime.

The Centers for Medicare & Medicaid Services (CMS) may waive hospice regulations, including temporarily removing the requirement that a nurse conduct a home visit at least every two weeks and expanding the allowable use of telehealth.

Create a system for evaluating this planning process and scoring its effectiveness for pandemic response planning.

---

residents have been known to tip their housekeeper to keep their secrets. Periodic inspections of housekeepers' work in the residents' apartments by the supervisor (at least quarterly) can help discourage this practice.

Most companies strictly prohibit the acceptance of tips by employees; violations can lead to disciplinary measures, including termination. When approached with a tip, employees should thank the resident for the gesture and remind the resident of the company's tipping policy. The employee might suggest that any contributions be made to the employee appreciation fund, so they can be shared by all the employees who work to ensure the resident's comfort and well-being.

(See chapter 6 for more discussion of establishing an employee appreciation fund.)

■ CLEANING RESIDENTS' UNITS

When a resident moves in, the housekeeping supervisor should meet with her to discuss the housekeeping service. The resident handbook, sales information, and other communications should spell out clearly the extent and limits of the service: residents should be advised to expect *light* housekeeping. They should also be told that the housekeepers are not on a specific time schedule, but rather are expected to perform a specific set of tasks in a number of apartments each day. New residents should be advised that apartments in their wing will be cleaned at set times, for example, on Thursdays between the hours of 8:00 a.m. and 12:00 p.m. or from 12:30 to 3:30 p.m., depending on the apartment's location on the hallway, and that the management prefers that the resident be there when the apartment is cleaned (or sign a waiver to permit access

to the apartment if the resident is absent), to protect residents and employees from the threat of theft. A routine will quickly develop so that the resident knows when to expect the housekeeper. Residents should also be asked to identify any valuable or breakable items

Exhibit 11.2	**Infection Control Daily Cleaning Schedule**
Task/Location	Responsible
Door handles (inside and out)	Housekeeping
Door handles (inside and out)	Caregivers
Flat furniture surfaces (tables, etc.)	Caregivers
Med carts and laptops	Nurse
Windowsills and other ledges	Caregivers
Light switches	Caregivers
Keypads on doors	Caregivers
Lamps, vases, decorative boxes	Caregivers
Remote controls	Caregivers
Piano and keys	Activities
Popcorn machine (outside)	Activities
Wooden chair arms (common areas)	Caregivers
Dining room tables and chairs and surfaces	Dining staff
Offices, computers, and phones	Managers
Activity storage offices	Activities
Activity supplies	After each use
Door handles (inside and out)	Housekeeping

that should not be cleaned, clearly informed that the management is not responsible for damage to or loss of valuables, and advised to obtain renter's insurance and any other coverage they deem appropriate for their possessions.

The Centers for Disease Control and Prevention (CDC) has released guidelines for disinfectant use in senior communities using products such as Lysol (EPA Registration number 675-55) combined with stare regulators who have suggested frequency (see exhibit 11.2).[1] Additional cleaning services may be offered to specific residents depending upon their isolation status; the resident should be advised of the type of services they can expect.

The frequency of housekeeping visits to residents' apartments largely depends on the level of care and diagnosis of the occupants: housekeeping needs increase with the level of care and communicable diagnosis. Independent living residents may require a visit every week or two. Assisted living residents may require a visit once or twice per week, and skilled nursing residents daily. Residents in isolation may require sanitation services several times each day. From a scheduling standpoint, it becomes important to preserve a distinction between independent living and assisted living residents as much as possible to promote the most efficient use of the staff. The cleaning schedule should include all nonresident apartments, including vacant units, guest apartments, and model units. The last thing the management needs is for a sales representative to show a vacant apartment to a prospect, only to find a big bug on the carpet.

Most independent residents do not require weekly housekeeping visits unless the competition for residents in the area dictates it. Bimonthly visits are more efficient and cost-effective. In most communities, in one shift a housekeeper should be able to clean seven or eight apartments (or nine or ten assisted living rooms) and vacuum hallway carpets, empty trash rooms, and coordinate linen replacement. Therefore, a 200-unit community should require 28.5 employee-days per week, or 114 employee-days per month, to clean all apartments weekly (including nonresident apartments such as guest and model rooms). The same 200-unit community cleaned bimonthly at five apartments per day (allowing 1.5 hours per apartment) plus the extras will require only 20 employee-days per week, or 80 per month.

Scaling back from weekly to bimonthly service is not easy in an established community, but one way to do it is to present the change as an alternative to increasing monthly fees. Options such as this have received widespread support among residents, especially those on fixed incomes. Some communities that have converted to bimonthly housekeeping offer it as an option at lease renewal. Obviously, communities that can offer the bimonthly arrangement from the start are at a distinct operational advantage.

Each community should establish cleaning specifications for resident apartments, guest rooms, and common areas along with the frequency of cleaning, estimated time for completion, and cost. At the end of each shift, the housekeepers should quickly walk the entire building with a damp rag and trash bag to ensure that the property looks fresh.

All staff members should be instructed to be especially considerate of residents. They should always knock before entering an apartment and greet residents as they are invited inside. This is particularly appropriate in a health care setting or a skilled nursing facility. Both in the apartment and in the common areas, staff members should watch their equipment and electric cords and courteously ask residents to move if they are in the way or at risk. The staff should be instructed on how to assist residents to move, including the body mechanics of lifting a resident if necessary. When floors are wet, appropriate warning signs should be posted. The staff should always be friendly and patient with residents and be reminded that ultimately they are employed by them.

The housekeepers should be instructed to follow a weekly checklist for each apartment and the adjacent public areas for which they are responsible (see exhibit 11.3). They should not touch or move breakable personal items. In addition, housekeepers should not move heavy pieces of furniture or turn mattresses. The housekeepers should supply all cleaning materials unless the resident wishes to supply special cleaning materials.

Residents often request spur-of-the-moment maintenance and housekeeping "favors" of staff members, who may find it easier to accommodate them than to argue over a chargeable service. The only way to manage this problem is to offer the residents service on a fee basis (often charged in 15-minute increments) and

Exhibit 11.3   Housekeeping Checklist: Weekly or Bimonthly

Kitchen

___ Clean refrigerator: handle, door, top

___ Clean backsplash, countertops, cabinets

___ Clean window and windowsill

___ Clean dishwasher door

___ Clean stovetop, range, and hood

___ Clean sink (do not wash dirty dishes)

___ Clean garbage disposal guard

___ Sweep, damp-mop floor

___ Remove trash

Living Room

___ Dust furniture and pictures

___ Clean windows, tracks, sills, and screens

___ Vacuum and spot-clean carpet

Bedrooms

___ Dust furniture and pictures

___ Vacuum and spot-clean carpet

___ Clean windows

___ Remove trash

___ Clean louvered doors

___ Change bed and ticket laundry

Bathrooms

___ Clean sink and counter

___ Scrub toilet

___ Clean tub or shower, including door tracks

___ Polish mirror

___ Polish all chrome fixtures

___ Remove trash

___ Clean louvered door

Public Areas

___ Clean elevator floors, walls, and ashtray

___ Clean fire extinguisher, inside box, and door

___ Clean hallway light fixtures and exit signs

___ Clean doorbell, door frame, and entry shelf

___ Vacuum hallway carpet

___ Clean handrails

___ Clean stairwells

___ Clean trash rooms

___ Clean housekeeper storage rooms and carts

___ Clean resident storage rooms

Porch

___ Clean porch furniture

___ Remove mildew

___ Vacuum away cobwebs

___ Vacuum carpet

___ Wipe down porch rails

Laundry Rooms

___ Damp-wipe washer

___ Damp-wipe dryer and clean lint trap

___ Clean floor

___ Clean louvered doors

Housekeeper: _____

Apartment: _____

Date: _____

Checked by: _____

provide incentives to housekeepers and maintenance employees to share in ancillary revenue generated (or else to schedule the employees so tightly that little time is available for such favors). For a special task, the resident should fill out a work-order request at the concierge desk. The housekeeping department can then contact the resident and arrange a time to perform the service.

It is the responsibility of the housekeeping supervisor to organize the staff for the most efficient operation. All housekeeping carts should have a list of supplies and be properly stocked at the beginning of each shift. Because most housekeepers have individual preferences for organizing their equipment and can become somewhat territorial, a cart should be assigned to each person. Lightweight Rubbermaid or other nonmetallic carts offer easy cleaning, mobility, and durability and usually fit easily into the housekeeping closet or storage areas.[2] Metal carts are heavy, tend to leave marks on hallway walls, can rust through, and are not easy to restore after they become worn. All mops, brooms, and ladders should be fitted with rubber caps on the handles to keep them from leaving marks on the walls.

SCHEDULING

The most efficient method of scheduling room cleaning is usually by floor. In this way, the housekeeper can vacuum the hallway carpet and clean fixtures and handrails as she or he moves from room to room. Housekeeping schedules often become disorganized in multilevel communities during fill-up, when occupants are scattered all over the building. It is critical to set a procedure early to maximize productivity. If housekeepers are moving randomly throughout the building, they may be able to clean only five or six apartments during a shift.

The housekeeping supervisor should assign each staff member a number of apartments and common areas to clean daily. A master housekeeping schedule should be posted at least a week in advance. This lets all staff members know how the workload is distributed, and arrangements can be made to cover for absences. The supervisor should keep a few on-call part-time employees on the payroll to cover vacations, sick days, and other unexpected staff shortages. This practice can save the department costly overtime and the use of expensive temporary agencies. Many communities also cross-train concierge, dining room, personal care, or transportation staff members to cover for staff shortages in different departments. It is important to charge their time to the appropriate department's budget. The cross-trained worker should be paid the same rate in each department.

It is a good idea to schedule one housekeeper Tuesday through Saturday, and one Sunday through Thursday so that a housekeeper is on the premises all weekend to handle any housekeeping emergencies. This is particularly important in communities that offer assisted living or higher levels of care.

SECURITY

Residents should be encouraged to secure their valuables during visits by employees or outside vendors and guests. As chapter 3 advises, new hires, particularly those who have access to the residents' apartments or provide direct resident care, should undergo a background check. This precaution is no guarantee against theft, however: it is often the long-term employee who learns the ways of the residents and how to take advantage of them.

Any missing item reported by a resident or family member should be investigated immediately by two or more community management staff and documented. If the loss is large, the management may recommend that the resident or family contact the local police with as much discretion as possible. Some effort should be made to determine whether the item has really been stolen or simply misplaced: it is human nature to misplace things as we grow older, especially for residents with dementia, and if this sort of disappearance is assumed to be theft, the rumor may spread, a wave of similar complaints may be lodged, and the community's reputation may be put at risk. The management should never reimburse a resident for lost or stolen articles, for this can set a precedent that is not easily reversed. Residents should, however, be reasonably reimbursed for any damages they sustain as a result of the community's negligence. All such matters should be fully investigated according to community policy and turned over to the local police and the resident's insurance agency. The community should also establish and follow clear key-control policies when issuing apartment keys to housekeepers. (See chapter 13 for more on key control.)

Many operators rotate housekeepers to prevent abuse of the housekeepers' time as bonds develop with residents and to alleviate boredom among the staff. Rotation has a number of advantages. It breaks the monotony of cleaning the same apartments month after month and may also improve performance: a housekeeper who cleans the same places repeatedly can overlook things that a new set of eyes may catch. In addition, rotation diminishes the possibility of residents forming such strong ties with staff that they suffer separation anxiety when a favored employee leaves the community permanently. It makes the employee turnover rate less apparent to residents. It also discourages favoritism on the part of both the resident and the housekeeper. Relationships are more likely to stay on a business level, and tipping, moonlighting, gossip, and cliques are discouraged.

Rotation has some drawbacks, however: residents are generally more satisfied if they have the same, familiar housekeeper each week. As people age, they feel more vulnerable and may distrust a new housekeeper. As a result, if valuables go missing, it may be difficult for the management to reassure the resident or identify the staff who might be involved. In addition, regardless of what may be on the task list, many residents are particular about how they like things to be cleaned, and it can take a new housekeeper weeks to learn these nuances.

COMMON AREAS

The management should develop a master housekeeping plan for cleaning all areas in both the front and the back of the house. The plan should specifically address how each room, furnishing, and fixture should be cleaned, how often, and which cleaning agents should be used. It is up to the housekeeping supervisor to take the guesswork out of the job and define specific expectations for the staff. Each cleaning activity should be identified and a study conducted to determine a reasonable time allotment for each job. Developing such a plan helps clarify the expectations of the management and employees alike. The management generally gains a greater appreciation of how much work it takes to clean a facility and can judge the needed time and resources more realistically. Employees better understand what the management expects of them and can negotiate any expectations that are perceived as unrealistic.

The housekeeping needs of a community change as the building fills. As the first residents move into the building, a variety of tradespeople attend to last-minute details. These workers often leave large, conspicuous messes that the housekeeping staff is expected to clean up. Many operators underestimate the amount of staff time needed to keep the property looking sharp during this critical time. They wrongly assume that without residents, only a skeleton housekeeping crew is required. In addition, all resident apartments need to be cleaned before they can be shown or occupied. Typically, the carpet installers are the last contractors to visit an apartment, and they rarely leave it in move-in

condition. During periods of heavy move-in activity, hallway carpets and corridors need more than weekly attention, as do elevator cars and back-of-the-house areas. Finally, as the project reaches full occupancy, the entire community needs to be inspected daily to keep it looking fresh. All staff members should be reminded of their responsibility to help keep the property looking its best and encouraged to take pride in the community.

Some areas—such as the dining room, kitchen, maintenance areas, and other back-of-the-house locations—may be cleaned by employees other than housekeepers. For example, the lobby may be the responsibility of the lobby attendant, the kitchen and back-of-house areas are usually cleaned by the utility staff from the kitchen, and the dining room may be cleaned by the servers. (See chapter 9 for detailed food-safety practices.)

CLEANING PROCEDURES

All housekeeping tasks must be performed in accordance with proper sanitary practices. These practices are defined differently in every community, according to the housekeeping supervisor's background and biases. In a senior community, more stringent standards of hygiene may be necessary to protect residents in frail health. The apartments and food service areas in particular must be kept clean and as free as possible of germs and other contaminating agents at all times, not just during the weekly visit. Staff should be trained in appropriate methods for cleaning, disinfecting, and sterilizing all areas, surfaces, and equipment as needed. In addition, regulatory standards may mandate special procedures and rules for the cleaning of apartments whose residents have contagious diseases, to prevent them from spreading to other residents.

The following definitions are usually applied in a health care setting, but they also apply to senior communities:

■ *Clean:* To remove dirt, impurities, or extraneous matter from a surface. *Examples:* Sweeping, mopping floors, damp-wiping, vacuuming, laundry. *Amount of bacteria removed:* Moderate.
■ *Sanitize:* To clean thoroughly enough to promote healthful surroundings. *Examples:* All of the above cleaning examples. Germicide may or may not be

used. *Amount of bacteria removed:* Moderate, depending on the cleaning agent and the thoroughness of cleaning.

■ *Disinfect:* To kill or inhibit the growth of disease-causing bacteria by cleaning thoroughly and then treating with a germicide. *Examples:* All cleaning tasks using water and detergent germicide, disinfectant spray, or boiling water. *Amount of bacteria removed:* Significant, depending on the strength of the germicide (disinfectant) used and thoroughness of cleaning.

■ *Sterilize:* To kill all living organisms on an item or surface by using intense heat or steam under pressure. *Examples:* Autoclaving, bedpan sterilization, dry heat sterilization. *Amount of bacteria removed:* All.

In health care facilities, a detergent or detergent-germicide combination cleaning product should be used in every cleaning-water solution. Although this is not usually required for residents' apartments, it is a good practice to establish. Disinfectant sprays should be used on all surfaces that cannot be cleaned with water and detergent germicide, such as cloth, upholstered furnishings, and mattresses.

Tile floors should be cleaned by first vacuuming or sweeping thoroughly, paying close attention to corners and areas near or under furniture, then mopping with water and added detergent germicide, and posting warning "Wet Floor" signs at both ends of the wet area. The same methods are employed when using a floor-cleaning machine; the staff should follow all directions posted on the machine. Following cleaning, a thin coat of floor wax can be applied. Only nonskid waxes should be used. Again "Wet Floor" warning signs should be posted until the floor dries. Wax should be stripped from the floors approximately every six months, following the manufacturer's recommendations.

The community should be equipped with a carpet shampooer. Before cleaning carpets, housekeepers should remove all furniture and vacuum the carpet thoroughly. Operators should fill the machine with the amount of water specified by the manufacturer and a carpet-cleaning product that contains some sort of detergent germicide. Dirty areas should be spot-cleaned first, and care should be taken not to saturate the carpet. Shampooing of common areas should be done during the evening, when most residents are in their apartments, to minimize slipping and tripping hazards and to allow the carpet to dry without tracking wetness to other areas. The staff must never vacuum wet carpets with a standard vacuum, or they may be electrocuted. Water leaks and overflow problems can be handled safely with a wet/dry or shop vacuum. Dry-cleaning systems can also be effective to spot-clean heavy-traffic areas during normal business hours. Staff should never use a bleach solution on baseboards above carpeted areas, as it may permanently remove carpet color pigments. Precleaners or spot removers are effective for cleaning heavily soiled small areas.

For windows and glass, the housekeeper can use a solution of water and nondetergent cleaning ammonia. Caution should be exercised because some ammoniated products are irritating to those with upper respiratory conditions; in such cases, an alcohol-based window cleaner can be substituted. The windows should be washed, rinsed, and dried thoroughly. Detergents or soap solutions not intended for windows or glass leave a residue. Squeegees and ammonia products should never be used on windows with tinted film.

For damp-wiping, a solution of detergent germicide in water should be used, following the instructions on the container. The staff should be instructed to dip the cleaning cloth in the solution and squeeze it out thoroughly to avoid dripping on and damaging adjacent woodwork or upholstery. They should pay particular attention to corners, ridges, and hard-to-reach areas by cleaning them first. The solution should be changed frequently. A small amount of concentrate and a measuring cup should be kept on each housekeeping cart to allow the housekeepers to refresh the solution without making return trips to the supply areas.

Public and private restrooms usually pose the greatest risk for the spread of bacteria. Extra attention is necessary to ensure proper disinfection of these areas. All surfaces should be cleaned thoroughly, especially the toilets and urinals, paying close attention to the sides and back and under the rim. All rust and stains should be removed, and all surfaces should be dried and the chrome polished. All other areas should be damp-mopped, and all dispensers refilled. In public washrooms, sealed soap dispensers are the most sanitary and economical to maintain. A cup dispenser is a convenience for residents who may need a drink with their medications, and a box of tissues can be helpful, as long as residents are not inclined to walk off with them.

Most common-area washrooms have floor drains to protect the outside areas from flooding in the event of a plumbing problem. Like all drains, they have a P-trap beneath the drain cover, which, when filled with water, creates a barrier to prevent sewer gases and insects from entering the bathroom from the drain. Over time, especially in dry climates, the water barrier in the P-trap can evaporate; bugs in the bathroom or a sewer smell are a sure signs that this has happened. The problem is easily resolved by pouring a cup of bleach solution down each floor drain. This practice may be used regularly as a preventive measure.

Usually the servers are responsible for cleaning the dining room, with the exception of polishing glass and mirrors and shampooing the carpets. The dining room should be vacuumed after every meal. Debris from chairs, tables, and table bases should be removed first. All tables should be washed and dried; all chairs should be damp-wiped and scuff marks removed from the legs. When vacuuming the dining room, the housekeeper should move all chairs each time and tables at least weekly to remove crumbs and other food debris. Failure to do so will result in insects in the dining room. If a problem already exists, a treatment of boric acid is effective. Boric acid is a nontoxic, odorless powder that is harmless to humans. It is usually applied to the floors and baseboards, using a bulb applicator, in the evening, and vacuumed up in the morning.

The kitchen area is generally cleaned by the kitchen utility staff; a deep cleaning of all equipment, walls, food storage areas, and floors should be performed at least quarterly with the help of the housekeeping staff. Kitchen cleaning parties (KP parties) can usually be coordinated after the evening meal; task lists for each worker should be prepared in advance. Many staff members will enjoy the extra hours, and the job will not seem too bad when 10 or 12 people pitch in to get it done. A pizza break can provide a morale and energy boost. During the takeover of acquired properties, we have conducted such parties to bring the new project up to our standards.

They are useful in communicating the management's expectations of sanitary standards to the employees, and they also help build camaraderie and weed out those employees who may not be committed to the community or the job. At the end of two or three nights of cleaning until the wee hours, you are left with an immaculate kitchen and a proud staff with a sense of accomplishment and the commitment necessary to keep it that way.

The housekeeping supervisor should attend all meetings of the infection-control committee, if the community has one. All housekeepers should be trained in proper methods for controlling infectious waste, including the disposal of such waste and appropriate cleaning methods. Soiled adult diaper waste should be disposed of after each changing using rubber gloves and double-bagged to contain any odors. Contaminated waste should be disposed of according to the procedures dictated by the county health department or by a licensed contractor.

■ TRAINING

Orientation to the specific job duties is critical to avoid communication problems and personal injury and to establish expectations for the job. Whenever possible, new employees should be paired with a senior housekeeper for at least one day to ensure that procedures, resident relations matters, and standards of cleanliness are thoroughly communicated and understood. In addition, the housekeeping supervisor should develop a departmental orientation checklist to ensure that all aspects of the operation are addressed.

It is not enough simply to review a job description and have the new employee sign it as understood. There is no substitute for one-on-one time with a new employee or an employee with a performance problem to set him or her on the right foot. Most people want to do a good job but may be uncertain of what a good job looks like. A thorough orientation and training program help clarify the supervisor's expectations and equip the staff member to deliver. If the supervisor is unclear about his or her own expectations, the executive director should review the orientation and training plan.

A well-conceived training plan should include an introduction to cleaning and safety procedures and instruction on specific tasks, relationships with other departments, sanitation and infection control, security, uniforms or dress codes, handling equipment and chemicals, location and use of supplies, and, most important, communication with residents.

Long-term, experienced housekeepers can benefit from a refresher course. The National Executive Housekeepers Association (NEHA) is a national organization of professional housekeepers that provides leadership and education and does research in the housekeeping field. It has a certification program and certifies professionals who meet all the educational requirements as registered executive housekeepers (REH).[3]

Other topics that should be routinely covered during in-service training include Occupational Safety and Health Administration (OSHA) rules and guidelines, safety, new equipment and methods for cleaning, understanding the aging process, recognizing health problems in residents, motivation, and the importance of communication with fellow staff members and supervisors. Because most laundry operations fall under the supervision of the housekeeping department, supervisors may want to include laundry employees in their training plans and staff meetings.

PURCHASING

Supplies, service contracts, and equipment expenditures usually make up about 10 percent of the housekeeping department's operations budget. For most communities, this combined cost should not exceed $10 to $12 per month per apartment cleaned. Service contracts should be kept to a minimum because of the staffing overhead already in place. When they are used, the executive director and housekeeping supervisor should keep copies of all contracts. All cleaning contractors should provide the facility with a copy of their certificate of insurance naming the facility as an additional insured. There should be at least two competitive bids on file, and all contracts should terminate annually to ensure competitiveness.

The housekeeping supervisor should maintain a current ledger of all vendor accounts organized by service function. The ledger should include account and pricing information with cut sheets of frequently ordered or inventoried supplies. All vendor supply accounts should be put out to bid at least annually. Although some account service representatives may

be friendlier or more attentive than others, the determining factor should be the price per unit. Proper planning and monthly inventory enable the supervisor to take advantage of bulk purchasing and the monthly special discounts offered by most vendors.

Premixed solutions (especially aerosols) may seem like a time saver for the staff, but they may not be an economy. Modern dispensers make it safe and efficient to mix chemicals properly. Some mixing can even be done automatically, but automatic mixing systems usually do not save enough time to justify the additional cost. The supervisor should consider the cost per gallon, per use, or per application when evaluating alternative chemicals. Vendors' offers of "free" automated mixing equipment should be evaluated critically; their cost is typically buried in the price of the chemicals or recovered through liberal mix settings.

The housekeeping supervisor should review and inventory all deliveries and check every purchase order against the packing slip and invoice. Supplies should be kept in a secure location. Each housekeeper should sign out all supplies from inventory as they are used, for control and to facilitate reordering. At least monthly, the housekeeping supervisor should perform an inventory of all supplies and send a copy to the executive director. Both managers should formally agree on the appropriate amount of inventory for the community's size and historical consumption. The value of this inventory should not exceed 10 percent of the annual supply budget unless the supervisor and the executive director wish to avail themselves of bulk purchasing discounts.

All housekeeping and laundry equipment should undergo routine maintenance. Much of this maintenance (e.g., cleaning and adjusting) can be performed by the housekeepers, leaving major maintenance and repairs to the community maintenance department. A small supply of cords, belts, brushes, and other frequently replaced parts should be kept on hand. The housekeeping supervisor can be trained to make simple repairs to equipment that will keep the department running without enlisting the services of the maintenance department.

The housekeeping supervisor should keep all equipment manuals, receipts, and warranty information together on file. All community tools and equipment should be inventoried by purchase date, purchase location, model number, and serial number and marked with the community's identification. Not only does this practice enable the supervisor to keep track of all equipment, it also provides useful information regarding the longevity and durability of equipment in use.

■■■■■■ SAFETY

All housekeeping staff members should be trained in the correct and safe procedures for using each cleaning product, device, or appliance. Some common precautions follow.

Check all cleaning machines daily to make sure they are clean, operating correctly, and free of defects such as broken locks, switches, cords, and plugs. Never operate power equipment with wet hands. Keep cords out of the path of travel of residents and other staff members. Always plug cords into the nearest outlet available, with a minimal use of extension cords. Never leave equipment unattended in a resident's apartment or a corridor.

Use scoops, measuring cups, or other containers to dispense soaps, detergents, bleaches, acids, or other cleaning solutions. *Never* use your hands. Measure and pour accurately according to the directions on the package or dispenser. Ensure that there is adequate ventilation when mixing or using cleaning chemicals. Never smoke or light a flame near these chemicals, because many are flammable.

Never pick up broken glass, china, or enamelware with your bare hands. Know the correct and safe way to empty trash receptacles, bags, or bins. Never dig into any trash container with your hands.

Many communities have significantly reduced the incidence of lower-back injury by issuing back support belts to housekeeping and maintenance personnel. These devices are lightweight and, when used properly, encourage proper body mechanics. Additional training can be provided to improve employee awareness regarding proper lifting techniques and promote awareness of the potential for back injury.

Regular safety classes or the development of a safety committee for the community can help identify vulnerabilities and implement precautions. OSHA rules are specific about the creation and maintenance of a safe work environment and should be posted and reviewed with the staff routinely. Postings in other languages should be obtained as needed for employees who are not proficient in English. In addition, emergency procedures should be posted in areas where chemicals are stored and mixed, and these areas must be equipped with eyewash stations.

All chemicals should be properly stored and labeled, and the staff must be fully trained in safe handling practices. An inventory of and emergency procedures for each chemical should be kept on file and accessible. Material safety data sheets (MSDS) must be on file for every product used, including products that have been discontinued. These sheets should be kept on file and accessible indefinitely.

Housekeepers who work with contaminated wastes that could host blood-borne pathogens should be encouraged to consider hepatitis B vaccinations for their own protection. Federal regulations governing OSHA encompass the management of employee exposure to blood-borne pathogens (Title 29 CFR 1910.1030). Compliance is mandatory for all those whose work involves potential exposure to blood or other infectious material. In senior housing, those positions could include housekeepers, laundry workers, nursing assistants, and other health care workers. The regulations place on the employer the responsibility for the following:

■ Developing an exposure control plan
■ Offering hepatitis B vaccine to employees at risk for occupational exposure
■ Record keeping and reporting of exposure incidents
■ Staff training[4]

All employees who could be exposed to blood or other infectious material should be trained in *universal precautions*:

■ Wash hands with soap and water or other antivirus or microbial cleaner before and after contact with any resident in the provision of patient care.
■ Under circumstances in which differentiation between body fluids is difficult or impossible, all body fluids shall be considered potentially infectious.
■ The anticipated contact with blood or other potentially infectious material requires the employee to wear protective gloves while engaged in this procedure.
■ Where it is not practical to anticipate contact with potentially infectious materials, protective gloves shall be worn.

All bins, pails, linen carts, or other types of receptacles intended for reuse should be inspected and decontaminated regularly, and immediately on the observation of visible contamination. Spills or splashes of blood or other potentially hazardous material should be cleaned up only by properly trained employees. Mopheads or reusable towels should be prepared for laundering immediately after the spill is cleaned and the area is decontaminated.

UNIFORMS

The use of uniforms for the housekeeping staff is at the discretion of the community's management. Although many communities feel the lack of uniforms creates a more friendly atmosphere, there are many good reasons for their use. First, uniforms allow the employees to look and feel more professional while relieving the supervisor of the need to monitor employee clothing for conformity with community dress codes. When employees are in uniform, they are also more easily recognizable by the residents and their families as employees, which alleviates possible anxiety about strangers. In addition, uniforms allow differentiation between community employees and private-duty aides or personal attendants. Finally, properly fitting uniforms can contribute to a safer working environment while allowing housekeepers freedom from worry about the effects of cleaning chemicals and crawling around on the floors on their personal clothes.

Uniforms should be made of material that can be easily cleaned by either the wearer or the community, preferably a polyester-cotton or wool blend that is wash-and-wear. Meta smocks can be ordered in many colors and are readily available from most uniform suppliers. All uniforms should be laundered and stored at the community. Do not allow employees to take uniforms home, as they will invariably be misplaced or forgotten.

Communities that require their employees to launder their own uniforms usually issue five sets so that a midweek wash is avoided. Communities that launder their own uniforms need to maintain only three sets for each employee.

NOTES

1. EPA, "About List N: Disinfectants for Coronavirus (COVID-19)," last updated May 24, 2022, https://www.epa.gov/coronavirus/about-list-n-disinfectants-coronavirus-covid-19-0.
2. Rubbermaid no. 6165 carts are large enough to use for laundry transport as well.
3. International Executive Housekeepers Association, PO Box 400, Westerville, OH 43086, 630-505-6771, https://www.ieha.org. Their trade publication is *Executive Housekeeping Today*.
4. Training materials are required, and videos with sample exposure-control plans are commercially available.

12

Laundry

The decision whether to set up a laundry operation within the community or to contract this service to an outside firm may be influenced by factors such as constraints of the water or sewer system, community water rationing (such as is common in California), shortage of space in the physical plant, and other mechanical barriers.

Commercial laundry services charge by the pound and will pick up and deliver. If the community contracts for laundry service, it should use the laundry company's linen as well. Contract services can be hard on linen because machine settings and chemicals may be designed to wash linen from a variety of sources, including nursing homes or hospitals, which have more stringent sanitary requirements. In addition, the residents' and the community's linen can become lost or mixed up with other customers' linen in a large commercial operation.

If dining room linen is sent out, all items should be inventoried as they leave and as they return. The contractor should be held accountable for any losses. When using an outside contractor, the community is not responsible for maintaining the linens, and typically the service company does not sort linens for quality or identify worn items for use as rags. This can be easily accomplished by the housekeeping supervisor when receiving the delivery. It is a good idea to assign the responsibility for dealing with the outside contractor to one department head, who can keep track of residential as well as dining room and other linen.

In many areas of the country, contract laundry services can be expensive because of a lack of competition in the business, the distance between the contractor's operations and the community, and the risk that the community's laundry will be priced at the nursing home or hospital rate. Typically, it is more economical to process laundry in-house. Many new communities plan for and construct laundry facilities, particularly if they intend to offer several levels of care, such as continuing care retirement communities. Phased communities, remodeled projects, and smaller communities may not have an on-site laundry.

A laundry operation, including the washers and dryers, an ironer, supplies, uniforms, tickets, mesh bags, and bins, can usually be set up from scratch to serve a 200-unit community for about $70,000, assuming that a suitable location and electrical service are available, and the facility does not require major reconstruction. (If a major plumbing or electrical modification is necessary, the costs can increase dramatically.) General operating supplies, soap and detergent, and repairs should cost about $6.00 to $8.00 per month per resident.

Usually, the higher the level of care provided at the community, the more intensive the laundry service needed. In skilled-nursing facilities, laundry service is governed by state and federal regulations.

For congregate or independent communities, however, many options exist. Services can include flat linens only, both sheets and towels using resident-provided or community-purchased linen, and even residents' personal laundry. There are advantages and disadvantages to each option.

SERVICES

Items that are usually serviced by the laundry department include:

- Residents' flat linens and towels
- Residents' personal laundry and coordination of dry cleaning (including pickup and delivery)
- Community and guest room linens, towels, and floor mats
- Kitchen rags and uniforms
- Housekeeping mopheads, rags, uniforms, throw rugs, and maintenance rags
- Dining room table linen, cloth napkins, chair cushions, and uniforms
- Other uniforms (the service can coordinate certain dry cleaning for employees)

The laundry department can also offer an alterations service and mend and hem clothing.

RESIDENTS' LINENS AND PERSONAL LAUNDRY

A community that accepts the responsibility for laundering residents' personal linen and clothing also accepts the problems associated with keeping it separated and stored, and the responsibility of washing it in accordance with the manufacturer's recommendations. Garments that are lost or damaged have a habit of immediately increasing in value! In addition, residents may misplace clothing, and employees may occasionally discard something that is soiled, for which the management will be held responsible. Some communities launder only flat sheets and pillowcases, while others also include towels and washcloths in the service package.

If the community intends to provide personal linen service, there are ways to minimize the risk. Computer software is available for counting, sorting, and inventorying, and this can cut down on paperwork and staff time. Residents' laundry can be collected by a member of the housekeeping or janitorial staff, who issues a laundry ticket in triplicate listing the items accepted. Whenever possible, the resident should complete the laundry slip and keep a copy. The other copies go with the dirty laundry, and one returns with the clean. Individuals' laundry can be placed in separate, washable mesh bags fitted with an identification tag that matches the laundry ticket. This way, several residents' laundry can be washed in the same load and be kept separate (although any potentially contaminated material should be washed in a separate load). All personal items should be marked with an indelible laundry marker. Some communities prefer to use apartment numbers rather than residents' names. Always use residents' names for residents with dementia, as some may remove articles of clothing from other residents' apartments. In dementia care units, a seasonal audit of each resident's closet and dresser is helpful in returning clothing to the proper owners.

Delicate items and those to be bleached should be placed in separate mesh bags and laundered on the appropriate wash cycle. Soiled laundry should be stored in covered containers for transport to the soiled-laundry storage area. Residents' soiled personal clothing should never be stored with the community's or service contractor's linen.

For heavily soiled laundry, any loose material can be disposed of in the resident's toilet and the laundry placed in a plastic bag to avoid cross-contamination. There are even plastic bags manufactured from a material that dissolves in hot water, so that the items do not have to be handled directly after being bagged. Laundry workers should wear latex or plastic gloves when handling laundry containing human waste. The laundry of residents who may have a contagious disease should be double-bagged. In skilled-nursing centers or assisted living special-care units with typically heavily soiled linen, the double-bag method helps contain odors. High water temperature is very important. Wash temperatures above 180°F kill most types of harmful bacteria and allow the fabrics to open up and expand for more efficient removal of soil. Cold water causes fabrics to contract, and soaps do not work as effectively in temperatures below 140°F. Families should avoid providing clothing for their loved ones that can be laundered only in cold water.

Housekeepers who clean the isolation rooms or handle contaminated linens should use the double-bag method. The double-bagged linens should be brought directly to the laundry room and not stored with other dirty linens. The laundry worker should avoid touching the contaminated linen and should wear plastic or latex gloves, a mask, and an apron. The laundry worker should open the outer "clean" bag, then pick up the inner soiled bag and shake its contents directly into the washer without touching the inside of the bag or the soiled linen. A germicide can be added to the load.

Mopheads, cleaning cloths, and other housekeeping service linens should be washed separately. Kitchen linen, towels, aprons, and cleaning cloths should be soaked in a degreasing presoak or detergent solution in the machine or sink for at least an hour to remove grease and stains before washing. Cloth hampers should be washed last, and cloth hampers that are from the isolation room or are otherwise contaminated should be washed separately.

The warm temperatures, high humidity, and limited ventilation typical of laundry areas are conducive to the growth of mildew, which is not easily removed from fabrics. To clean mildew from hard surfaces, use chlorine bleach to remove stains, then follow up with a disinfectant to kill the spores.

Laundry should be processed on the day it is collected. This is especially true of nursing home linen. The longer a stain sets, the harder it will be to remove. Pretreating can be effective. Treat stains as soon as possible and avoid allowing soiled items to come into contact with other soiled pieces to avoid transferring stains. The heat of the dryer can help set stains, so linens should be checked as they are removed from the washers and washed again if stains have not been removed, or they can be discarded. Perspiration stains can be removed with ammonia or alkaline products. Bleach does not remove perspiration stains and should *never* be mixed with ammonia, because this combination creates toxic vapors.

Laundry should be picked up during the weekly or bimonthly housekeeping visit and returned clean to the resident at the next visit. Offering same-day laundry service is not a practical option for senior communities. The laundry can be folded and stored in a clean area near residential apartments, where the housekeeper can pick it up at the beginning of each shift. Many communities have found that shrink-wrapping each order with the ticket on top keeps washed laundry clean and separate. A shrink wrapper is a relatively inexpensive tool that can serve for other community laundry jobs as well.

In some smaller communities, housekeepers launder residents' linens using washers located on the resident floors. This practice is not recommended, and it is illegal in most health care facilities. The washing machines in the residential areas are usually connected to the domestic hot water system, in which the temperature should be set no higher than 110°F to avoid the possibility of scalding the residents. Because water temperatures of 180°F are required to kill most bacteria, a community laundry facility equipped with a booster heater is required to protect residents from the spread of disease. If operators choose to use washers in the resident buildings as part of the laundry service, then chemical sanitizers should be added to the wash cycle as a minimal means of infection control.

Residents' linens should be rotated rather than delaying remaking the bed until the linens are laundered. In other words, when the room is made up, clean linens should be immediately placed on the bed, and the laundered linens should be returned when they are clean.

■ COMMUNITY-PROVIDED LINENS

There are many advantages to communities' providing flat linens and towels to residents. The complications of sorting and storing personally owned linens are eliminated, and in some circumstances it can be more cost-effective to contract this service. Community-provided linens are, however, more expensive to maintain. Except in skilled-nursing facilities, residents should be encouraged or required to use their own linen. Among other benefits, using linens in patterns and colors of their choice makes residents feel more at home than the all-white institutional linens.

To minimize loss, housekeepers should double-check that the dirty linen picked up matches the replacement request. Three changes of linen per resident in assisted living and nursing homes is usually adequate, including linen in use.

■ LAYOUT OF THE LAUNDRY

Dirty laundry should always be separated from clean to avoid cross-contamination. Hampers should be clearly labeled "Clean Linen" or "Soiled Linen." Dirty laundry should come into the laundry area through one set of doors, and clean laundry should exit through another. Ideally, the laundry flow should be set up in a circular pattern. A separate sorting room for receiving laundry can help contain the soiled laundry. Residents who may be infected with a communicable disease must have their laundry handled using infection control procedures and handled by staff wearing personal protective equipment (PPE). Soiled linen should be transported in a closed container that does not permit airborne contamination.

When soiled laundry enters the laundry facility, it can either be kept separate in mesh bags or, if items are properly marked with the residents' identification, be sorted into tubs of like variety and temporarily stored in plastic bins. These bins can then be wheeled to the washers, washed, removed from the washers, and put into the dryers. Once the dirty-linen bins are unloaded, they should be disinfected, then wheeled into the drying and folding area. A wash cycle usually takes 15 to 20 minutes, depending on the selection, and roughly double that time to dry. Therefore, the efficient laundry facility should be equipped with more drying capacity than washing.

The drying and folding area is the clean side of the operation; here clean laundry is dried, ironed or steamed, folded, wrapped, and temporarily stored. To prevent infestation by rodents and insects, the laundry room door should never be left open. It is a good idea to provide air conditioning for employee comfort and to prevent the growth of mildew. Ceiling fans are a must in humid climates.

Rubberized tile floors are the easiest to clean and disinfect and provide the most standing comfort for employees. Laundry that comes into contact with cement floors is subject to increased staining and contamination because cement is porous, making it impossible to clean and disinfect properly.

Equipment needed varies according to the community size and service package. Commercial washers are rated by maximum capacity, in pounds, for a single load. The laundry should include some combination of 50- to 75-pound-capacity washers, plus one or two domestic-size washers for delicate items and personal clothes; a gas-fired ironer; a steamer or steam cabinet for steaming uniforms and other items; irons and ironing boards; 75- to 110-pound commercial dryers; and folding tables. (The color scheme should be based on tan, which is easiest on

the eyes; white can cause headaches.) Most modern washers are capable of up to 30 programmable cycle formulas and come with 10 preprogrammed cycles. Machines with capacities larger than 50 pounds usually have two motors: one wash motor and one extract motor, typically 1.5 horsepower. The smaller 35-pound washers usually have only one two-speed motor. All washers should be capable of spinning at a speed of at least 500 RPM to remove as much water as possible before the drying cycle. The more efficient the extract cycle in the washer, the less drying time is needed. Employees should be advised not to overload washing machines; doing so reduces efficiency and can damage the machines.

The folding tables should be waist high to keep employees from bending over. Some laundry bins can be fitted to rise as laundry is removed. Polyfilm wrap (36 inches wide) can be used to wrap the clean linen with heat-sealing hand irons. Commercial plastic wrappers are also available to automate this task. Clean linen should be stored in a clean, well-ventilated closet, room, or alcove used only for that purpose.

Pressing can be done with an electric presser capable of processing 40 pounds per hour, or with a gas-fired flatwork ironer. The Chicago Champ gas-fired ironer has a 60-inch usable ironing width and an 8-inch-diameter heated roll. These machines are the best choice for processing dining room and guest room linens (napkins should be spray-starched before ironing). Electric flatwork finishers also do the job but can be expensive to operate. Most physical plants operate equipment with gas because it is both more efficient and cheaper.

Steam cabinets can be cost-effective for removing wrinkles from employee uniforms. The system uses a steam cabinet and a booster heater to generate the additional hot water needed. The steam cabinet can finish approximately 140 garments per hour, compared with 10 garments per hour in a hand-ironing operation. Even wash-and-wear uniforms need to be touched up before use, and dining room uniforms should be pressed. The steam cabinet system can easily handle permanent press, woolens, loosely woven fabrics, flannels, tweeds, knit dresses, and double-knit suits as well as all poly blend uniforms. When compared with the cost of hand processing uniforms, the payback period to cover the capital expenditure is usually less than one year for communities larger than 200 units.

Most communities provide laundry rooms for residents' personal use. Residents with any symptoms of communicable disease must not use public laundry rooms to wash or dry their laundry. Washers and dryers generally operate at no charge to the resident. Heavily soiled linens should be washed only in the central laundry facilities, where any fecal material can be removed and proper operating temperatures can ensure infection control. Operating instructions for the washers and dryers should be posted in the laundry rooms. Also, large signs should be posted for visually impaired residents to denote common settings for machines. Laundry rooms should be open 24 hours a day, but residents should be encouraged to remove their clothing as soon as each cycle is completed. Because residents often forget their clothes in the machines, laundry baskets or carts should be provided so that other residents can unload idle machines. The residents should be reminded of their responsibility to clean the dryer lint traps after each use, and the laundry room should be supplied with a wastebasket for this purpose. Communities that provide ironing boards should also provide self-shutoff safety irons that can be checked out at the concierge desk, with a charge assessed if the iron is not returned. The laundry rooms should be cleaned and disinfected weekly, and a disinfectant-solution spray bottle and paper towels should also be available in the room for residents to use. Resident aides and family members should never be allowed to use the community laundry machines for their own purposes. This could lead to the introduction of pests into the community and causes resentment among residents who are inconvenienced by busy machines. All resident laundry rooms should be fitted with a floor drain, especially if they contain a laundry tub or sink.

■■■■■ CHEMICALS AND SAFETY

Dispensing chemicals into the laundry machines can be done either manually or automatically. Automatic dispensers have several compelling advantages over the manual system. They are fed by dispensing tubes that siphon the chemicals from five-gallon buckets in preprogrammed amounts, and the supplies can be stored in a secure location. This system virtually eliminates the need for employees to handle chemicals. The automatic dispensers are usually pro-

grammed to dispense chemicals for a full load, so some waste is possible when processing partial loads.

Manually dispensed chemicals are usually added to the top of the machines, generally at eye level. Employees should be instructed to use scoops, measuring cups, or other containers to dispense soaps, detergents, bleaches, and other chemicals. They should never use their hands. It is up to the employee to determine the correct amount of chemical needed and to take appropriate precautionary measures when handling and dispensing the products.

Five categories of chemical solution are used in the laundry operation:

■ **Softeners.** These soften terrycloth and cotton, reducing the buildup of static electricity in the dryer and wear on the dryer drum and the linen itself. They also freshen fabrics.
■ **Sour.** This reduces the iron content of water. It also reduces the alkalinity that causes stiffness in linen and can contribute to skin breakdown.
■ **Destainer.** This bleaching agent whitens and removes discoloration.
■ **Emulsion detergent.** This detergent with a wetting agent breaks up (emulsifies) and removes grease and heavy soil. It conditions water by suspending calcium and magnesium to keep stains down and reduce graying. (XP is an additional wetting agent that is commonly used for restaurant linens. It helps detergent penetrate the linen better to release food soils.)
■ **Oxygen bleach.** The main difference between oxygen bleach and chlorine bleach is that oxygen bleach contains sodium percarbonate and the active ingredient, whereas chlorine bleace contains sodium hypochlorite as the active agent. It does not remove colors but removes stains, as chlorine bleach does but is environmentally safe.

A material safety data sheet (MSDS) for each product must be kept on file and accessible to employees. These can be ordered from most manufacturers in several languages. The law requires an employer to keep an MSDS even for a product that has been discontinued. The MSDS details hazardous components, recommended first-aid measures, handling data, protective measures, and storage recommendations. Employee orientation and training programs should in-

---

> **Exhibit 12.1   Laundry Orientation Checklist**
>
> ❑ Job description
> ❑ Sorting
> ❑ Protective clothing and equipment
> ❑ Formulas for washers and operation instructions
> ❑ Disinfecting procedures: carts and counters
> ❑ Inventory procedures
> ❑ Residential versus health care laundry
> ❑ Proper folding techniques
> ❑ Separate containers used for transporting clean and dirty linen
> ❑ Cleaning lint screens on dryers morning and afternoon
> ❑ Supply inventory and control
> ❑ Ironing: what is ironed and what is not
> ❑ Drying: what is dried and what is not
> ❑ Wrapping and storage procedures
> ❑ Schedules
> ❑ General safety precautions
> ❑ MSDS instruction
> ❑ Handling isolation linens
> ❑ Uniforms
> ❑ Use of back-support belts
>
> Date: _____
>
> Employee: _____

clude information on the proper handling of chemicals. (An orientation checklist is shown in exhibit 12.1.) All MSDS sheets should be reviewed at least annually to ensure that all employees are fully aware of the risks associated with exposure and of appropriate first aid. OSHA requires that eyewash stations capable of 8 to 10 minutes of continuous flow be installed in chemical use and storage areas. All spray bottles containing cleaning chemicals should be appropriately identified and labeled. Empty bottles should be triple-rinsed and punctured before disposal.

Biohazard waste receptacles should be used in laundries for the disposal of isolation bags and sharps that may have been accidentally thrown in with dirty laundry. These are picked up and delivered by a specialized contractor with disposal authorization. The staff should exercise caution when sorting dirty laundry from health care components of the community to avoid possible contamination. Gloves, masks, and vinyl aprons should be worn when handling soiled linen, which should be carefully sorted piece by piece. Back-support belts are also recommended for employees who lift heavy loads of laundry.

Employees should never open a laundry machine or touch its surfaces when it is operating. These machines run at high temperatures, and workers can easily be burned or scalded.

In health care communities, the linen and laundry services are inspected and evaluated by the state health department or other regulatory agency. The evaluation usually determines whether the community's laundry and linen services comply with state regulations and federal conditions of participation pertaining to laundry services and infection control, which normally states something such as: "The facility has available at all times a quantity of linen essential for proper care and comfort of the residents; and linens are handled, stored, processed, and transported in such a manner as to prevent the spread of infection."

MAINTENANCE

Expensive service contracts for maintenance of laundry equipment are generally unnecessary, as the machines are relatively easy to repair, and parts are readily available. The maintenance department should establish a preventive maintenance schedule for the laundry machinery. This should include routine oiling, balancing, replacement of gaskets and belts, and cleaning of the lint trap and removal system. A washer that goes out of balance can vibrate violently enough to shake the building and bend the machine's cam shaft, which is expensive to replace. Modern commercial washers are equipped with a shutoff switch to prevent this damage.

Most small repairs and seal replacements can be accomplished by the facility's maintenance staff. Gas-fired dryers typically fail because of a faulty igniter. Replacements can be purchased from the manufacturer and replaced easily. Many appliance parts can also be purchased online from discount appliance-parts vendors at substantial savings. It is wise to stock a few frequently used parts, such as dryer door seals, washers, fuses, and belts to minimize downtime in the event of a breakdown.

13

Maintenance and Capital Improvements

The maintenance department is responsible for providing a safe environment for the residents and staff and for the long-term protection of the physical aspects of the building, including the equipment, furniture, and fixtures. It ensures that building systems are configured and operated to provide a comfortable environment at a minimal cost. Finally, it maintains the public areas as well as occupied and vacant apartments and responds competently and reliably to residents' requests. Standardized procedures and systems can help the staff to accomplish these goals.

The tasks of the maintenance department usually fall into two basic categories: maintenance and repair. Maintenance is the day-to-day, periodic, or scheduled work required to preserve the community's physical assets. It includes work to prevent damage or deterioration that might be costly to repair. Prompt maintenance is essential to operating efficiency. Repair is the restoration of a system to a condition that allows it to be used for its designated purpose. The repair may involve overhauling or replacing parts or materials that have deteriorated because of use, age, or the lack of proper maintenance.

Minor repairs and maintenance of the building systems can be considered part of the upkeep of the property. The costs of such repairs are usually budgeted on the basis of past expenditures and projected requirements. For the overhaul or replacement of major building systems, the maintenance director must take a more detailed approach. He or she should study the overall economy of the system, its cost of operation, and the desired operational efficiency. Factors for the management to consider and evaluate on an ongoing basis include the following:

- The cost of replacing the system in relation to the expected life span of the system and to the cost of repairs
- Operation and maintenance costs of the old system versus those of a new system
- Possible obsolescence of the system and availability of parts
- Present and future availability of maintenance funds
- Operational hazards of downtime for the resident population if the system fails

Some of these costs are more easily estimated than others. The maintenance director can perform the basic financial evaluation, but it is up to the executive director and ultimately the owners to assess the long-term availability of capital for maintaining the building systems at their best, and the possible risks to the residents and to investment of deferring maintenance. Many major system failures can be delayed or averted with an ounce of prevention.

NEW INSTALLATIONS AND PREVENTIVE MAINTENANCE

The objective of any preventive maintenance plan is to reduce the costs of operation and replacement. When equipment and systems are properly maintained, they function more efficiently and are less expensive to operate. Clogged air-handler filters and heat exchangers operate at reduced capacity, which means they must work harder and will wear out sooner. Properties that have deferred their maintenance work over the years must invest large amounts of labor in repairs. It is much less expensive in the long run to make repairs as they are needed than to allow problems to accumulate. If the deferral is due to budget constraints, the maintenance director should take these issues to the owners for resolution. Deferred maintenance will ultimately result in a decrease in the overall value of the property. It will cost much more to bring in contractors to complete the deferred projects than to have facility staff handle them.

The building's major systems should be checked on a regular schedule. The maintenance director should keep a running status report of the regular maintenance and repair work required to ensure proper operation of the systems. The details of the process will vary according to personnel and skill levels.

The maintenance director and executive director should set priorities for the preventive maintenance plan. Of utmost priority is equipment affecting the life and safety of the residents. These systems include but are not limited to fire suppression and alarms, the domestic hot water system, the heating and air conditioning systems (HVAC), emergency power generators, emergency lighting, and emergency response systems. The temporary failure of any of these critical systems can pose risks to an aging population.

The second priority is proper maintenance of the most expensive equipment of the property. This includes the chillers, air handlers, recirculation pumps, major valves and shutoffs, boilers, and elevator equipment. This equipment, when properly maintained, should serve the community for many years.

Manufacturers' operations manuals usually include recommended preventive maintenance schedules, and these manuals should be filed in the maintenance office and followed. In new buildings, these are provided at the time of installation. Some general con-

tractors or project managers make a video recording of the orientation and service recommendations from the installer before the manufacturer's representative leaves the job site. This gives the maintenance department a visual record of each of the building's major systems that can be easier to understand than the operations manual; it will also take account of any modifications specific to the property. Videotaping expensive maintenance and repair procedures performed by outside contractors or manufacturer's representatives can also help to minimize downtime in the future. The maintenance director should also keep a set of blueprints of the building for use when soliciting bids for service work, with all valves, clean-outs, and major equipment locations highlighted.

The turnover of the building from the general contractor to the management should cover all required construction and operating permits and a description of the permitting process, along with requirements of the building inspector or fire marshal. Blueprints and "as-built" drawings detailing all of the building's utilities, including location in the building and materials used for water, electric, gas, sewer, phone, and fire alarm systems, are invaluable in the event of a major breakdown. All contractors (electrical, fire alarm, plumbing, mechanical, HVAC, painting, mill working, landscaping, flooring, and so on) should provide the following:

- Specifications for materials used
- Information on where to purchase parts on 24 hours' notice
- Instructions on operating all of the equipment
- Schedules and instructions for preventive maintenance on all equipment
- All warranty and guarantee information
- A complete walk-through for all equipment installed
- Emergency contacts and schedule of emergency repair charges

The third priority for a preventive maintenance program is the maintenance of equipment and finishes affecting the appearance of the building and, ultimately, resident satisfaction. To residents and visitors, the overall appearance of a community signals its financial health and the competence of the management. Usually, operators attend most carefully to the appearance of the common areas and the exterior of the building, which are most readily visible to residents, guests, and owners' representatives. This attention to the "finish" of the building, however, often comes at the expense of safety and major-cost equipment, which is typically located in non-public areas. A strip of loose wallpaper may be noticed and repaired before anyone ever notices the badly worn bearings on the recirculation pump that distributes hot water throughout the building.

The fourth priority is the maintenance of equipment that promotes a more efficient operation, such as systems for water or air handling. These require frequent attention and cleaning to function optimally and prevent breakdowns.

The best way to organize a preventive maintenance system is with a computerized maintenance management system (CMMS).This software allows the community maintenance director to organize and track preventive maintenance, work orders, inventory, costs, and vendors. Not only will this system track manufacturer-recommended preventive maintenance and schedule the tasks, it will also maintain OSHA, ASHE, and state fire code or life safety compliance. It can easily produce reports for management, insurance auditors, or surveyors detailing maintenance that is needed or has been performed. The system will also simplify billable resident maintenance requests. Normally new residents are allocated approximately 1 hour of maintenance time upon move in to assemble and move furniture, hang pictures, and connect smart tvs, etc. Time requested by residents or families beyond this allowance is generally tracked and billed each month to the resident's account. The unit log includes a report for each apartment that records all maintenance visits. Information recorded should include the date of the visit, description of service, any special comments about the job, and the name of the person performing the service. Visits to the apartment responding to work orders as well as for preventive maintenance should be documented. This log documents when the apartment was last painted, the carpet changed, the toilet serviced, and so on, allowing the management to track such information as the life span of carpets and paint and the last preventive maintenance session, and to use the information to plan a replacement schedule for apartment fixtures.

Some routine preventive maintenance should be performed whenever a maintenance staff member visits an apartment. This way, the department makes the best use of its time in each apartment, and the resident sees that the maintenance department is on top of its preventive maintenance program. As with any department, maintenance needs to manage the residents' expectations. Routine preventive maintenance for each unit should include running a short cycle of the washer and dishwasher and checking for leaks; verifying that the refrigerator doors seal completely when shut; checking the sink cabinet for insects; checking for mold and mildew; flushing toilets and checking the floor around the base for leaks; running all faucets; noting any water marks or leaks on exterior walls and around window casings; and testing locks on all windows and doors. In addition, staff members should replace the filter on the apartment's heating and cooling unit and visually check the condensate drain pan. These drain-pan tubes can become clogged with dust or algae, causing them to back up, which in turn can cause significant water damage to the ceiling of the room below. It is a simple procedure to clear them with compressed air.

The maintenance director should conduct a complete inspection of all public areas and the exterior of the building at least quarterly and set a schedule for needed repairs. It is also a good idea to maintain a log for all the filters in the building. Clogged or dirty filters can cause equipment to be overworked and can contribute to premature failure. The air filter log should include the type of heating, cooling, and ventilation systems; type of filter(s) installed; manufacturer and manufacturer's instructions for cleaning and replacement; ASHRAE efficiency rating; manometer reading; and location of all the filters within the community.

Exhibit 13.1 shows a suggested preventive maintenance plan.

■ WORK-ORDER SYSTEM

Work orders are a key element of operating the maintenance department. The functions of the system are as follows:

■ To provide a standard, centralized system for requesting and performing maintenance work
■ To provide written records of maintenance requested, to whom it was assigned, and by whom it

Exhibit 13.1 Preventive Maintenance Plan

Daily Checklist:

Checklist Item	S	M	T	W	T	F	S
Clean common area furniture, floors, walls, windows, pictures							
Furniture in the correct place in all common areas, including library and corridors							
Lights in common areas have been checked and are all working							
Public restrooms are clean and stocked with toilet paper, towels, and soap at 9:00 am							
Public restrooms are clean and stocked with toilet paper, towels, and soap at 3:00 pm							
Dining room floor is clean							
Private dining room floor is clean and room is organized							
Discovery room is clean and organized							
Library is clean and organized							
Front entrance doors have clean windows							
Rug in front entrance has been vacuumed							
Laundry rooms are clean, mopped, and organized, and lint is cleaned out of the dryers							
Washers and dryers have been wiped down							
Trash is removed from laundry room							
Front porch is blown and clear of clutter and debris							
Front porch furniture is organized							
Front porch tables are wiped down							
Walk around the property picking up trash all the way to the Kroger road							
All external lights are in good working order							
All external fans are in good working order							
No vehicles are parked on the lawn or in no-parking areas							
Offices are clean, dusted, vacuumed, and trash is removed; furniture is in good repair							
Rehab area is clean, dusted, vacuumed, trash is removed, and furniture is in good repair							
Dining room tables are in good working order							
Dining room window coverings are in good working order and consistent throughout							
Dining room temperature is between 72 and 78 degrees							
Dining room floors are not sticky							
Fountain is clean and no water lines are visible; no bleach smell							
Employee break room is cleaned thoroughly, refrigerator is cleaned out							
If applicable, back porch is clean, and furniture is organized							
Activity room is clean and organized, trash removed, lights work							
Living room is clean, organized, and lights work							
Stairwells are cleaned							
Hall between employee break room and kitchen is cleaned, mopped							
Work orders completed							
Housekeeping closets kept locked at all times							
Laundry room doors kept closed at all times							
No portable heaters or extension cords used							
Corridors are clear for egress							

(continued)

Exhibit 13.1 Preventive Maintenance Plan *(continued)*

Weekly Checklist:

Checklist Item	Wk.1	Wk.2	Wk.3	Wk.4
Front porch and ceiling clean and free of debris				
Exterior lights checked and in good working order				
Furniture in common areas checked for scratches and in good working order, repairs made as needed				
Touch up paint in all common areas				
Touch up walls in all common areas				
Inspect lawn and make recommendations to lawn company				
Plants in common areas are in good shape; report any problems to the plant carer				
Water plants in common areas that belong to the community, two planters in front and fresh flowers in lobby				
Unloading dock behind the kitchen is cleaned with pressure washer				
Pressure wash areas around the building that appear dirty				
Staircase should be vacuumed				
Stairwells should be cleaned				
Complete weekly unannounced inspection of the resident rooms to inspect housekeeping standards				
Wash up to 10 wheelchairs per week (at night)				
Trash area free of debris and clean				

Monthly Checklist:

Checklist Item	Jan	Feb	Mar	Apr	May	Jun	Jul	Aug	Sep	Oct	Nov	Dec
Conduct safety meeting												
Check secured doors to ensure proper working order												
Check emergency lighting throughout the community												
Inspect water temps throughout the community												
Hot water at:												
Lavatories and in resident rooms not to exceed 120 degrees												
Hot water at dishwasher and kitchen not to exceed 180 degrees												
Hot water at washing machines not to exceed 160 degrees												
Fire extinguishers are present and checked in good working order, including van												
Walk grounds with the ED to inspect grounds and building												
HVAC units checked												
Touch up paint in common areas												
Elevators inspected to be in good working order and cleaned												

Checklist Item	Jan	Feb	Mar	Apr	May	Jun	Jul	Aug	Sep	Oct	Nov	Dec
In-service for staff members												
MSDS books are up to date with all chemicals used in the community												
Participated in QA program												
One 2-A:10-BC fire extinguisher within 25 feet of all exits												
One 20-BC type fire extinguisher in kitchen												
Flammable liquids properly stored												
Smoking area, if applicable clean and ashtrays empty												
Ensure comfortable furniture in outdoor areas for resident use												

Quarterly Checklist:

Checklist Item	1st quarter	2nd quarter	3rd quarter	4th quarter
HVAC units inspected and filters changed				
Fire drill in Memory Care				
Carpets should cleaned in all common areas				
Touch up paint on exterior of the building				
Stove hood cleaned professionally				

Biannual Checklist:

Checklist Item	Jan–June	July–Dec
Exterior windows washed throughout community		
Windows in resident rooms washed		
In storage areas, items stored no higher than 18 inches between the top of the items and the bottom of the sprinkler head		
Stored items are on pallets, not directly on the floor		
If mechanical rooms are used for storage, the items are stored away from the mechanical equipment		
Winterize/recharge vulnerable waterlines		

Annual Checklist:

Checklist Item	Initial and date
Gutters cleaned	
Generators checked	
Sprinklers and fire alarm system checked	
Elevators inspected by licensed professional	
Wiring inspected by licensed professional	
HVAC system inspected by licensed professional	

was completed, along with the date and duration of the work

■ To provide a means for managers to screen and prioritize maintenance requests

■ To facilitate staffing assignments by providing a readily visual and traceable record of work needed

■ To provide document requests for services by residents for billing by the accounting department

Work orders can be initiated by the reception desk, department heads, or maintenance personnel. A log of requests initiated and completed should be kept current on the computerized maintenance management system for quick reference and tracking. All current or outstanding work orders should be printed out in a report and provided to the concierge so that she can respond to resident and family inquiries. The maintenance director should then assess the priority given to the request and assign the request to a staff person for completion. If more than 30 minutes will be required to complete work in a resident's apartment, the resident should be called to schedule a maintenance appointment. On completion of the work, the completed work order can be checked off in the CMMS system and record if it is billable back to the resident. At any time, a resident or department head can check the status of a request at the front desk.In the absence of a computerized system, a manual system can be used. A work-order board in the maintenance department is a convenient way to keep track of the assignment progress and of work orders. The board should have several hooks for orders at different stages of progress. The first is the "Work to Be Completed" hook. The work order tickets can be sorted here according to who is assigned to do the work: maintenance personnel, housekeeping staff, or an outside contractor. If parts need to be ordered, the work order ticket can be put on a "Parts on Order" hook on the board. The director of maintenance should confirm that the appropriate parts have been ordered and then contact both the receptionist and the resident to inform them of the expected delivery time. When the parts arrive, the work order ticket can be assigned to the appropriate person. Any work order that has been delayed by the ordering of parts should be reassigned top priority once the parts have arrived. Once the work orders are completed and signed off by the assigned

staff and the resident, they can be transferred to a "Work Orders Completed" hook and then passed to the evening receptionist and recorded as completed in the work-order log book, completing the cycle.

All interested parties can use the work-order log to monitor total requests, completion times, and requests that have stalled. The log is also useful for revealing patterns of maintenance issues that may require further investigation or different troubleshooting procedures.

Preparing an apartment for a new tenant should be given priority over all except emergency work orders. Any necessary painting and repair work should be scheduled in advance of the lease ending date, and permission should be sought from the resident or responsible party to enter the apartment for this purpose. The need to order parts or fixtures for the unit should be anticipated. The vacant apartment should be thoroughly cleaned immediately after maintenance is finished and should be left in a showable condition. Each day that the apartment remains unoccupied because of maintenance work, the cost of completing the work dramatically increases because of lost revenue potential.

■■■ CAPITAL IMPROVEMENTS

Fixed-asset capitalization, also known as capital improvement, is a process of addressing the current and projected physical needs of a property, establishing the costs of maintaining or modernizing it, and creating a strategic plan for addressing those needs within financial constraints (see chapter 2). This process is also easily tracked and managed using most computerized maintenance management system (CMMS) programs. The first step in developing such a plan is to conduct a comprehensive inventory of the community's physical systems, both mechanical and aesthetic. Managers have a tendency to focus on major systems such as the boilers, roof, in-unit components, and finishes. But the little things that may be left neglected, such as a broken thermopane seal, window caulking, and upholstery, can add up and need attention all at once. With careful and comprehensive planning, the community's capital resources can be allocated in a deliberate fashion.

The inventory should quantify things as specifically as possible. For example, the make, model, and size of mechanical equipment, square feet of paving, roof, and common area carpets, and counts by type and size of windows and furniture should be noted precisely for easy reference when soliciting bids and budgeting repairs or replacements. Architectural plans generally yield accurate information about building dimensions and can make this part of the job much easier than measuring by hand.[1]

The life span of any given system, fixture, or equipment is a function of age, design, material type and quality, nature of use, maintenance, and environmental conditions. The estimated life for each item in the inventory can be derived from the manufacturer's warranty, actual experience, industry standards, and estimates by the community's maintenance staff and outside contractors. In some cases, upgrades and replacements may be prompted by changing market conditions or new competition.

Cost for repairs and replacements can be estimated with local contractors through a bidding process. In established communities, the management can often draw on direct experience for estimating certain costs. For complex estimates, such as those for larger mechanical systems, historic information may be available from other properties of similar design.

All cost estimates should include materials, labor, freight, and tax. Typically tax and freight are approximately 12 to 15 percent of the cost of goods. For projects involving contracted labor or construction, bids for the work completed, a signed standard construction contract for each company providing the labor, certificate of insurance, and a signed general waiver and release of lien rights should all be included in the submittal.

Having identified expected capital needs, ascribed costs to them, and projected when they are likely to occur, the next step is to project the effect of these costs on the bottom line. A 10-year capital spending plan estimates total capital costs for each year. Spreadsheet programs permit this calculation to be done quickly and accurately and facilitate adjustments for inflation. In this way, it is possible to review annual anticipated needs and allocate the resources appropriately over time. In most cases, a capital reserve of 2 or 3 percent of the gross revenue from opening should be more than adequate to keep the community in good repair and looking its best. For larger, costlier projects, it may be necessary to spread the work out over time. But the advantages of staggering the costs need to be weighed against lost economies of scale. When emergency capital needs arise, it may be necessary to reallocate funds budgeted for other projects.

Priority

The priority system should be defined to establish a comparative relationship between capital needs to facilitate informed decisions during the budgeting process. For example, those expenditures that are required for health and safety reasons normally would be assigned top priority. Second priority could be assigned to projects that facilitate a more efficient operation, thereby reducing the cost of operations. Third priority could be assigned to projects designed to meet company standards. Fourth priority could be reserved for major renovations, and fifth could be assigned to elective projects that may simply promote community enhancement or "wish list" items. Payback periods should be calculated on all items (including installation) that are intended to save operating money. The payback period is the time it takes for the cumulative operating savings to exceed initial total costs (calculate by dividing the initial cost by the annual operating savings).

Estimated Life

Enter the estimated life of the *current* equipment; if it is at the end of its life, use "EOL." Determination of the estimated life for each item in the completed inventory can be derived from the manufacture warranty, actual experience of the subject site or like site, industry standards, and the first 10 estimates made by community maintenance staff and outside contractors.

Run to Fail

Some mechanical systems can be operated until they fail without affecting resident safety or comfort. For these systems, it must be determined if replacement parts and equipment are readily available so that operations will not be unreasonably disrupted or cause a safety risk upon failure.

For projects involving contracted labor or construction, actual bids for the work completed, a signed standard construction contract for each company providing the labor, certificate of insurance, and a signed "general waiver and release of lien rights" should all be included in the submittal.

One final word regarding capital improvements. Its is important to avoid making promises to staff or residents regarding approved improvements until the process is completed. Soliciting bids and allocating funds will be very fluid and can change the allocation dramatically. Staff should not make any representations to other employees, families, visitors, or regulatory officials regarding the process status of a capital improvement or replacement item unless the plan has received written approval from ownership.

■■■■■■ STAFFING

As a rule, one full-time maintenance person is required for every 100 units of a congregate or assisted living property in good condition. If the property has a history of deferred maintenance, or if it is new, with construction and punch-list work still to be done, more staffing may be required.[2] Usually, new projects are less demanding of the maintenance staff because of the lack of residents, but as the population increases, both the marketing department and new residents will place more demands on the maintenance department. Continuing care retirement communities require at least one additional maintenance person to handle the specialized needs of the nursing home, as they may be subject to certain conditions of participation and state licensing requirements.

Generally speaking, few executive directors have the expertise required to ensure proper management of building systems. Maintenance expertise also tends to be specialized. For example, an individual may be an excellent electrician but have limited knowledge of plumbing or HVAC systems. Conversely, a generalist who is capable of fixing just about any minor problem may have to call in expensive outside contractors when major systems fail. The key is to find a generalist who can handle most routine repairs and who knows when to call in the specialists and at what price. Many operators are now using pre-employment skills exams to better evaluate a candidate's general knowledge and skill level. These exams can assess the candidate's knowledge regarding electrical, mechanical, plumbing, or basic building maintenance. This process can help identify maintenance candidates who can actually make their own repairs rather that simply triage breakdowns to various outside vendors before they are hired.

Clearly, the maintenance director's level of expertise must be appropriate to the complexity of the physical plant. Many large continuing care retirement communities can afford to employ people with specialized training in plumbing, electrical work, and heating and air conditioning. Communities with golf courses or other extensive grounds may need to hire specialized crews to keep their landscaping well groomed.

The successful maintenance director must be able not only to oversee routine and emergency work but also to get along with residents, who can be demanding and unforgiving regarding their maintenance needs. Some may also be lonely and look for excuses to interact with the management or a favorite maintenance person. The skilled maintenance director will balance the needs of these residents, and the attention they expect and deserve, with the demands of maintaining the physical plant in top condition.

In some ways, residents' perceptions of the maintenance department can be a popularity contest. Residents will compliment the department if they receive the attention they desire and, conversely, make the maintenance director's job stressful if they are not satisfied. The residents, of course, see only a small portion of the maintenance director's job, as most of the equipment is located in the back of the house. The successful director will manage residents' expectations and communicate maintenance priorities to them. Most residents will understand that the repair and maintenance of the major system components relating to their safety have priority over minor work-order requests. More challenging is balancing demands from residents to fix their apartment problems with demands from the marketing department to attend to vacant or model apartments; these seem unimportant to the current residents but represent revenue for the community.

For large communities (more than 200 units), it is a good idea to stagger maintenance shifts to cover evenings and weekends. Not only does this schedule allow for responses to emergencies, but these are times when vacant apartments can be renovated with little interruption from the residents. The maintenance director should also outline a number of typical maintenance problems and provide the concierge desk with simple instructions for dealing with them so that he can avoid being called after working hours for minor problems. The list should identify each problem, suggest a solution, and attempt to distinguish between real emergencies and jobs that can wait until the following day. For example, simple instructions on how to fix a clogged or overflowing toilet can be left with the concierge and carried out by other management employees or housekeepers. Often, quick action on the part of an informed non-maintenance employee can prevent considerable damage and save the maintenance director a trip back to the facility.

CONTROL OF KEYS

The control of keys in the community is an essential element of the building's security: if poorly managed, it can expose the community to significant liability. One person should oversee the control of keys and locks. This is usually the responsibility of the maintenance director, with the approval of the executive director.

There are two types of key system: traditional hard keys and electronic keys. Hard keys are more readily accepted and understood by residents, but electronic systems can be more convenient and flexible, as they can be programmed to track each entry and allow the management to monitor key use by both staff members and residents. Because electronic systems are usually much more expensive to install and maintain, the management must weigh security needs against this added cost.

Uncut and unissued keys should be kept in a locking key cabinet, with access limited to the maintenance director and executive director. Department operating keys can be kept in a locking box at the concierge's desk and should be signed out and in.

Apartment keys are usually issued according to the following procedures:

1. Resident move-ins are confirmed by the marketing department. A notification is issued to all managers that states the move-in date as well as other pertinent information.
2. The maintenance director prepares two apartment keys, one mailbox key (if different), and one exterior door key (if applicable) for the new resident. These keys are attached to a key ring labeled with the resident's name and apartment number and are kept secure until the day before the move-in.
3. One day before the move-in, the maintenance director hand-delivers the new resident's keys to the office manager. Both sign a form to acknowledge transfer of the keys.
4. The office manager keeps the new resident's keys secure until move-in. This policy is necessary to prevent unauthorized access to the community and to prevent unauthorized work on community apartments by residents or family members.

Control of keys is much easier to accomplish with employees than with residents. Many residents give their family members copies of their keys, which allows nearly unlimited access to the building. Key duplication should be discouraged, as it can allow unauthorized access to the building and expose the community to legal liability. Clearly, electronic key systems can minimize these risks, but this advantage needs to be weighed against higher installation and maintenance costs.

The community should have a variety of master and submaster keys, or sets of keys, for employee use. Only the following department heads should have a grand master key: the executive director, the maintenance director, the marketing director, and the director of housekeeping. Issuance of this key must be noted on a personal property form. On termination, the employee must return the key.

An emergency (E) key should be kept at the concierge desk. The E key is a special master key that operates all of the locks in a system at all times. There should be only four E keys on the property: one should be on the executive director's key ring, one at the concierge desk, one in the emergency supply cabinet, and one available only to the fire department (to be kept in the "Knox Box" for fire department use near the main entrance).

All departmental keys and locks should be issued according to the following procedures:

- When locks or keys are needed, the appropriate manager completes a maintenance request form, giving the reason for the request.
- The executive director approves and signs the maintenance request.
- The maintenance request is submitted to the maintenance director.
- When locks are installed, a key is given to the department head, and a copy is kept in the maintenance director's key cabinet.

- All departmental keys must be kept on the same ring, and that ring must be clearly labeled (e.g., food service keys).
- All departmental keys must be kept at the concierge desk. These keys must be signed out and in. The sign-out log should record the date, time, name, and department of the employee, purpose for signing out the key(s), and initials of the concierge on duty.
- Departmental keys must not leave the property. Medication cart keys must not leave the property.
- Staff members who are authorized to sign for and hold keys may not, under any circumstance, pass their keys to another employee.
- If keys must be passed from shift to shift, they must be signed in by the employee going off shift and then signed back out by the next authorized employee.
- Under no circumstance should an employee have in his or her possession keys that have not been properly signed out. Any other keys found in the possession of an employee should be considered unauthorized.
- No person may use a key to enter an area that he or she is not authorized to enter or to allow another unauthorized person to enter.
- At no time should a person use a building key to enter an area other than the area designated in his or her work schedule.
- Any outside employee (e.g., from the cable company or phone company) who requests building keys must obtain authorization from the maintenance director. These keys must be signed in and out by the outside employee, who should be held accountable until the keys are returned and signed in. The concierge should not keep extra keys for this purpose.
- Employees must report misplaced or misused keys to their supervisor. This notification must be accompanied by documentation and their key logs. If the keys are not found, the supervisor must notify the executive director of the loss. The executive director will decide whether to rekey the lock.

■■■■■■ SERVICE CONTRACTS

Service contracts on large and expensive equipment that requires specialized training for maintenance and repair can be good insurance against the risk of a catastrophic breakdown and expensive repairs. Equipment such as the elevators, fire suppression and alarm systems, emergency call system, and other critical systems that ultimately affect residents' safety should be contracted out for routine maintenance and servicing. In urban areas, a number of vendors have this expertise. It is a good idea to solicit bids from contractors who are dealers or service representatives for the specific brand of equipment in the building. It is in their best interest to service their own equipment and to demonstrate to other clients how cost-effective their equipment is to maintain.

As many vendors deal in similar equipment, it is imperative to solicit at least two bids for major service contracts. Most contractors place an "evergreen" clause in their contracts so that they automatically renew at the end of the term. Arranging for the contracts to terminate each year will keep the contractors' prices competitive. Whenever prices are increased, the contract should be put out to multiple bids. Most service contracts and prices are negotiable. All you need to do is shop around and compare.

The maintenance director should keep a ledger with a one-page summary of each of the community's service contracts. The summary should include the contractor's name and address, contact name, home and work telephone numbers, the essential elements of the contract, whether parts are included, and a short description of when and when not to call. Contractors usually charge a premium for visiting the property on holidays and after hours, so it is important to understand what constitutes an emergency and what can wait. With access to this information, anyone can locate help when a system fails and can quickly understand the key terms of the service contracts. The ledger should also include a list of all vendor accounts, technicians by service area, and contact people.

Any time an outside contractor is called to the community, a written statement should be collected from the service technician. This statement should include the date, the item serviced, a detailed description of the work performed, the present operating condition of the system serviced, and any additional repairs that may be required. Thorough documentation of each contractor's visit can save considerable confusion as invoices are received and processed. Copies of all current service contracts should be kept on file and should have at least two bids. Certificates of insurance naming the community as an additional insured should accompany these contracts and be updated as they expire.

TOOLS AND EQUIPMENT

Any well-equipped maintenance department will have the tools and equipment necessary to effect repairs and perform routine maintenance. Although some maintenance directors prefer to use their own tools, the community should stock some basics. If the maintenance director possesses special skills, such as those required to maintain and recharge air conditioning systems, appropriate tools and parts should be stocked. The cost of basic equipment to perform these functions is quickly amortized, considering the cost difference between contract labor and in-house employees.

When considering the purchase of major tools and equipment, the maintenance director should balance the cost against the expected usage and compare them to the alternative cost of associated downtime and contracting out the service. The payback period is the true test of the correct business decision. But it is also important for the maintenance director to be able to keep his or her skills current, and employee satisfaction plays a role in the decision.

The cost to equip a new facility with basic tools should not exceed $3,000. The equipment can be purchased either at once, using start-up funds, or on an as-needed basis, through the usual budget process. Regardless of the timing, it is a good idea to mark each tool, using an electric pen, with the community's identification, and to number them sequentially and record them in a logbook. This way, the maintenance director can sign for them at the time of hiring, and an inventory can be done on employment termination to protect the community's investment. Also, tools engraved with community identification are less likely to disappear and are more likely to be returned when lost. This is especially true for large pieces of equipment, such as lawnmowers, compressors, and snow-blowers.

NOTES

1. T. E. Nutt-Powell and D. P. Whiston, "Capital Planning for Repair and Replacement," *Journal of Property Management* (September 1991): 48–50.

2. A punch list is compiled by the general contractor and the owner and itemizes unfinished detail work on new construction that is substantially complete.

III

Marketing and Sales

Marketing

define *marketing* as the planning and processes designed to generate interest in and attract prospects to the community. *Sales* can be defined as the process of converting these prospects into residents. The success or failure of these processes, which are fundamental to the survival of the community, depend on a well-planned and well-executed strategy to which every aspect of the community's operation must contribute.

Marketing is a priority in the management of a senior community. Residents and employees must all be marketers. The residents should be taught to recognize that a fully occupied community is a financially sound community and that the referrals they make are critical to its stability. Employees on all levels need to understand the importance of marketing to their own success: this applies equally to the housekeepers, the executive director, and the president of the company. *Everyone* must adopt a marketing mindset.

Having a marketing mindset, though, is not enough. All employees must be committed to delivering a high-quality product. If operations cannot deliver on the promises of the sales counselors, the community will end up sabotaging its own marketing success time and again. If you do not have a good-quality product, you are wasting your marketing dollars attempting to create demand for something that people do not want.

Quality is the difference between what people expect and what they get. If the employees are personally committed to exceeding the residents' expectations, then the community will be perceived as a good-quality operation. This commitment to service does not come easily. It is the result of continual, painstaking training, motivation, and employee recognition. When employees believe that what they are doing is special, it shows. Employees who are convinced that they are the best in the business will deliver the best service. Families, visitors, and referral sources will notice their performance and talk about it to others. (See chapter 3 for more on managing and motivating employees to promote the community.)

Marketing work begins at the earliest stages of planning a community. The following sections describe all phases of marketing, from initial analyses to promoting a facility that has reached stabilized occupancy.

ANALYSIS OF FEASIBILITY

The analysis of feasibility for senior living communities is a two-step process. First and foremost, a financial analysis needs to determine the minimal absorption (fill-up) rate that will meet investment expectations for return or, for nonprofits, allow the community to break even. (See chapter 2 for more on financial projections.) Second, it must be determined whether sufficient demand exists in the marketplace with the demographic profile that the community is intended to attract. This can be done by analyzing market penetration and market share. Some flexibility in the concept and design of the project may broaden its appeal and increase the absorption rate.

There is a direct relationship between the rate of fill-up of a community and its financial performance. Generally speaking, the quicker the fill-up, the better the return on invested capital. For example, an $11 million 100-unit community with a 75 percent loan-to-value ratio and a 20-year, 9 percent mortgage will require approximately $74,000 per month in amortizing payments. Let us assume that meeting operational cash flow requires 50 percent occupancy and that to service the debt will require 86 percent occupancy (86 units). At a net absorption rate of 8 units per month, it will take 11 months to reach cash flow (86 units ÷ 8 units per month). This means that for 11 months the project will need to borrow working capital to meet operational shortfalls, and interest will also accumulate on working-capital funds. Usually, after this point is reached, the surplus balance will be used to pay down the more expensive working-capital loan. Only after this is achieved will the project be able to realize any return on invested capital. Should the net absorption rate be actually only 4 units per month, then it will take approximately 21 months to reach cash flow after debt service.

To illustrate the financial consequences of this difference, consider the $74,000 per month in debt-service payments alone from month 11 to month 21, or the $750,000, plus interest, that will need to be financed as a result of the slower fill-up rate. This will add at least another $81,000 per year to the amortizing payment just using the 9 percent initial interest rate, and not including additional operational shortfalls incurred during this slower fill-up period, which could easily total $500,000 or more. The addition of $81,000 per year in debt service translates to $7,290 per month. At an average rent of $2,500 per month, it will require 3 more occupied units to reach cash flow after debt service, or 89 units—89 percent (not including the additional cost per month to service these additional residents). Add in the debt service on the additional operational shortfalls of $3,750 per month and 1.5 more units to cover this amount, and the figure rises to 90.5 units, or 90 percent, before investors will see any return. This leaves only 4.5

units at 95 percent stabilized occupancy for return on investment, capital improvements, principal reduction, and coverage for unexpected contingencies. This small margin is further eroded if the inflated cost of operations each year cannot be passed on to the residents, who are usually on fixed incomes.

The larger the project, the faster the fill-up necessary to achieve the same financial goals. A 200-unit project may have $7 million more in debt service (100 additional units × $70,000 per unit project cost) than its 100-unit competitor. This project will need to fill at 8 net units per month in 20 months to reach the same 80 percent operations plus debt-service cash-flow threshold.

The accumulation of operational shortfalls during the fill-up of projects is usually postponed by marketing before or during construction. In fact, many states require that a project meet a presold threshold of up to 70 percent before construction begins. Prudent developers are now test-marketing proposed communities well before putting a shovel into the ground, using community focus groups, seminars, and mail surveys and even by building a model unit and opening a local sales office.

Another factor affecting the financial feasibility of the project is the effect of absorption on project financing. Construction or bridge loans usually bear a higher interest rate than the permanent loan that will replace them. The longer the construction loan remains outstanding, the greater the interest expense the project bears. The permanent mortgage financing will usually replace the construction financing after the operating net income of the project is sufficient to cover the debt service of the permanent loan by about 10 to 20 percent. Therefore, for each month that the occupancy fails to reach this threshold and the construction loan remains in place, the project incurs a higher interest expense than was projected in the financial pro forma, which in essence becomes a construction cost overrun.[1]

The absorption and continued occupancy rates are clearly the most critical factors affecting the financial feasibility of senior living (and other multiple-family) real estate projects. The combined effect of the costs associated with a slower than projected fill-up rate of the project can quickly deplete any contingency funds built into the pro forma and turn an otherwise well-conceived project into a financial disaster. The developer's inability to meet projections is the single greatest factor contributing to the financial failure of projects. These projects are then recapitalized by their new owners at the expense of the original mortgage holder and investor's equity. Not only does such failure severely damage the developer's financial position and reputation, but it can also have a devastating effect on the project's residents, whose lives and property investment become entangled in the developer's problems.

ASSESSING DEMAND

Before structuring a marketing plan and strategy, the company must assess the demand for the project in the chosen location and market. If the project already exists, the evaluation of market size and existing penetration will determine the marketing approach. Such studies must be carefully done, as initial indications may be misleading. In the early 1980s, burgeoning health care costs associated with the aging baby-boom generation generated considerable media coverage and overstated the anticipated growth of the population over 65. New developers in senior housing interpreted the fact that more than 5,000 Americans turned 65 every day as proof of unlimited growth in this apparently underserved market. This optimism spurred rapid development, mostly of rental communities. When these communities were completed, it quickly became evident that the profile of those who were attracted to the new projects differed considerably from demographic projections. Consequently, absorption fell significantly short of developers' (and bankers') expectations. We now know that seniors are not attracted to senior housing communities merely by their affinity with others of similar age. The market, in fact, is much more need-driven than developers anticipated: as health care and other services are more easily accessible to seniors in their homes, they are less likely to choose a senior community, and developers are now more cautious about their absorption projections.

There are many ways to estimate demand, including absorption rates of existing communities, demographic statistics sorted by an age and income threshold, the availability and cost of home health services, economics, lifestyles, and migration trends, to mention a few. It is advisable to define the target market for a community as specifically as possible by

age, income, and anticipated level of care on entry. The target might be, for example, upper-income active, middle-income frail, or affordable housing. The target market should also be identified by proximity to the community. For rural communities, the primary market may encompass a 15-mile radius; in a large urban setting, it might be limited to a 10-block radius. The project should be at least 80 percent justifiable by demand in the primary market area.

The pandemic disruption in all its forms continues to test and challenge the senior housing sector. It is also likely that society will face additional variants of existing diseases as well as new outbreaks in the future. But the level of agility, preparedness, and responsiveness among senior housing operators has never been higher and remains a tailwind for senior housing demand, as measured by the change in occupied stock.[2] Independent living and assisted living have experienced differential impacts. While the impact of the pandemic weighed heavily on assisted living, occupancy contraction remained relatively small in independent living. This is largely due to the difference in health status, where assisted living residents are generally more frail with multiple comorbidities and vulnerable to pressures from new diseases. During the height of the pandemic, many assisted living communities were closed to new admission, thereby generating a "pent-up" supply. This phenomenon could reflect a more rapid recovery since assisted living residents are more need-based, where independent living communities are more choice-based.

RESIDENT AGE AND INCOME PROFILES

The rapid expansion of the industry during the 1980s, primarily by for-profit developers, was built around the independent-living congregate model. These communities were attractive to seniors seeking alternatives to costly nursing home placement. The average entry age of 80 years was in sharp contrast to the 70-and-over demographic projections of early developers. Providers are now marketing these projects to the 75-and-over demographic profile.

Children who agonize over sending aging parents to nursing homes play a major role in the decision. According to a national study of 4,800 older adults conducted by James R. Lumpkin, of the University of Southwestern Louisiana, more than half (53.6%) of those living in senior housing indicated that a daughter helped make the decision to move, followed by a son (47.9%), spouse (34.2%), family doctor (17.1%), friend (17%), minister (12.2%), grandchild(ren) (10.5%), and sibling (10%).

Experience now shows that prospective residents are less attracted to the community itself than to the idea of avoiding a nursing home. Nursing home scandals have fed these concerns, but more often the core issue is the fear of a life sentence to mental and physical imprisonment; for many, the greatest fear is confinement to an institution in which they retain little control over their lifestyle. Lumpkin's qualitative focus-group research found that the senior housing industry "suffers an abysmal image" among elderly people owing in part to project failures, hardships created for existing or prospective residents, poor management of facilities, and lack of affordable products. Focus-group participants agreed that personal care and assistance in daily living were the most valued services a senior living community could offer.[3]

To qualify financially for rental communities, an individual should need to apply no more than 60 to 70 percent of his monthly income to the fees for an independent living community, or 75 to 80 percent for assisted living. The lower the financial prequalification percentage at entry, the easier it will be for residents to absorb increases in rent or service fees during their stay. Over several years in rental communities, residents may incur annual 5 percent increases.

Many homeowners who expect to finance their senior living with the proceeds of selling their homes may face a substantial shortfall. The example below assumes $100,000 net proceeds invested at 7 percent interest; this income will cover only about three months of service fees. Therefore, an additional annual income of $25,000 will be required to provide a safe margin for the new tenant. The income qualifier for the lowest rent at this project would be approximately $32,000 to $35,000 (see table 14.1).

Sales and marketing personnel need to understand the financial limitations of seniors on fixed incomes. The interest earned on cash or near-cash investments can drop significantly over the resident's tenancy, even as operational costs continue to escalate. Many residents routinely experience cash shortfalls of $400 to $600 per month. They are forced to finance their housing by tapping their principal, which in turn erodes their income-generating potential. Some are eventu-

Table 14.1   Income Qualification

Income qualification	Independent	Assisted living
Lowest rent assumption	$3,000	$4,500
Percent of income for housing and meals	60	80
Annual income requirement	$60,000	$67,500
Home sale net proceeds	$150,000	$150,000
Assumed safe interest rate on principal (%)	4	4
Additional income required from homeowner	**$54,000**	**$61,500**

ally forced to seek accommodation elsewhere, which can be unpleasant for residents and providers alike.

The majority of nonprofit providers offer endowment or equity models that offer a full range of health care services on a single site, giving residents access to progressive levels of care as they age in place and their needs increase. As seniors become more informed about living options, they are turning in growing numbers to this life-care concept, and it is also being embraced by for-profit developers and their financial partners. This scenario is confirmed by the growing reluctance of lending institutions to underwrite simple rental projects. Typically, life care attracts a younger prospect, averaging in the mid- to upper 70s at entry, as compared to the 80-year-old rental prospect. In endowment or entrance-fee projects, operators usually require a prospective resident's net worth to exceed twice the amount of the accommodation or entrance fee and the prospect's guaranteed monthly income to be at least equal to the total monthly service fee plus $500, or 1.5 times the annualized monthly service fee, or to have 30 or 35 percent of assets remaining after paying the one-time entrance fee. Some communities use a sliding scale, reducing the income qualification as the age of the applicant increases. Obviously, the amount of remaining assets required to cover the monthly fee depends on the amount of the fee and can be affected by the prevailing return on the resident's investments. Occasionally residents move into these communities and become financially insolvent. Usually this problem is handled through a resident hardship fund established by nonprofit sponsors or by allowing residents to draw against the refundable portion of their entrance fee.

The extent to which a prospect relies on the selling price of a home to fund entrance fees carries a great deal of weight for communities who charge advance fees. Some residents may have sufficient financial resources to finance the entrance fee without selling their home. It may be advantageous for them to transfer their assets to heirs who can inherit the home based on its stepped-up value rather than sell the home and pay the capital gains taxes on that increase in value. On the average, fewer than 50 percent of prospective residents need to sell a home to finance entrance fees.

ADMISSION POLICIES

Most newer senior communities are residential rather than institutional properties. To succeed, they must continue to be perceived as residences rather than as glorified nursing homes, which means that residents must be able to function fairly independently. Moreover, nobody is well served if a new resident turns out to require more care than the community or chosen level of service can provide. Most providers therefore establish medical criteria for admission to senior living communities. Usually, they require that the applicant be capable of independent living based on the evaluation of the medical director, who uses a confidential medical application completed by the applicant's personal physician. The application, together with a complete medical history, can be evaluated by the community's medical review committee. Frequently, the medical director will consult with the applicant's physician, or the executive director will conduct a personal interview with the applicant to assess her ability to live independently. Residents, physicians, and family members may misrepresent the applicant's abilities, even with the best-intentioned medical screening. Managers should be wary of family members who seem to be in a hurry to make the placement on their relative's behalf or who express an interest in signing an agreement before the applicant has even toured the community.

There have been several successful court challenges to medically based admissions policies. The courts have found that providers cannot deny admission on the basis of disability. The Americans with Disabilities Act (ADA) and the Fair Housing Amendments Act (FHAA) have implications for

senior living communities both on the resident's admission and during subsequent operations. Some attorneys believe that the ADA applies mainly to employment, because senior communities are not, in the meaning of the law, "public accommodations operated by private entities," except possibly for their health care facilities and some public areas, or communities that may lease space to outside businesses.[4] The FHAA allows people with selected health problems to be excluded from participating in the health care benefits of a community, but admission cannot be denied unless a person has a contagious disease "which can pose a direct threat to others." Renters can modify their own living units at their own expense to accommodate their special needs. But the operator can require the tenant to restore the unit to its original condition on the termination of residency and can require the establishment of an escrow account to provide for such restoration. The FHAA also states that covered facilities cannot deny or limit services, and their management cannot require residents to occupy a special section or floor. In fact, both acts require that communities make reasonable accommodations under rules, policies, practices, or services to afford equal opportunity to use the dwelling, including public and common use areas.

Many life-care providers offer amended residency agreements for frail prospects who may be attracted by affordable access to skilled nursing services. Usually, medical screening in senior living communities is not challenged by unsuccessful applicants if operators have made the effort to find an alternative solution or a more appropriate setting elsewhere. The key to avoiding legal disputes is to position the sales counselors and the management as problem solvers interested in finding the optimal level of care for prospective residents. Providers who represent themselves as advocates for the prospects and who take an interest in their well-being are rarely criticized for suggesting more appropriate settings.

Healthy residents may react negatively to the admission of frail prospects or be frightened by the sight of disabilities that remind them of their own vulnerability. Residents constantly remind the management that they were attracted to the community because of its active, independent image and accuse the sales staff of relaxing standards to generate sales. They will ask, "How can you attract younger, active residents to the community if you let in people who use wheelchairs or walkers?" Salespeople will even complain to the management at times that their prospects walk into the building, look at the frailty of the resident population, and tell them, "I'm not ready for this." These are among the most challenging issues for providers to deal with on a daily basis. They should keep in mind that residents must not be allowed to set the community's admissions standards and should endeavor to manage residents' (and prospects') perceptions and attitudes so that supportive devices are seen as tools allowing independence, not advertising dependence.

The toughest sales job is to convince a long-term resident of a rental community (and their family) to move to a higher level of care. Fortunately, most providers are able to handle these delicate issues with good family and physician counseling combined with naturally occurring peer pressure. After first passing through the denial and bargaining stages, most people eventually understand and accept the limitations of their deteriorating health. Providers must anticipate problems well in advance so that they can lay the groundwork for discharge or transfer with the resident, the family, and the resident's physician. In most states, continuing care retirement communities (CCRCs) require people to transfer to higher levels of care based on their needs as perceived by the management or the medical director, a policy that clearly violates the intent of the FHAA. It is not clear that there will ever be any rules to govern these situations because of their political sensitivity and the need for case-by-case assessment. Communities must establish their own criteria, which may change over the life of the project, to manage these sensitive issues effectively. Providers who can keep open communication channels will be most effective at avoiding legal proceedings, which could set precedents and ultimately limit their options.

Using various assessments to track a resident's functional status and meeting quarterly with the family or responsible parties can not only allow nursing to spot alarming trends and apply immediate interventions but also educate and sensitize the family to normal declines in functioning that they can expect and observe as their loved one's health challenges become increasingly complex. See chapter 17 for additional details on assessments and interventions.

MARKET PENETRATION AND ABSORPTION

The percentage of age- and income-qualified prospects in the primary market area needed to fill existing and proposed senior living communities to stabilized occupancy (95%), assuming that 80 percent of units are filled by prospects from the primary market area, is usually referred to as the *market penetration rate*. Statistics sorted by age, income, and zip code are available from actuarial firms such as the National Data Planning Corporation or Claritas. This information is primarily derived from census information and can be projected from historical growth in the area. These growth estimates can also be compared with projections by the local chamber of commerce. The number of gross qualified households should then be reduced by the number of existing competitors' units, regardless of their occupancy rates. The number of households should also be adjusted for competitors' units either planned or under construction. Planned units under construction can be discounted by the probable number of units to be built. The market penetration rate is calculated by dividing the total number of stabilized units in the primary market area into the *gross* number of income-qualified noninstitutional households.

The *project penetration rate* is calculated from the *net* number of qualified households after existing and planned competitive units have been deducted. Calculating the penetration rate helps to measure the degree to which the primary market is underserved or saturated. The higher the penetration rate, the longer the potential expected time to fill the community.

High penetration rates are not necessarily a wholly negative factor. They may indicate a well-educated and highly accepting market for senior living projects, and underserved niches that may still exist in certain market segments. Many investor services use the guidelines in table 14.2 for analyzing penetration rates.[5]

The penetration rate differs from the *market absorption rate,* which is the percentage of existing units in the primary market area that have become occupied over a specified period. A sample calculation of penetration rate is illustrated in table 14.3.

The *project absorption rate* is generally defined as the total number of months it will take for a project to reach stabilized occupancy, beginning with the first month the project is offered in the marketplace. This

Table 14.2   Analyzing Penetration Rates

Penetration rate (%)	Opinion
<5	Good
5–10	Some concern
11–15	Significant concern
>15	Material concern

Source: E. C. Merrigan, *Rating Guidelines for Nonprofit Continuing Care Retirement Communities*, Fitch Health Care Special Report, Fitch Investor Services, Inc., June 1994.

Table 14.3   Calculating Penetration Rates

(200 planned units; market area radius of 10 miles, sorted by zip codes)

Age bracket	≥75	70–74	65–69
Income qualifier	$35,000	$35,000	$35,000
Gross number of qualified households	3,122	4,132	6,594
Percentage absorbed, by age group	85	10	5
Age- and income-qualified prospects	2,653	413	330
Gross number of age- and income-qualified	3,396		
Less existing competitive units	450		
Less competitive units under construction	0		
Less planned competitive units	250		
Discount by	15%		
Anticipated number of planned units canceled	38		
Probable competitive units	212		
Net number of qualified households remaining	**2,734**		
Project planned units	200		
Stabilized occupancy (%)	95		
Percentage of units filled from primary market area	80		
Number of units supported by primary market area	152		
Penetration rate (%)	**5.56**		

includes the preopening period. Absorption can be equated to occupancy only if there was no sales activity before the project was ready for occupancy. As discussed earlier, acceptable absorption rates vary depending on the community size, capitalization, preconstruction marketing, and other factors. Therefore, caution should be exercised when comparing national absorption rates to site-specific performance.[6] Absorption in excess of double the national average could still fall considerably short of investment expectations.

The number of occupied units of a community expressed as a percentage of the total occupied units in the primary market area is referred to as the *market share*. This is simply a measure of the strength of each competitor in the primary market area. As additional participants enter the marketplace, the market share of existing providers decreases. Generally speaking, the greater the market share of an individual provider, the greater the opportunity to manage revenues and ultimately bottom-line profitability. Larger, well-established, good-quality providers can command an advantage in a limited marketplace with little competition. Many savvy owners watch market-share percentage closely. Downward trends of 10 percent or more can trigger a need for repositioning or remarketing to differentiate their product from the competition's.

OVERVIEW OF COMPETITORS

Comprehensive information on the market and industry is necessary for deciding how to approach a specific market strategically, operationally, and organizationally and to predict performance. Information about competitors in the primary market area enables a provider to identify the threats, opportunities, and likely future direction and responses of each key competitor and thus to improve a community's competitive advantage.

The competitor overview should include such information as location, year opened, percentage occupancy, owner or management company, entrance fee, number of units, and floor plan. Pricing information should be gathered by unit type and compared to your own community by monthly fee per square foot. If an inventory of apartments by unit type and occupancy can be gathered, then market preferences can be assessed, and strategies can be developed to market less-desirable unit types. In some cases, it may be possible to predict a competitor's financial performance and sensitivity to discounting prices.

Other useful information includes a comparison of each competitor's service package and amenities. The analysis should identify which services are included in the monthly service fee and which are billed separately. This information enables sales counselors to assist their prospects in identifying hidden costs and to analyze the value of each competitor's offering. The comparison should itemize the community features (art studio, swimming pool, wellness center, beauty salon, private dining, on-site rehabilitation, and the like) of each competitor.

Another essential component of the competitor overview is the collection of all promotional material. This information is most effectively gathered by a clipping service. These services will perform searches of all or a select number of publications in the local area or nationwide and are inexpensive in relation to the value of the information collected. Community brochures and other promotional material can be collected by employees, relatives, or even residents. In addition, it is useful to have a representative of the community attend competitors' special events or seminars to evaluate their effectiveness and presentation. Former employees of competitors are also an excellent and often untapped source of information regarding offerings and, more importantly, what may be missing.

The final component of the competitor overview is an analysis of the sales presentation at each competing community as well as your own. This can be accomplished through a "mystery shopper" visit, in which a representative of the community poses as a prospective resident. This common practice not only provides a valuable assessment of the sales skills of the competitor's marketing counselors but can also offer some insight into how they are representing your property to their prospects. Many companies routinely review their own staff with the same technique. Mystery shopping is best accomplished by someone with an eye for detail and an understanding of the sales process. Real estate agents or professional shoppers are the most objective and will perform this service for a reasonable fee. Some experienced sales counselors can detect a mystery shopper, but they may not know whether the shopper represents their own company or a competitor.

To make the most accurate assessment, the mystery shopper should arrange the tour and presentation with an official sales counselor, not the activity director or office assistant, and should ask how long the counselor has been employed at the community. She should assess first impressions and greeting, tour, close, confirmation, physical features of the property, and overall impression. It is also important to recognize that everyone can have a bad day: even if the competitor's presentation is unimpressive,

your sales representatives should not let down their guard. The information gathered should be compared to your community's performance, and strategies developed to strengthen your weak areas.

After collecting all pertinent information about the competitors in the primary market area, prepare a summary of the strengths and weaknesses of your community compared to all competitors. Specific strategies can then be developed for the overall marketing and sales plan and tailored to take account of the competitors' resources and strategies. Market and industry intelligence allows you to align your community's capabilities with the needs of the primary market area to ensure appropriate marketing funding, a coherent strategic vision, and realistic expectations.

PLANNING MARKETING

An effective approach to marketing must take the guesswork out of finding what works and what does not. The "shotgun" approach—test marketing a wide array of strategies, hoping that something will bring in prospects—often yields mixed results at best. Generally, seasoned, results-oriented professionals prefer a more targeted, statistically based approach.

The statistical approach employs the use of the lead-to-lease conversion-rate analysis for each type of advertising medium and marketing strategy. The lead-to-lease conversion rate is calculated by dividing the average new leads per month generated from each marketing strategy by the average gross leases or sales from those strategies. For example, a community with an average of 200 new leads per month from media placements with an average of 10 gross leases per month from those placements will have a lead-to-lease conversion ratio of 20:1. In other words, the community can expect one lease or sale for every 20 new leads. Note that sales are also generated from the site, resident referrals, and nonresident referrals. Each of these lead sources also has a conversion rate and should be considered separately when allocating marketing dollars. The inclusion of these other lead sources when calculating the community's conversion rate will inflate true marketing results.

To express the lead-to-lease conversion rate as a percentage, divide the lead-to-lease figure into 1 and multiply by 100 (in our example, $1 \div 20 = 0.05 \times 100 = 5\%$); see table 14.4.

Table 14.4   Marketing Conversion Rates

Lead-to-lease conversion rate	Conversion rate as percentage	Performance level
10:1	10	Excellent
15:1	6.7	Very good
20:1	5	Good
25:1	4	Fair
30:1	3.3	Poor

Table 14.5   Sample Annual Unit-Sales Forecast

	Number of units
Projected year-end occupancy, planning year	250
Projected year-end occupancy, current year	150
Gross unadjusted sales	100
Plus projected move-outs at 2 per month	24
Minus outstanding sales pending move-in	–15
Plus projected cancellations at 1 per month	12
Total annual gross sales required in the planning year	**121**
Units to lease or sell per month	**10**

Following this analysis, the strategies with the highest lead-to-lease conversion rates are allocated proportionally higher shares of the marketing budget. This approach allocates funding to the most efficient strategies first, with the remaining funds allocated to try new innovations or ideas that the marketing staff or management consider potentially effective. The lead-to-lease conversion rate is a combined measure of prospects' attraction to the type of medium and the perceived value of the service package, as well as the skill of the marketing staff at converting inquiries into sales. If the conversion rate seems low, each of these separate components must be evaluated and corrective measures implemented. The statistical approach can be refined each year as more information about the market is gathered.

Equipped with these statistical tools, the marketing planner can design a realistic marketing plan for an individual community. The plan should not be based on a single strategy, as conditions may change: a well-balanced approach that distributes the marketing budget among a variety of proven strategies is less risky. Ultimately, the marketing planner can become skilled at predicting the response to and conversion rate for each strategy, and marketing budget requirements can be forecast more accurately.

ANNUAL FORECASTS

Before developing any specific marketing strategies, the marketing planner needs to determine the number of units that must be leased and the corresponding volume of leads and leases required. The projected net occupancy for the end of the current year, based on current trends, needs to be estimated. Usually the owners establish the projected year-end occupancy for the following year. The difference between year-end occupancy next year and year-end occupancy during the planning years is the unad-

justed gross leases required during the year. The next step is to review the year-to-date move-out activity and use these data to project move-outs per month for the following year. The resulting figure is added as the first adjustment. Next, any outstanding sales pending move-in are subtracted, and, finally, projected cancellations are added to yield the total gross leases required. Table 14.5 shows an example of the annual unit-sales forecast.

A specific budgeted occupancy for the month implies that the budgeted number of units will generate full revenue for the entire month. If the community allows proration of rents and fees for midmonth move-ins or vacancies, additional sales may be required per month to offset these revenue losses.

The *annual lead forecast* calculates the number of new leads required in the planning year to achieve the forecasted gross leases or sales. To derive it, the lead-to-lease conversion rate for the current year should first be reviewed to determine whether it represents a realistic forecast for the planning year. To obtain gross leads needed in the planning year, the gross leases required are divided by the lead-to-lease conversion rate. For example, 121 gross leases required in the planning year × a 4 percent lead-to-lease conversion rate = 3,025 gross leads. Subtract from this number the existing active leads in the lead bank and add lead deletions to yield the total new leads required in the planning year. Table 14.6 details a sample annual lead forecast.

The marketing planner can now begin to develop specific strategies to generate these leads. Proper market positioning of effective collateral material should be designed to inform, create an image, be a tangible representation of the community and the owner, shape expectations, motivate the prospect, and ultimately

Table 14.6   Sample Annual Lead Forecast

Total annual gross leases or sales required in the planning year	121
Lease-to-lead conversion rate	4%
Gross leads required in the planning year	3,025
Minus active leads in lead bank	−1,000
Plus lead deletions (75 per month)	900
Total annual new leads required	**2,925**
Total monthly new leads required	**244**

create a dream. The development of effective marketing materials requires insight into the value systems and sensitivities of today's wary seniors.

■ UNDERSTANDING THE MARKET

The decision to move into a senior living community can involve many people (the individual's spouse, children, grandchildren, and friends), and it is emotionally charged and personal. Seniors and decision influencers have various opinions and biases about senior living. Marketers need to be aware of these biases and deliver messages that are sensitive to them.

To succeed with any target market, marketing planners must show that their community and its services reflect the values of that market. There has been a tremendous amount of research into the lifestyles and values of older adults. Although opinions differ, some general conclusions can be drawn. Seniors want to be seen as active, interested, and involved, and they see themselves as at least 10 years younger than their chronological age. Their anxiety about aging is closely connected with an aversion to the associated health complications which will eventually limit their personal freedom. They are looking for ways to live fuller lives and stay in control longer. They are generally private people, especially about their finances; they are comfortable with themselves; and they are more experiential and less materialistic than their children. They see themselves as morally conservative and intellectually liberal; they are more aware and educated than previous generations of seniors and consider learning to be a lifelong experience. With age, seniors often develop a greater interest in spirituality and altruism. They are among the greatest donors of time to volunteer causes. They are particularly interested in helping other, less-active seniors. They are spouse- and family-oriented, proud, and independent.

Seniors control more than 50 percent of the nation's discretionary income while constituting only 26 percent of the population. Although they have significant buying power, they are reluctant to exercise it. They are thankful for what they have and know the meaning of a dollar. They are particularly interested in passing on their assets so that their heirs will not face deprivation. And they live off their social security supplemented by interest generated by their investments.

The typical prospect is over 80, female (10% are men or couples), and needs assistance with two or more activities of daily living (ADLs). Prospects generally live within 10 miles of the community or have family who do; 50 percent are homeowners, and 83 percent of those homes are owned free and clear of any mortgage. They may be slightly confused, but they are clear about the danger of outliving their funds and about the escalating costs of health care and services. Most inquiries can be categorized into a desire for services, need for companionship and security, and access to health care as the individual's lifestyle needs change. Above all, they are interested in options and value. Seniors may want a high-value item, but they want to pay as little as possible to get it. They want a deal.

Seniors generally need the services and conveniences that a senior living environment has to offer long before they acknowledge that need. Usually, the decision to inquire about senior living alternatives is precipitated by a change in health or lifestyle—for instance, the loss of a driver's license due to failing eyesight, the death of a spouse or friend, or the onset of a degenerative medical condition. Prospects are typically under stress. The decision to move into a senior living community can be a long process. The earlier the prospect is contacted, the better, and frequent contact is important to the relationship-building process (see chapter 15).

The ultimate decision to move is generally made by the senior, but in 80 percent of cases it is strongly influenced by children and in-laws, particularly women. The average woman in the United States today will spend more time caring for her parents than for her children. Adult children may recognize the need for an assisted living environment long before their parents do. Unlike the parents, they are probably receptive to marketing messages. Family members can quickly see the benefits and value associated with the community; they will, however, worry about pressuring a parent to make a decision that might not work out and so will scrutinize the community's stability, reputation, and management. Adult children want to free themselves of the guilt surrounding their inability to be the primary caregivers in their parents' time of need. The decision among family members is rarely unanimous.

The decision-influencing adult child is typically a 45- to 65-year-old married female who lives and works in the area. She usually has children living at home, in college, or with families of their own; she may thus feel sandwiched between the needs of two generations. Such women are prone to guilt, sensitive to their own aging, and concerned with preserving their parents' estate and conserving their own funds.

When developing ad copy and collateral materials designed to attract seniors, marketers need to keep in mind that they are selling a lifestyle, not real estate. Ads should attract seniors' attention with pictures that tell a story, showing real people who are active and involved, people they might like to meet. The headline should state the benefit, and the copy should demonstrate it.

The ad should offer straightforward answers to common questions and concerns. Hard-hitting is good; mystical copy or overly subtle implications will fall flat. Clever is good; contrived is not. Fluff will hurt your credibility.[7] Seniors sense that if something looks too good to be true, it probably is. The single most important question for most seniors is whether the community will enable them to maintain independence, privacy, and control of their lives. They will reject ads that seem to offer a catered lifestyle, as the idea of being catered to implies a loss of control. Seniors are interested in fact-oriented material that shows a community where they can plan and choose their own activities and lifestyle.

Individually tailored marketing strategies require insight into the target market's awareness and understanding of your community. In spite of massive amounts of previous advertising, seniors may still be unaware of exactly who the community is and what services it provides. Or they may be aware of the community's existence but remain unconvinced that it will benefit them directly. The concept of senior housing is still widely misunderstood. Seniors may persist in thinking your community is some type of old folks' home for people with dementia.

A particular challenge for marketers promoting a community under new management may be the negative image of the project under the former management, especially if it failed for financial reasons. Whatever the case may be, the more completely and accurately marketers can identify market sensitivities and levels of awareness, the better equipped they will be to design strategies to address them.

The best way to understand the market is through research. Strategies include direct mail surveys and focus groups.

Focus Groups

A focus group is a small gathering of people in the target market who meet for an informal discussion about the likes, dislikes, fears, and motivations with which they approach the community. Separate focus groups should be made up of current leads, age- and income-qualified prospects, decision influencers, family members, residents, and even employees. Each group should be interviewed separately so that you can draw specific conclusions from each target audience. Having an outside consultant conduct the focus groups is likely to yield more informative results: people like to be helpful and, if community representatives are in charge, will tend to say what they think the management wants to hear. Conversely, they may be reluctant to express their concerns or criticism to the management for fear of misinterpretation or retaliation. Many people have now become very comfortable with video conferencing online from their homes using a platform such as Zoom or FaceTime. It is easier to recruit participants from these types of groups and at considerably less expense.

Prepare a list of the information you are seeking so that the discussion leader will cover all those topics during the session. The discussion might start with an icebreaking discussion about senior living communities, then probe for the group's awareness of each senior living community in the primary market area. Next, it might attempt to gauge the group's awareness of their own costs of living in comparison with what they think is offered at the community. The facilitator should describe the services and amenities of the community in detail and solicit specific reactions to each.

A slideshow, drone footage, or Video 360 tour of the community and models can set the stage for the next discussion, that of the associated costs. After the tour, the group should be asked to estimate the cost of living at the community. Most will overestimate, having just completed the exercise to determine their own current cost of living. At this point, the group should be developing a solid appreciation for benefits, services, and amenities the community offers and is primed to discuss the general pricing, along with the entrance fee, price comparison with the competition, fee increases, security deposits, nursing home deductibles, and other details. Specific reactions to every aspect of the financial package should be solicited. Then the positive features and opportunities should be brought up, as well as the challenges to marketing that the community may consider eliminating or neutralizing. The discussion leader might also start a discussion on the continuum of care and the choices the community offers for addressing residents' increasingly complex needs: for example, participants might be invited to discuss their concerns about accessibility of health care and their reactions to assisted living, home health care, and long-term care coverage.

At the end of the session, the location, physical features, ownership and management, services and amenities, and overall perceived value of the community should be evaluated by each group member privately then by the group. Finally, the discussion leader may choose to do a "trial close," asking under what circumstances the individuals would consider a move to the community and in what time frame. The leader should also ask them if their perceptions of the community changed as a result of the focus group, what they would tell others to convince them to move into the community, and what it would take to convince them. Discussions that take off in an unexpected direction are worth paying attention to. Participants may be expressing concerns and motivations that have not occurred to the management or marketing team. Videotaping the sessions can be informative for the management, as they provide documentation of the meetings and allow review and analysis of the group's response. Most videoconferencing platforms offer a recording option, but be sure to advise participants that the session will be recorded in case they choose to opt out. Reviewing each session with the discussion leader can serve as a basis for exploring sidetracks and refining subsequent sessions.

The discussion agenda can be tailored for different groups, but the objective remains the same: to solicit feedback on key attributes of the community while communicating its benefits and demonstrating its value. Not only will a well-planned and focused discussion provide critical information about the perceptions of the market, but it can also be a powerful selling tool. Many participants have been converted to residents through focus groups. Even for established communities, annual focus groups are valuable for gauging reactions to the community.

Surveys

Researching the target audience by survey allows polling of a much larger group and can help verify the accuracy of focus-group results. The survey should incorporate many of the questions from the focus group. A good survey opens with a screening question that prevents wasting time with people who are not the target audience. This should be followed with a simple but engaging question to get the respondent interested in completing the survey. Start with easy questions that can be answered quickly and suggest that the survey will be quick and easy to complete. Group like questions together in a logical manner. Save psychographic and demographic questions for the end, as many seniors are reluctant to provide this information and will do so only after they have already gone to the trouble of completing the rest of the survey. Questions about prospects' income should come last.[8]

MARKETING STRATEGIES

Advertising works by capturing attention, holding interest, luring the reader, prompting action, and leaving a lasting impression. Effective marketing materials include three main elements:

1. A thorough description of the product or service and its benefits
2. Testimonials from residents
3. Third-party reinforcement of your message, such as an endorsement from the Alzheimer's Association, a local geriatrician, or a satisfied family member

Develop a few good concepts and stick with them. Be patient: it may take some time for the market to absorb the message. Often there are no significant incremental results; only when media exposure has passed a certain threshold will responses start arriving in numbers.

Keep the advertising campaign consistent. Frequent changes in the message or appearance of new ads confuse the market and waste your advertising budget. Of course, if results are totally flat, more research and testing on senior prospects are warranted.

Plan the ad campaign around one idea. Ad copy should have a single objective and a single message. If the message needs reinforcing with other ideas, keep them in the background. If you have several messages, use a different ad for each one and run the ads over several weeks or months.

Never assume that you know what will appeal to seniors: they are not a monolithic market, and you can see the world only through the prism of your own experience. Base your advertising on the community's strengths and competitive advantages, then *test them* on age- and income-qualified prospects. Identify what distinguishes your community in the eyes of this audience and highlight those features. Although this process does not guarantee success, it may help you eliminate concepts and layouts that do not appeal to your market. Seniors usually know what they like and what they do not.

Online Marketing: Websites

The World Wide Web has become the main source of information for virtually every product and service. People who have access to a computer will look online for elder care options in their area more than they search any other source of information. Print media and professionals refer prospects to company websites to obtain additional information. Attracting good-quality, high-volume leads to your marketing department through a well-organized and user-friendly website is cost-effective and efficient. Your website is a virtual brochure and should demonstrate the community's mission and expertise while supporting your marketing plan and goals.

Online or web-based marketing is by far the most efficient, targeted, and economical method of reaching a large number of seniors. It allows you to control not only the message but also the level of exposure. More people search the internet now than ever before—almost 80 percent of Americans have a social media account. Web-savvy population demographics are continuously evolving to reach older and older populations as the internet expands and users age into it.

People are looking for services online all the time. This means there is a potential for them to find your business when they go looking. Many successful business owners will tell you that word-of-mouth advertising is the best advertising. Businesses are built on relationships; online marketing allows you to strengthen your relationship with existing families and referral sources and build new ones. When people search for a service on Google, the search engine results page (SERP) returns paid ads, organic (nonpaid) search results, Google's Business Profile listings, social media accounts, reviews, and information from other sites.

Effective websites feature a home page that allows the visitor to quickly discern whether the site is of relevance or interest. The community's home page should mirror its other advertising material in its look, message, and function and provide quick links to the company history, community locations, services offered, activity programs, a photo gallery, frequently asked questions, career opportunities, and contact information. The company history and mission pages should outline the company's philosophy of care and its core values as they relate to both residents and employees. For corporations with multiple locations, the site can feature a map with links to each community, along with photos and contact information. The "services offered" pages should detail what makes your community different from the rest. The care delivery setting, innovative approaches, and leadership in the field are all factors significant to decision makers. Most family members concerned with a parent living alone are keenly interested in seeing what sort of activities are offered. A sample calendar and photos of resident activities can help reassure everyone that Mom will have things to do that are much better than sitting home alone. Management profiles should focus on the managers' extensive qualifications for providing care and managing these types of facilities, not on how rapidly the company has grown or what financial milestones have been passed. In addition, it is useful to establish reciprocal links with suitable related sites by including a links page on your own site and asking to be included among the links on other relevant sites, such as those of the Alzheimer's Association, the Assisted Living Federation of America, and the National Association of Professional Geriatric Care Managers.

A virtual tour can be an effective way to give web visitors a look at the property. This is a sequence or panorama of photos that can be linked into an animated presentation to give the impression of walking around the property. It gives viewers a good idea of what to expect on the in-person tour and also gives out-of-town family members a look at the community. As with all promotional materials, it's a good idea to include endorsements from families and professionals.

To attract visitors from search engines (like Google), the site's descriptions and keywords should include a number of frequently searched terms that relate to your business. This is because every major crawler-based search engine uses link analysis in its ranking algorithms. The more meaningful and relevant the site's links, the higher its search engine rankings will be. Link analysis is not about popularity but rather about creating links to selected, good web pages that are relevant to your marketing efforts. Google Ads is effective because it allows companies to reach prospects who are actively looking for specific products and services by using keywords. Keyword searches can even be divided by intent to target the most motivated customers. Specific curated landing pages and ads are created to motivate those interested customers to click your links to redirect them to your website or specific pages. With pay-per-click (PPC) accounts, businesses can designate when and where their ads will appear in the search engine results page (SERP) with a varied cost depending upon popularity. This way the business only pays when a customer actually clicks through to your link. Google Analytics is a free service that tracks and reports website traffic. It can collect and analyze a website visitor's demographic, location, time on the site, bounce rate, engagement length and type, and other session statistics. It is a very valuable tool for market planners to determine which promotional and informational materials they post are attracting the most interest and engagement. This way future placements online can refine customer preferences over time to maximize return on investment for the money spent.

It is possible to track activity on the community's website to determine when, for how long, and how often it has been visited, which pages are most popular, which keywords or phrases were used to find your site, and which links attract visitors. This information can be useful in keeping your website responsive to areas of interest while at the same time evaluating the effectiveness of your advertising in directing people to the site. Most advertising agencies offer web design and development services. These professionals can ensure that the website efficiently displays a facility's features and benefits and ultimately leads the visitor to a guest book, which generates an email to the marketing department with appropriate contact information to appeal directly to the appropriate customer.

Having your business online is only part of the puzzle. Email marketing is one of the most effective marketing channels because it allows you to automate your communication so that your contacts are touched in a timely manner and with relevant information. Automation ensures that you are following up with the right people at the right frequency. Soliciting email addresses from prospect inquiries can supercharge your follow-up process. Emails should be sent about once a month with invitations to seminars and workshops, unit availability, or staff and community achievements. It should be designed to inform, motivate, excite, and build a sense of belonging.

Social Media

You can reach your target audience not only by advertising on search engine platforms but also on social media. People find your business online through search engines like Google or Bing, or social media platforms such as Facebook, LinkedIn, Twitter, Instagram, or even Yelp. The more exposure or "reminders" you can give your business, the more top of mind, the higher the likelihood that you will connect with someone who may be seeking out what you provide. The key to effectively advertising on social media is to choose the social media platform that your target audience frequents. In Facebook's news feed, you will be competing with friends, family, and local and world headlines. You will be able to respond to questions from potential customers, drive sales by letting people know about upcoming events and seminars, and increase awareness by posting content that your target audience may be attracted to and engage with by liking, commenting, or sharing. LinkedIn is a professional network that is great for business-to-business communications and recruiting staff.

Here you can share a video about a new program you are running, respond to support questions to solve issues, or drive action by sending people to your website for more information. Instagram is a highly visual network where people can see what's happening with your business. Here you can increase awareness and let people know about your events and accomplishments, respond to direct messages from customer responses, and also drive action by sending people directly to your website. Twitter is more of a public news feed of what's happening now. Twitter allows you to let followers know about other social media channels. You can respond to questions and drive action by letting followers know how to take advantage of specials and availability.

Social media helps you engage with people so that you can ultimately redirect them to your website. It also enables you to build a list of email addresses to send targeted and automated marketing messages.

Listings and Review Sites

There are a variety of websites that provide specific information about businesses. Sometimes these listings are automatically generated, or your customers may create them. You will want to take control of these listings by claiming them. This can be a simple as clicking to submit a request, then sending relevant information about your business. Once you have claimed the listing, you will be able to update the information and respond to comments and reviews. Google Business Profile allows you to claim the page on your business and provide accurate and compelling information about your story. Google Business Profile results appear on the righthand side of the SERP, which is a prime placement.

Many people use sites like Yelp to find businesses that other people have reviewed. Similarly, you can claim your Yelp listing and provide attractive information about your community. When you receive a family compliment about your community, it's a very good practice to send them a link to your Google Business Profile page and ask them to add a review while their experience is still fresh. The more positive reviews, the better. Families looking to tour a senior living community will often look it up on Google and read the reviews first to learn about existing customers' experiences. YouTube is also a great way to post your audio and video content. This site allows the user to create their own channel. Often families are hungry for content on how to deal with problems they are facing and want pragmatic and free advice to enable them to recognize the risks of aging and changes they are seeing in their loved ones. Providing narrated video presentations created from your senior seminar series PowerPoint presentations can help educate families and demonstrate your knowledge of these issues, while offering pragmatic solutions. My Caregiver Coach is one of these channels, with over 200,000 views and over 1,000 subscribers.[9] The channel also offers training videos for caregivers who work both in their homes and at senior living communities.

Blogs

Families often begin researching information about senior living options after their loved one has experienced a serious medical challenge, been diagnosed with dementia, or observed to be struggling with hygiene or meal preparation. They will often turn to the internet to research specific topics. When you are producing the type of content that your audience is searching for you will have more people finding it and sharing it with others, all which leads them to your website. Content online is king. Search engines will find your content, which can result in free traffic to your website without going through pay-per-click (PPC). A blog is an easy way to post your content on a regular basis. If the content is good enough, people will subscribe to it and be alerted each time you post new material. If you host a blog without promotional material, the visitor to your blog will see you as an information source and even a public service. My blog called *The One Minute Caregiver* was specifically created to respond to continuous questions on senior lifestyle and aging related topics from families.[10]

All online advertising is intended to create opportunities for you to connect, experience, entice, and engage people who are searching for or interested in your services. When your connections engage with you on social media, forward your emails, or share your content with their contacts, each of those interactions creates more visibility for your community.

Magazine Advertisements

Like social media, magazines are highly psychographically targeted. Numerous magazines with large readerships, such as *AARP,* published by the AARP seniors' association, are targeted specifically to seniors. In fact, *AARP* boasts a readership that exceeds that of *Time*, *Newsweek*, and *U.S. News and World Report* combined! Unfortunately, their advertising rates are prohibitive for the typical senior living community. Local senior publications, church bulletins, hospital newsletters, and financial or real estate magazines can all be effective outlets. Like newspapers, most magazines know exactly the profile of their readership, so it is worth doing some research to learn which publications have the greatest circulation among your target audience.

Although magazines can be expensive, they can also be one of the best ways to reach a highly selective target market. As a general rule, you can expect to receive 90 percent of your total responses within three weeks when advertising in monthlies.

The reproduction capabilities of most magazines are high. The layout or picture that disappointed you in the newspaper will look better here than in any other print media. Detailed photographs of the community interiors or exterior lend themselves nicely to magazine advertising.

Ads in a local tourist magazine can effectively target the out-of-town decision influencer who may be in town for a local convention. Other events that attract decision influencers and seniors are golf tournaments and estate and Medicaid planning seminars.

Magazines typically require a much longer lead time than newspapers: the material must be prepared and ready for press months ahead of time. Planning is thus critical. Production costs can also be expensive: whereas newspapers generally provide some assistance in putting an ad together, magazines require camera-ready artwork or computer files.

Space in periodicals is usually sold in fraction-of-page units, such as full page, half page, quarter page, half column, and quarter column. Most rate cards translate the page unit sizes into actual ad size. Discounts may be available based on the season, frequency of insertion, or amount of advertising purchased. Some media buying services establish umbrella contracts under which they reserve space with given publications and can offer discounts even for one-time ads. The *Standard Rate and Data Service* (SRDS) research covers radio, television, direct mail, advertising and magazine rates, circulation figures, and general coverages. Top US ad agencies use SRDS for their media campaigns, searching among 125,000+ media properties, categorized by media type, market, and geography. It also specifies whether special geographic inserts or customization are available. Some magazines feature a classified section with its own rate structure.

Guidelines for magazine ad placement mirror those for newspaper advertising. The closer to the front of the magazine and the more visible the ad, the better. Research has shown that an ad in the first seven pages of a magazine produces a significantly better response than the same ad in the back half, the only exception being the back cover. For insert cards, too, the best position is closest to the front. "The pull of position is as inexorable as the pull of gravity."[11]

Advertisement in Business Directories

People who use directories have already made up their minds about the benefits of senior housing and are psychologically ready to be convinced.

The challenge, then, is to purchase an ad that is larger or more attractive than a competitor's ad but not larger than you need. The ad should cover just the facts, preferably in bullet format. The senior housing industry lends itself well to larger display ads, which are competitive, attention grabbing, and aimed directly at the needs and questions of the potential resident and his family. A boldface listing or a listing that gives extra lines within a regular listing, surrounded by a border, may be all that is required to differentiate one community from the competition.

Choosing a listing category can sometimes be important. Competitors usually list their ads under "Retirement." Rather than listing your community in other categories, such as nursing or assisted living, you might be able to get a cross-reference in each and thus avoid paying for three separate ads.

Specialty directories, such as *The Source Health Care Directory*, published by Data National Corporation, list local health care resources intended for use by physicians and therapists. These are usually inexpensive to advertise in and allow exposure to potential professional sources of referrals. Professions, associations, and special interest groups also publish directories for their members, who can be highly targeted. Many accept only standard listings, but some allow display ads. Check rates and circulation to determine cost effectiveness.

Radio and Television Advertisements

Radio and television advertising can promote interest in senior living, as long as they reach the target market. It requires a large enough budget, however, to present your message to the target audience at least three times within a week to expect any response. Some communities have successfully used this medium to advertise the opening of new developments or additions to currently established communities.

Radio advertising is relatively inexpensive, and stations may offer seasonal or frequency discounts. Seniors generally find one or two radio stations that provide the type of programming they enjoy and stick with them for years. Most radio stations provide assistance with ad production and offer suggestions about copy and content of the ads. In addition, they identify specific time slots when the target audience is likely to be listening. It is best to determine the time of day that attracts most of your target audience and concentrate your spots at that time. This way, you are likely to reach the same individuals each time rather than different sets of ears at various times of the day.

The major disadvantage of radio is that it does not have a shelf life: listeners are not afforded the opportunity to sit back and evaluate the details. Radio also tends to be regarded as a background medium. Listeners generally do not give it their undivided attention, as they would a direct mail piece or a newspaper insert.

Radio advertising time is usually sold in spots, with a premium charge for popular time slots. The SRDS has separate volumes for radio and television that describe the area of coverage, the format of each station, and rates. Drive time, during morning and afternoon rush hours, is usually the most expensive time to advertise, followed in order by daytime, evening, and overnight. Most seniors are early risers and typically listen to the radio in the kitchen over breakfast and lunch. Because breakfast falls within the most expensive drive-time slot, advertising during lunch may be the most cost-effective. In addition, adult children may hear lunchtime ads while listening at their desks.

Many radio stations offer sponsorships for specific program features such as the weather, news, health watch, and the like, which for a slightly higher rate will lead people to associate the community's message with regular programming they enjoy and may also generate goodwill for its support of the program. Sponsorships of National Public Radio programs such as *Here and Now* and *All Things Considered* on local PBS affiliate stations have been especially productive.

As with print advertising, radio ads must be produced with the physical needs of the target audience in mind. As we age, and particularly after the age of 40, we lose hearing acuity. Radio spots aimed at seniors should use speech that is clear, undistorted, and presented without competing noise. They should avoid the use of background music, rapid speech, or special effects.[12]

Many talk radio stations are always looking for content that would interest their audience. Especially if you are advertising with the station, they are often receptive to bringing you in for a live interview regarding some topic of general interest to seniors or their families. Don't worry, you can prepare for this in advance and supply the host with a list of questions to ask you that you are prepared to respond to brilliantly! This is a great way to highlight your expertise in the field and build rapport with an audience that may already be searching for your services. Posting a recording of your interview on your website or social media platform can increase your electronic footprint online while building credibility and demonstrating your commitment to serve the senior population and create new connections and inquiries.

Television differs from radio in that it is a prestige medium. Television advertisers are perceived by viewers as significant entities, and the audiences are large. In consequence, television advertising is very expensive and may not always be cost-effective. Although seniors tend to watch TV frequently and may schedule their meals around favorite programs, only the largest of senior living communities can afford to produce and air a broadcast TV ad, and then only for new developments or grand openings. Some cable stations offering programming that may be specifically targeted at seniors may have more affordable rates.

Many of the recommendations for radio and print advertising apply to television as well. Keep the message short, sticking to the facts. Show the interior and exterior of the community, particularly garden areas, and people who look like they might be fun to get to know. Resist the temptation to use special effects. Seniors do not respond well to cute or clever messages. Stick with what you know will work or, better yet, try out your spots on a test audience.

Pick one format for your TV and radio advertising and stick to it. Using the same style of graphics or the same audio format helps people recognize your ads quickly. One effective radio campaign featured a 10-year-old boy who described his frequent visits to his great-grandfather in a senior community. The spots were aired on a news/talk radio station on which most listeners would not expect to hear a young voice. The ads grabbed attention and triggered numerous inquiries each time they ran. They told a continuing story about life in the community, much as the successful Taster's Choice coffee ads on television did. The campaign was so well thought out that it inspired a following among listeners.

Direct Mail

In many markets, direct mail can be a great lead generator. It has good shelf life as people who think they might need it someday tend to hold on to these mailing cards. With the types of advertising discussed so far, the costs are largely determined by the medium. Using direct mail, the advertiser controls the expense (generally expressed as cost per thousand pieces) by designing the mailing and deciding on the size and frequency of the distribution.

The greatest advantage of direct mail is that it can be precisely targeted. Mailings can be tailored to a specific age- and income-qualified audience, even specific neighborhoods. The main disadvantage is the average cost. A high cost per thousand to reach the qualified target market will be justified, however, if the responses are converted into sales at a higher rate than responses from alternative, less expensive forms of advertising.

Three main types of list are used for direct mail campaigns. House lists, the marketer's own leads, are the community's most valuable asset, although they never appear on the company's balance sheet. These individuals are presumably already age- and income-qualified and are likely to be categorized by interest level. The lead bank is often neglected as marketing representatives look for fresh leads to work, but these leads have already been bought and paid for, and can represent an investment of $100 to $300 each. Responses from the lead bank are generally better qualified and generate higher conversion rates, especially from prospects who contacted the community through its website (see below). Direct mail is also a good vehi-

cle for resurrecting old leads. A high response may indicate that the sales staff is deleting leads too quickly.

Families of current residents are important sources of referral and should be included in any direct mail campaign. It is also a good idea to send the families a monthly postcard announcing events at the community that they might enjoy, such as speakers, seminars, or entertainment, and any community newsletters.

Next in importance after those who have responded to your promotional efforts are those who have responded to someone else's targeted efforts. These are the mailing lists of other companies or organizations, such as the local Retired Senior Volunteer Program (RSVP), a hospital mailing list of senior consumers, patient lists from local optometrists or gerontologists, elder law attorneys, geriatric care managers, and long-term care insurance vendors, and even a list of seniors from the state's department of motor vehicles. Many will gladly trade lists with you. These may all be sources of individuals who match your psychographic criteria.

In addition, thousands of mail-order lists are available from firms targeting senior hobbyists and their adult children. These lists are commonly rented through mailing list brokers. Usually the people on the list have a history of responding to direct-mail appeals. List brokers do not own these lists; rather, they act as agents for many companies who rent their lists for a fee. These lists cannot be photocopied or be used more than once without extra payment.

The mail-order list of names is generally the poorest producer of responses, but the best for potential volume. Compiled lists come in a great variety and are generally developed from several sources. They can be sorted by zip code, age, income qualification, and other criteria. Sometimes large lists are merged from a number of sources; a sophisticated list developer should be able to eliminate duplicate names. Information gathered from such lists is reliable most of the time. But many nuances exist, such as a widow who continues to use her deceased husband's name to protect her anonymity but may be offended by receiving mail addressed to him.

With the rising cost of postage, it is increasingly important to target direct mail to the best-qualified prospects. Although many communities mail to their own lead banks, few investigate the option of using others' house lists and may choose to mail to a compiled list instead. Planning a direct mail campaign to allow for the use of bulk mail and designing the piece to conform to post office size standards can help reduce postage costs. Check with the post office regarding the insertion of appropriate barcodes in the address fields, and make sure that the address panel is correctly positioned for post office optical reading equipment. Pieces that jam the equipment or require manual repositioning incur extra charges.

Direct mail pieces can range from postcards to multiple-piece packages. Postcards, which can be effective and inexpensive, are suitable for mailing to a compiled list. They can be of high quality and can include a response coupon. Response rates can be increased and interested prospects identified with the offer of a low-cost incentive to those who return the coupon: for instance, a free informational brochure or article, such as a guide to planning a move, selling a home, or conducting a yard or tag sale. Seniors like to send away for free information, particularly if it applies to their personal situation. This piece must be of good quality, as it represents the community. Postcards can also be used as coupons: the prospect is asked to bring the card to the community to receive a free gift or handout—along with a tour, of course. It is a good idea to put an expiration date on the offer to prompt a response. Postcards are not appropriate for communicating complicated information. When announcing a grand opening, special event, or seminar, however, they can't be beat.

A self-mailer is a brochure (usually number 10 size) that is folded so that the recipient's address can be printed on the back, thereby eliminating the need for an envelope. An 8×8-inch tripanel brochure can double as a direct mail piece and community brochure. The size allows ample space to communicate your message while still fitting nicely into a presentation folder. Folding can be done by machine, which eliminates costly labor. Self-mailers can be multicolored or one color and can include a reply card or other insert. Single-sheet flyers are an effective and cost-saving alternative to more elaborate, professionally printed brochures.

Consider seeding your direct mail list with staff or corporate addresses so that the community can receive and track the mailings of organizations with whom you may have shared your list or who "borrowed" it from you. Finally, it is a good idea to send each direct mail piece to your home address to track delivery time. Bulk-rate postage can legally sit in each post office on its journey for up to three days, and this can be an important consideration for time-sensitive material.

Newsletters and Email

When the staff of senior communities are respected and trusted by residents and their families, they may find themselves being consulted on many aspects of aging and related issues: the tax deductibility of assisted living costs, the liabilities of hiring a home companion, depression, nutrition, dealing with guilt and stress, recognizing changes in a loved one's condition, Medicare and Medicaid, and insurance coverage for prescriptions. This relationship is worth nurturing not only for the satisfaction and reassurance it gives current members of the community but also for its value as a marketing resource.

One effective way to share information and present the community's staff as a valuable and reliable source of expertise is through a regular newsletter. In one example, a two-page newsletter that was developed to educate several hundred families is now emailed as a PDF file to a list of more than 3,000 subscribers! Not only is the newsletter distributed to families who in turn forward it to their friends and relatives, it is also sent to all networking contacts and referral sources as a resource for their clients. These contacts include geriatricians, geriatric care managers, hospital outplacement staff, clergy, elder law attorneys, counselors, case managers, social workers, therapists, and other health care professionals. These are the professionals who influence seniors or make care decisions on their behalf. The newsletter must be positioned as an information source distributed as a community service, and accordingly it should contain no advertising. It must be viewed as totally objective and not a platform for selling. At the same time, it should be clearly identified with the community through its name and logo.

People will be more likely to read a newsletter, whether in print or electronic form, if it meets the following criteria:

■ *Informative:* The newsletter should cover topics of interest to a wide audience of those dealing with elder care issues. The information should be concise, to the point, and well researched and documented.

Most people tend to skim newsletters, so critical points should be highlighted and articles kept brief, not exceeding two pages. The key to keeping subscribers is to make each newsletter predictably relevant, so that people anticipate good-quality information and take the time to read it when it comes.

■ *Purpose driven:* The newsletter should be presented as a community service and not an advertising gimmick. It should indicate that it has been created in response to family inquiries and aims to benefit other readers as well.

To survive, newsletters need to give users specific information that helps readers—whether family members or professional advisers—resolve the elder care issues of their loved ones and clients. A newsletter that fulfills this purpose will be widely read by subscribers and shared with others. This trickle-down effect is a key component of the community's overall marketing strategy.

While referrals are a critical part of successful marketing and sales, they are often also the most challenging aspect. Referral building can be time-consuming as well as tiring, and targets of such efforts are likely to be courted by competitors as well. A regular newsletter allows the community to deliver its name and message to thousands of potential referral sources every month without sending its marketing representatives out pounding the pavement. The company is "in their face" in a highly desirable and distinctive way, providing an altruistic community service. A good newsletter is a marketer's dream, providing top-of-mind brand recognition that increases issue by issue while leaving the marketing staff free to focus on what they do best. The company is positioned as an elder care advocate in the larger community, and this advocacy will yield referrals and help people make informed choices.

Although some segments of the target audience may still need or prefer to receive the newsletter in printed form, email is by far the most efficient means of distribution. Sources of email addresses can include business cards exchanged while networking, people who visit the community's website, people who inquire through senior resources guides distributed widely in the community, referral sources whose clients give their email addresses when requesting information, directories published by industry advocacy groups (such as the Register of Clinical Social Workers), and hospital discharge planning departments (who will share their lists if you ask for them and demonstrate the value of the newsletter).

The power and reach of email are also increasingly becoming its drawbacks. Information overload and the fear of spam can deter users from subscribing to email newsletters. And once a newsletter arrives in the user's inbox, it may be deleted by a spam filter before ever being read. Moreover, if users perceive that a subscription may generate unwanted email, they will unsubscribe. The fight for inbox survival therefore leaves room for only the most useful, highly targeted newsletters. But your newsletter has a future if it can establish a relationship with users and continually deliver benefits.

Newsletters, of course, do not write themselves, and budget consideration should be given to the associated costs of researching, writing, and editing the monthly articles. In addition, email subscriptions need to be kept current and maintained to eliminate duplicates, add new subscribers, and allow readers to unsubscribe. These features can be automated on the sponsor's website or can be contracted out to a vendor who specializes in newsletter production and email distribution.

Special Media

Nontraditional forms of advertising, such as outdoor advertising, transit advertising, posters and displays, community vehicles, and even business cards and letterhead, may have a place in a community's marketing plan. These types of visual media can create a vivid image of your community and establish your logo and colors in the minds of the general public. Such advertising can usually be done well at minimal cost and provide a wide degree of flexibility.

People are rarely prompted to buy after seeing a billboard or logo; rather, these sources provide exposure for the community and familiarize the general public with its existence. They are the least demographically targeted and can sometimes be a turnoff: billboards, for example, may be perceived as environmentally insensitive. In some markets, billboards can really drive walk-in traffic. They are also useful to announce a newly developing community, program, or service the facility is offering.

One important advertisement is the entrance sign to the community. This is effectively the property's business card. An elegant sign that is easy to read by day and by night can speak volumes about what is inside and the financial stability of the organization. An entrance sign that is in bad repair, dirty, full of birds' nests, or covered with weeds is unlikely to attract prospects. The colors used in a sign should complement the community's business colors, logo, and even interior design. The Equal Housing Opportunity designation must be included somewhere on the sign, as required by law.

Temporary sign or "A" boards that invite passersby for a tour of the community can boost your walk-in traffic, particularly in new developments where the locals have watched the community being built and are curious about the end result. Banners and flags can also attract attention. Especially in townships with restrictive signage regulations, a large mailbox with your logo, a descriptive banner, "Open" flag, or a flagpole flying the American flag above the company flag will let people know who you are and usually circumvent these restrictions. Mailbox posts can be fitted with a waterproof brochure holder, such as those used by realtors to hold fact sheets or brochures. You may get a lot of tire kickers, but often it takes only one referral to make a sale.

Marketing Events and Seminars

Active seniors are often seminar junkies, and they love a good party. Many newly opened communities organize marketing events to attract prospects to the community. These events can be expensive to produce: the combined cost of equipment, supplies, and food can easily top $10,000. Marketing events can be useful to introduce the community or to celebrate anniversaries or reaching occupancy thresholds, but they rarely lead to sales. Usually the marketing staff is so preoccupied with producing the event that there is little time to visit with prospects. The sales staff, too, is often involved with planning these events, which takes away from valuable sales time. Marketing events should be carefully planned, and their value analyzed and compared with alternatives.

All major parties (other than the grand opening) should be limited to the top 50 most likely prospects. This limit will minimize the disturbance to the current residents, keep freeloaders out, and allow salespeople at least some opportunity to mingle with the guests. Although they may recognize the need for some sales events, residents can sometimes feel as though the activity budget is being spent on marketing rather than on them.

Seminars, by contrast, are inexpensive to produce and can be designed to attract a specific audience. The seminar curriculum can be developed by the executive director and marketing staff to encourage prospects from the lead bank to visit the community and meet existing residents. The residents often welcome the opportunity to help host these events and are receptive to the concept. They see value in these seminars for themselves and often invite friends living outside the community to attend. To promote public awareness of the facility and educate the elderly and their families to key health-related topics, monthly seminars throughout the year can be conducted, covering subjects such as the following:

- Senior nutrition
- Senior fitness and exercise
- Podiatry and foot care
- Understanding and managing cholesterol
- Skin cancer awareness
- Women's or men's issues
- The many faces of dementia
- Long-term care insurance
- Medicare eligibility and coverage
- Medicaid planning
- Wills and estate planning
- Trust planning

Guest speakers can be engaged to deliver these talks on a pro bono basis. They may be local professionals interested in doing business with the resident population. Light refreshments should be served. Attendees can be encouraged to tour the community and meet the residents. Programs such as these can draw large crowds, especially if advertised with a direct mail flyer, and the cost is minimal. If well managed, they can position the community as the hub of senior activity and education in the local community. These seminars can also be recorded, or the presentation saved with narration and added to your social media platform.

Resident Referrals

Resident referrals are your greatest marketing tool. There is no recommendation more reliable than one from a satisfied customer. Residents and their families will represent the community favorably to their friends if the following conditions are met with some consistency: (1) the service package matches their expectations and the promises of the sales representatives, (2) the management is consistently fair in its treatment of residents and employees, (3) the owners are viewed as stable and fiscally responsible, (4) fee increases are generally in line with the health care cost of living and those of competing communities, and (5) the food is good. Residents will tolerate reasonable fluctuations in most of these categories and will generally give the management the benefit of the doubt. But if you miss the mark on any one of these criteria consistently or if residents begin to identify a negative pattern, referrals will come to an abrupt end. Herein lies the symbiotic relationship of operations and marketing. Operations depend on marketing to fill the building and cover attrition. Marketing can succeed in doing so only if operations can deliver on the promises made, either real or implied. To that end, the management should remind all employees that marketing is ongoing and that every time they provide a service to a resident, they are in effect making a sales presentation.

The typical senior living community evolves through several stages from first opening to stabilized occupancy, starting with blind optimism on the part of the developer through to the euphoria of the grand opening, then on to operational "can do," followed by marketing panic, investor panic, and finally the reality of balancing everyone's objectives. The number of resident-referred leads should increase as the community reaches stabilized occupancy, then stabilize or even fall off.

During the fill-up stage of the project, the excitement and energy generated by the marketing department usually spread through the community. Residents see their community promoted in the media and may even be the subject of media coverage themselves. During this period, they usually encourage their friends and acquaintances to visit. The management needs to learn to anticipate residents' needs and increase their variable expenses, such as staffing and food services, slightly ahead of new resident demand. It should resist the temptation to shower the first move-ins with attention, as that attention will have to be diluted as the community fills, leaving the early residents feeling discounted and resentful.

If the management consistently delivers the service that residents expect, referrals should continue to grow as occupancy approaches capacity. Resident referrals may fall off in mature communities with a very old or frail population because of resident apathy or lack of friends outside the community. Ultimately, however, a well-run, stabilized community should be able to rely on 15 to 20 percent of its new leads coming from referrals (for assisted living, this number should be closer to 50 percent).

Many communities offer financial incentives for residents' referrals. Small rewards may be appropriate, but large incentives may erode the perceived value of your services or even cause alarm. This strategy can also backfire on the resident who encourages a friend to move into a community that subsequently suffers from operational or financial difficulties. If you do offer financial incentives to your residents for referrals, be sure to include a reminder on the monthly statement.

Assuming that residents remain satisfied with the community and its services, there are many ways to market to your residents internally at little or no cost to the community. Test resident satisfaction with surveys of the operations, referral surveys, and resident focus groups. (See chapter 6 for more information on developing, conducting, and interpreting resident surveys.) Establish resident-referral goals and spread the responsibility for their solicitation to the executive director, resident relations staff, and other employees. Offer guest passes for residents to bring their friends to lunch or coffee, or allow them to use meal credits for qualified guests. Form a resident marketing committee to test marketing concepts and solicit advice on how referrals can be generated. Develop contests with incentives between salespeople and other company communities. Develop doorhangers to kick off resident-referral contests or raffles. Develop your own attractive change-of-address cards that new residents can send to their friends. Using flyers and monthly reminders in the newsletter or activity calendar, explain to the residents how referring their friends increases companionship, occupancy, and financial stability in the community. Let them know that resident referrals are the least expensive way to market the community—a task that their monthly fee supports. Offer special distinction to residents who have given referrals, such as special meals or wine with dinner, a corsage or lapel pin, personalized note cards, or a small donation to their favorite charity. Use their photo and testimonial in your ads or direct mail pieces if appropriate. Another good source of resident referrals is direct mail to the clubs and organizations they belong to outside the facility or to a directory from their former apartment building. Many senior apartment buildings have evolved into naturally occurring retirement centers (NORCs) and can be a bonanza of new leads.

Most important, simply ask the residents for their referrals or ask what you can do to earn them. Many residents do not see themselves as a potential source of referrals. Teach them to recognize their sphere of influence.

Public Relations

Positive journalistic coverage of the community is free promotion from a trusted source that validates the image the marketing department works to project. Establishing a symbiotic relationship with the local press is the first step in earning publicity. Most editors are constantly looking for newsworthy stories of general interest to their readers. Your public relations program should be designed to disseminate information through the news media to increase public awareness of the existence and benefits of the community.

Employee stories featuring a new hire, a promotion, an unusual accomplishment, or an act of valor in an emergency are always worth notifying the press about. Changes such as opening a new wing or adding services—home health, long-term care, or the opening of a specialty store or delicatessen—help to keep the community's image fresh.

Resident marriages and anniversaries are popular subjects, as are stories about a resident's accomplishments or continued contributions later in life. Generally, anything out of the ordinary that underscores the abilities and independence of seniors makes for good reading for other seniors and their families. Organize a panel discussion with the National Council on Aging and invite residents or local spokespeople to participate. Involve the local media when a resident receives an award or recognition for contribution to local service organizations or charities. Or organize your own Senior Hall of Fame program and seek nominations from senior groups and organizations who would like to honor seniors for contributions to the community at large.

Create your own news by hosting special events. One community in Dallas hosts an annual gingerbread-house competition through the local chefs' association. The houses are auctioned off, and the proceeds go to needy seniors in shared housing. Tap into the creativity of the activity program to promote intergenerational programs, senior fitness clubs, aquatic aerobics, volunteer programs, or programs that coincide with hot topics such as recycling and nutrition. Also consider a joint project with nonprofit groups such as Senior Olympics or host a senior costume contest. Nonprofit groups usually attract more attention in the media than for-profit groups. Some residents have been volunteering and fundraising for organizations their entire life. Steering resident activity toward fundraising in town for favorite causes can provide the residents with a very meaningful opportunity to continue their advocacy but also communicate to the general public that seniors at your community remain active and engaged in their community even after they move into assisted living. For example, a local animal shelter brought many of their animals to the community for an adoption fair which was newsworthy and highly successful. Frequent announcements of seniors giving back to their community and enjoying life can have a big impact on families who care for their isolated loved ones at home.

The best publicity comes from events that offer visual interest. The newspaper may not have a lot of space available or want to assign a reporter to a story, but they will often send a photographer if there is something worth seeing.

The best way to pitch a story about the community to the press is through the editor who usually handles the type of story that you propose. Stories that feature residents celebrating their hundredth birthday, intergenerational programs with schoolchildren, or seniors serving their community usually make it into print. A public relations office should have already laid the groundwork with local editors, but if not, simply call the organization's switchboard and ask for the appropriate editor. Summarize your story idea or upcoming event in a fact sheet or press release and review it briefly with the editor over the phone. Always follow up in writing and check in by phone just before the event. The fact sheet should cover just the facts: the who, what, why, where, and when of your story. Always include contact information.

A survey of newspaper editors identified seven factors that most often prevent them from using material from press releases: the information is not newsworthy, the release contains too much advertising fluff, the information is not of local interest, the release arrived too late to be used, the release is too long and cumbersome, the release is poorly written, or the contact listed is not accessible. Anticipating the needs of the editor can go a long way toward getting stories into print. Stories issued as "mat releases" are more likely to be picked up by smaller community newspapers. This ready-to-use article format is used by thousands of community newspapers across the country that do not have sufficient staff to produce all their material in-house.

If you have an employee who writes well, take advantage of the press release to tell your story in detail. Do not be overly concerned about using the right journalistic style, as reporters rewrite most press releases anyway. It is a good idea, however, to ask for the opportunity to review the final copy for accuracy and presentation so that it conveys the intention behind the story. Essentially, the press release paints a portrait of your fact sheet.

To improve the chances of a press release's being used, follow the commonly accepted format. Place your name and phone number in the upper right corner and the name and title of the editor in the upper left. Give your story a short, descriptive title in all caps and include a release date. Double-space the copy with one-inch margins, and add "more" at the bottom of the page if the story is longer than one page. Write the release with the goals of stimulating interest and generating inquiries. If the story is rejected, it may be worth pitching it again from a different angle.

Newspapers prepare editorial calendars that plan feature articles well in advance. Ask for a copy early in the year so that you can offer timely and appropriately targeted submissions.

Any event, advocacy, performance, seminar, or historical event is a chance to increase awareness on all of your social media platforms. Promoting the events online can help drive participation at your community, and videotaping activity and entertainment segments demonstrates to the community that things are going on at your community.

Community Outreach

A senior living community is an integral part of the neighborhood and depends on the support of local businesses and professionals to communicate its reputation; they, in turn, benefit from the custom of the residents and their guests. The community outreach program should be designed to generate continuous referrals from the various interest groups and agencies who have regular contact with the community's target market.

Community outreach is often a two-way street. Not only are you attempting to disseminate information in the local service area, but you are also aiming to refer residents to local resources who can provide superior services to elderly people. One of the best approaches is to create a directory of senior services in your community. Contact all the potential senior resources in your community and invite them to participate. Most will gladly cooperate and may even offer to help underwrite the directory by purchasing an ad. The background research involved will give you great insight into the business and professional community, provide a reliable source of information about senior services for both seniors and their relatives, and encourage referrals to your community.

Any community outreach effort should be organized and thorough. Start by searching the internet by Googling businesses in your area for senior services organizations and inquire about lists of services available in your community. Next, categorize the results (see exhibit 14.1). Then create a fact sheet for each resource describing its services and costs. As you contact these sources, tell them what you are organizing and ask for help in collecting information about their services. Always follow your fact-finding visit with a letter to the owners or managers of the services thanking them for their time and interest, and informing them that you have selected them as a referral source for your residents because of their quality of service and commitment to elderly people in your community. When referring residents to fee-for-service sources, always give at least two different organizations to limit your liability for inappropriate direction or advice.

Exhibit 14.1   Priority Based Outreach Plan

Priority 1	Capacity to refer immediately and ongoing	Twice monthly	Hospitals, psychiatric physicians, rehabs, cardiologists, orthopedists, geriatricians, neurologists, oncologists, APFM, Caring.com, geriatric care managers, senior living private agencies, area agency on aging, discharge planners, geriatric specialty physicians, pharmacists, skilled nursing centers, social workers, pulmonologists
Priority 2	Capacity to refer every 60–90 days	Monthly	Family general practitioners, adult day care centers, hospice agencies, home health agencies, Alzheimer's Association, chiropractors, elder-law attorneys, financial advisors, investment advisors
Priority 3	Capacity to refer annually	Every other month	Chamber of commerce, churches, alumni associations, Council on Aging, family counselors, funeral directors, grief support centers, women's clubs, Jewish Federation, moving companies catering to seniors, Red Hat Society groups, senior centers, Veterans Affairs, golf clubs, emergency services, UPS drivers

Relationship

Green	Reliable and consistent lead source with committed relationship
Yellow	Potential to become a consistent lead/referral source but not reliable currently
Red	Potential to become a referral source but currently unresponsive

	Leads or Contacts	Contacts per Month	Contacts per Week	Contacts per Day	Frequency
Prospecting Outreach		75	18.8	3.8	Monthly
Priority 1	450	900	225	11	Twice per month
Priority 2	50	50	13	1	Once per month
Priority 3	75	38	9	0	Every other month
Total		1,063	266	16	**Total**

Many community outreach efforts fail because they are too broad, and lack prioritization. An effective community outreach campaign can be very labor intensive, so it is wise to create a plan to identify the most likely referral sources and evaluate the community's relationship to each.

Some referral sources have the capacity to refer a qualified resident to the community on a regular basis. These include hospitals, psychiatric physicians, rehabs, cardiologists, orthopedists, geriatricians, neurologists, oncologists, APFM, caring.com, geriatric care managers, senior living private agencies, area agency on aging, discharge planners, geriatric specialty physicians, pharmacists, skilled nursing centers, social workers, and pulmonologists. These are the community's Priority 1 referral sources. These can be further classified based upon the quality of relationship and consistency of referrals. Using a color-coded system, they can be classified as green (a reliable and consistent source with a familiar and consistent relationship), yellow (has the potential to be a reliable and consistent source but not reliable currently), or red (currently unresponsive to or unaware of your community, its marketer, or the services offered). Clearly, the goal is to move the relationships of your primary potential referral sources to Priority 1. Face-to-face contact with these sources will help to identify any impediments to your community earning their referrals. These relationships should be contacted twice monthly.

Priority 2 referral sources have the capacity to refer a qualified resident to your community every 60 to 90 days depending on their volume. These include family general practitioners, adult day care centers, hospice agencies, home health agencies, the Alzheimer's Association, chiropractors, elder-law attorneys, financial advisors, and investment advisors.

Priority 3 referral sources have the capacity to refer a qualified resident to your community at least annually. These include the chamber of commerce, churches, alumni associations, the Council on Aging, family counselors, funeral directors, grief support centers, women's clubs, Jewish Federations, moving companies catering to seniors, Red Hat Society groups, senior centers, Veterans Affairs, golf clubs, emergency services, and UPS drivers.

As with Priority 1, the outreach representative will attempt to make a personal connection and establish rapport and trust in moving each of the potential referral sources to green status.

Another component of the community outreach program involves inviting professionals to conduct seminars and presentations. The objective is to promote word-of-mouth advertising of the community. Some communities sponsor senior fairs at which a variety of businesses are invited to set up booths or displays or give presentations. Many communities develop networks of senior care professionals and arrange mixers and seminars at which their members can network. Often people who participate in these organizations are eager to help each other and will actively promote your organization if you take an interest in theirs or do some business with them. The local chamber of commerce is a good networking source.

Another possibility is to offer the community's conference space to drug companies hosting continuing education seminars. These seminars, often arranged and conducted by a local pharmacy, are held on a variety of health and medical topics for local health care professionals. They are usually held in local hotel conference rooms and poorly attended. If the seminars are held at the community instead, the community benefits from the exposure to visiting professionals—and from catering a hot lunch for the participants that is paid for by the pharmacy and the drug company at a 30 percent premium. Attracting resident referral sources to the community has now become a profit center!

Assisted living and dementia care communities should not overlook local hospitals as a source of referrals. Many acute care hospitals have a geriatric section. Discharge planners and nurses work to relocate patients who no longer need acute care to other settings to make room for new acute care patients. Consequently, many skilled nursing, rehabilitation, and subacute care facilities employ recruiters whose job is to identify potential patients for their units and who are well known to the hospital staff. Assisted living communities can participate, although it is more difficult for them because most do not offer Medicaid-reimbursable services. But assisted living patients and patients with dementia in the hospital (or their families) are often convinced to consider skilled nursing facilities, sometimes prematurely, because of the influence these nursing home recruiters have on the doctors and hospital staff anxious to free up beds. Assisted living operators are well advised to visit their residents in the hospital and communicate with families about returning their loved ones to the community after hospitalization. If a resident can return to the community from the hospital, a potential turnover is avoided.

Marketing Materials

The information packet should be an attractive brochure or presentation folder containing all the information necessary for a prospect to evaluate the community. If the prospect calls in advance to make an appointment, the marketing department should take the time to personalize the information packet by printing his name on the outside cover or on a personalized letter inside. The inquiry thank-you letter should provide a friendly introduction to the services and amenities of the community, thanking the prospect for his interest and highlighting the reasons why residents are happy living there. It should also itemize all the materials in the packet and invite the prospect to call and ask questions about any of the materials or information provided.

The rate sheet should include all possible community charges: the basic charge and what is included, plus any optional services and their charges. If the community offers several financial options, it is best to present them in chart form so that they are easy to compare.

If the community distributes a monthly newsletter, bulletin, or activity calendar to the residents and it reflects the quality of the community, then it should be included. Never include an unprofessional in-house communiqué in a finely printed brochure packet. The differences in the two pieces may communicate to the prospect that marketing and operational materials receive different amounts of care and attention, depending on who is on the receiving end.

Reprints of any favorable articles or press releases published in the local media about the community or its residents help validate the claims outlined in the brochures. Newspaper supplements or tabloids can also give prospects the impression that people are talking about the community and that it is attracting attention. Mentioning any national awards received by the community or company helps demonstrate industry leadership. Finally, reprints of articles from local and national media giving positive information on choosing a senior living community and the benefits of the lifestyle in general can be convincing.

The information packet can be designed with a pocket in the back or inside to allow the addition of supplementary and customized material. This can be one way to present costs, providing a cost-effective alternative to reprinting the entire brochure whenever the service packages or price structures change.

Digital Printing versus Offset Printing

Preparing printed marketing materials requires a basic understanding of commercial printing methods and their relative advantages and costs. Many printers offer both digital and offset printing, and it is wise to discuss the job with the printer ahead of time to ascertain which method will better satisfy your quality and budget requirements. In addition, the printer can offer valuable advice on preparing material for printing, particularly color images, which can be challenging to reproduce accurately and attractively. As in obtaining all kinds of services, it is prudent to obtain multiple bids for large-scale projects and to evaluate them on the basis of quality as well as cost.

Digital printing is a direct-to-paper printing process that requires little set-up and no printing plates. The cost per copy of digital presses is generally higher than that for offset presses. But the set-up charges on offset presses are substantial, and these must be included in the total cost. Thus, the general rule is that digital presses are better and faster for smaller quantities, and offset presses are better and faster for larger ones. The break-even point varies depending on the specifications of the job. Digital presses also offer more precise and consistent quality control. The first copy printed on a digital press will look exactly like the last copy. This is not necessarily true for offset printing, as ink densities must be adjusted until an acceptable copy is produced.

Digital presses can accommodate only limited paper thickness and finishes, and generally offer printing only on smooth, bright white papers. Most digital printing houses do not have the binding and finishing capabilities that offset printers do, so effects like complex folding, die cutting, foil stamping, and embossing may not be available. Large formats are also not generally available with digital presses, with the current limit being about 20 inches wide.

With offset printing, the printer always allows for extra materials to ensure that enough acceptable copies are produced to meet the quantity ordered. It is difficult to produce a precise quantity, and most printing agreements allow the printer a 5 percent leeway above or below the ordered quantity. The additional copies, known as "overs," are usually billable to the customer. Conversely, if the printer fails to produce the ordered quantity, the customer is credited for the number of copies short.

Unlike digital presses, most of which can print only in four-color process, offset presses, depending on which models the printer has, can print up to eight colors at one time (with a corresponding increase in cost for each color). Offset presses can also print color images at a higher resolution (more dots per inch) than digital presses can, resulting in smoother and more intense color. Traditional offset presses can accommodate a range of paper sizes and thicknesses, permitting more innovative and creative projects.

■ MEDIA SCHEDULES

The media schedule and calendar are the planning tools that coordinate all marketing strategies and projects, establish their frequency, assign their priority, and allocate the budget. Essentially, they summarize where and how the community will advertise for the year, broken down by month. Whether employing print or online media, there are three main scheduling strategies to consider, depending on the stage of occupancy, turnover, and budget of the community.

New developments that need to generate public awareness and a large volume of leads commonly use *continuous advertising*. Their media schedule is always full, and they advertise every week using a variety of media. This type of strategy tends to be expensive and is generally not practical or necessary for more established communities. In fact, it may not work to the new community's benefit either: when new communities enter the marketplace with a big splash, they attract considerable attention to senior living in general, and their advertising can therefore benefit established, competing communities. Indeed, communities in some markets have reached stabilized occupancy by riding the wave of awareness created by a new community.

A variant of continuous advertising is *pulsing*. This involves running a small base of continuous advertising that increases in intensity during peak periods and before significant events. This strategy works best for communities in the fill-up stage that still need a large volume of new leads each month. Such communities generally experience an ebb and flow of marketing activity. Sometimes this is related to external factors such as holidays, the economy, or elections, but often it is linked to internal factors such as employee morale, management, departmental politics, financial thresholds, employee productivity, and, especially, move-outs. Any of these factors can trigger an acceleration or pulse in marketing activity.

The third strategy is usually practiced by established communities at or near stabilized occupancy that are already well recognized in their primary market area. This strategy is called *flighting*: the marketer concentrates the frequency and maximizes the influence of the marketing exposure with a minimal investment. Using this strategy, ads are placed for short periods at a high frequency as needed, depending on the size and quality of the lead bank and the number of projected vacancies. Wary marketers learn to anticipate fluctuations in their lead bank and understand that it may take at least 60 days to convert new leads to sales, with another 60 days before move-in. By flighting media placements 60 to 90 days before the hot and warm leads are converted (see chapter 15) or on receiving news of pending move-outs, they can stretch their budget dollars. This practice works well when complemented by lead generation from resident and professional referrals. Flighting is even more cost-effective when media purchases are concentrated to qualify for bulk discounts.

All effective media plans should be based on four concepts: reach, frequency, cost per thousand, and lease-lead conversion rates. *Reach* is the average number of people who are exposed to your advertising message at least once. Reach helps to develop awareness and understanding of your community. The response to reach advertising, also known as attitude or image-building advertising, is harder to measure because sales are usually generated long after the ad has appeared.

Frequency is the number of times the average person in your target audience is exposed to your message. The frequency of ads generally determines whether prospects and interested parties will inquire further once they have become aware of your community. New developments that blanket the media are trying to create awareness. Established communities are generally interested in prompting qualified inquiries. The desired media mix strikes a balance between reach and frequency at the most cost-effective rate, as demonstrated by the lease-to-lead conversion ratio. Exhibit 14.2 shows how to build a media schedule to maximize the results from chosen media.

Fine-tune your media schedule by developing a calendar for media placement. This calendar should also schedule special events and deadlines for production work necessary for placements, such as a photo shoot or production of ads and direct mail pieces. The media calendar should itemize all activities in each strategy for each month and note the percentage of the total budget that will be allocated to each for the month. As you progress and develop statistics on responses, you can adjust ad size, placements, and frequency as needed. Always save some funds for contingencies. Having to ask for additional marketing funds midyear exposes flaws in your planning.

Exhibit 14.2   Developing the Media Plan

1. Collect all media information.
2. Price each media strategy according to cost per thousand.
3. List strategies by lease-to-lead conversion rate.
4. Choose the medium that has the highest conversion rate for the dollars invested.
5. Choose the second and third best media strategies that will coordinate well with your top strategy.
6. Assign a percentage of your total advertising budget to each medium according to results.
7. Determine which scheduling strategy to adopt: continuous, pulse, or flighting, according to occupancy projections.
8. Schedule media placements on a calendar.
9. Estimate the number of leads that will be generated from each strategy each month based on historic results.
10. Allocate a monthly budget to each placement by media type; include production costs.
11. Calculate the cost per lead.
12. Multiply the cost per lead by the appropriate closing ratio to get cost per sale.
13. Summarize the total leads, cost per lead, total leads, and projected conversions by month, by year, and by media type.
14. Include lead and sales estimates from special media, seminars, resident referrals, and other forms of outreach.
15. Refer to the annual unit-sales forecast and annual lead forecast to determine the leads and sales required each month or for the year and compare to your summary. Adjust if necessary.

The media schedule provides the management and owners empirical justification for the amount and allocation of the marketing budget. Statistical analysis depends on the collection of accurate lead-response data and conversion ratios. This is not an exact science, as the responses may be the result of a number of placements in different media. Keep the marketing plan flexible. Turnover and fluctuations in staff productivity can affect lead-generation strategies. Conversion rates will grow with the refinement of each strategy and as sales skills improve.

The marketing planning process is only as good as the sales representatives whose job it is to convert the leads into sales. Good salespeople are the foundation on which the success or failure of the community rests. The next chapter explores the management of the sales function.

OFFENSIVE VERSUS DEFENSIVE MARKETING

Traditional approaches have employed "defensive" marketing tactics to sustain occupancy once the community is full. Defensive marketing, a reactive strategy for managing turnover, is widely employed in the industry. It assumes significant cuts to the marketing budget, minimal staffing, and minimal levels of sales compensation once the community is full. The potential disadvantages of this strategy, however, can outweigh the obvious cost-saving advantages. Financial balance in the marketing program will help ensure longer-term success.[4]

As marketing and advertising expenditures are scaled back, fewer leads are generated for a community. If the leads and subsequent closing ratios on each type of lead are insufficient to cover resident turnover, several serious problems can result:

■ Insufficient leads may result in longer time frames for sales and move-ins, thus reducing apartment revenue. Difficulty in obtaining leases is likely to lead to price concessions, which can further reduce revenue. More important, vacancies restrict the community's ability to command rate increases.

■ Communities may try to retain frail residents longer than is appropriate, raising ethical and regulatory concerns regarding the provision of care in the most appropriate setting. Frail residents may also erode the image of the community, jeopardizing resident referrals and attracting frailer new prospects.

■ Smaller marketing budgets often force the sales staff to work harder with fewer resources and lower compensation. Staff members are then attracted to competitor communities, resulting in the loss of the time, energy, and money invested in training the top salespeople. This loss is complicated by the need to train replacements and orient them to the community's assets and character.

Whereas defensive marketing manages turnover, "offensive" marketing is designed to proactively manage the profitability of a community. Offensive marketing tactics seek to minimize marketing expenditures without compromising a community's ability to maintain a stable occupancy and maximize revenue. Offensive marketing provides the following assurances:

- The generation of new leads keeps pace with the turnover. Sale and move-in time frames are minimized, thus achieving or exceeding apartment revenue projections.
- Residents' levels of care are optimized, so that frail residents are placed in the most appropriate setting. By retaining an active image, a community is better positioned to compete with new communities. This is particularly important for congregate rental communities that do not have the option, as continuing care retirement communities do, of transferring a resident from independent living to assisted living or nursing care.
- Increases in monthly fees on vacated units are maximized. Increases in monthly fees on lease renewals can also be aggressively managed because vacancies can be filled quickly.
- Price concessions are minimized because efforts to generate leads increase demand and build a strong waiting list.
- Top sales producers are retained because they have the resources to generate sufficient new leads to offset the turnover and receive compensation that is competitive. The costs of recruiting, training, and orienting new sales staff members are avoided.

Offensive marketing reduces a community's financial exposure by proactively managing turnover. Specific strategies include maintaining a marginally larger staff to work existing leads adequately and minimize burnout. The lead bank is part of the community's current assets, and, with the exception of resident referrals, each lead represents money invested in advertising or other media. Some communities have spent thousands of dollars to build their lead banks and their presence in the marketplace. Reducing staffing levels too aggressively at stabilization may compromise these investments. Operators should reduce staffing levels slowly as the size of the lead bank diminishes over time. At stabilized occupancy, lead banks are usually at an all-time high. All leads must be worked monthly to keep them fresh. Keeping a "baseline" presence in

the media to avoid rebuilding awareness from scratch protects the community's position in the market.

Operators should guard against losing their top talent (and possibly many hot prospects) by maintaining a competitive compensation program. In addition, ongoing sales training helps reduce sale and move-in time frames and keeps the staff motivated and challenged. (See chapter 15.)

An alternative way of examining this issue is to analyze the opportunity cost related to marketing defensively. Vacant units will result in lost cash flow and ultimately lost investment value for a community. For example, if 75 percent of the monthly fee is typically needed to cover fixed operating expenses and debt service, then each vacant unit reduces the contribution to those costs. A 200-unit community that stabilizes at 94 percent rather than 99 percent represents an opportunity cost of $180,000 in lost revenue, or $1,500,000 in lost value for the investment at a 12 percent capitalization rate: (200 units × 99% = 198 units) − (200 units × 94% = 188 units) = 10 units × $2,000 per month × 12 months = $240,000 × 75% contribution to fixed operating expenses and debt service = $180,000 ÷ 0.12 = $1,500,000.

Communities have traditionally focused on reducing operating and marketing expenses as buildings mature. But only so much value can be added to the investment by cutting expenses. The more aggressive the cuts, the more apparent their effects will be to the residents. They will notice that the service package is being reduced while the rent goes up, and they will react negatively, which will reduce referrals and perhaps even lead to voluntary discharges. In other words, at some point efforts to cut costs yield diminishing returns. Communities that focus on a defensive expense-management strategy combined with an offensive revenue-enhancement strategy are more productive in the long run. Even a modest combination of $50 per unit per month in increased revenue or decreased expenses yields $10,000 per month, or $120,000 per year for a 200-unit project. At an 11 percent capitalization rate, the enhanced product value is more than $1 million. Most communities can make this type of adjustment with a minimal impact on residents or the marketing budget.

In summary, offensive marketing is a revenue-enhancement strategy, whereas defensive marketing is an expense-management strategy. Although both are important, the potential benefits of revenue-generation opportunities clearly outweigh those of aggressive cuts in the marketing budget for a stabilized community.

NOTES

1. A. J. Mullen, D. Cwi, and D. Yulish, "An Analysis of Nationwide Absorption Rates: The Critical Element in the Feasibility of Senior Living Projects," unpublished report, 2.

2. B. Mace and O. Zahraoui, "Assisted Living Demand Bouncing Back Relatively Swiftly," *NIC Notes: Insights in Seniors Housing and Care*, March 17, 2022, https://blog.nic.org/the-pandemic-weighed-on-assisted-living-demand-is-bouncing-back.

3. J. R. Lumpkin, M. J. Caballero, and L. B. Chonko, *Direct Marketing, Direct Selling, and the Mature Consumer: A Research Study* (Westport, CT: Quorum Books, 1989).

4. C. H. A. Hoskins, "The ADA and Retirement Communities: Time to Be Proactive," *Retirement Housing Business Report* (1993): 6–10.

5. E. C. Merrigan, "Rating Guidelines for Nonprofit Continuing Care Retirement Communities," *Rating Guidelines for Nonprofit Continuing Care Retirement Communities*, Fitch Health Care Special Report, Fitch Investor Services, June 1994, 8.

6. E. C. Merrigan, "Rating Guidelines for Nonprofit Continuing Care Retirement Communities," *Rating Guidelines for Assisted Living Facilities*, Fitch Health Care Special Report, Fitch Investor Services, October 1996, 4.

7. S. Brooks, "Who Is Our Senior Housing Client? Marketing and Public Relations Ideas That Hit the Target," presentation to the National Association for Senior Living Industries, December 1994.

8. C. W. Wallace, *Great Ad! Low Cost Do-It-Yourself Advertising for Your Small Business* (Blue Ridge Summit, PA: Liberty Hall, 1990).

9. My Caregiver Coach, a YouTube resource to support caregivers and staff who work with the elderly, http://www.mycaregivercoach.com.

10. The One Minute Caregiver Family Education Blog, http://oneminutecaregiver.blogspot.com.

11. B. Stone, *Successful Direct Marketing Methods* (Chicago: Crain, 1979).

12. C. D. Schewe, "Marketing to Our Aging Population: Responding to Physiological Changes," *Journal of Consumer Marketing* 5, no. 3 (Summer 1988): 67.

15

Sales

S elling senior housing is different from selling anything else. It involves selling not only the residence but also the services and intangibles that go with it. Often the buyer is shopping out of need rather than choice, and the decision is almost always emotional. An effective sales program must be designed around building relationships and trust with a client facing dramatic change. Salespeople must be familiar with all the assets of the community and able to establish rapport with prospects and their families.

A top sales director was asked by the sponsoring board of directors how she filled her building. Her response was, "One person at a time." Although it is important to have a plan and strategy for marketing the community, there are no shortcuts to building trust and inspiring confidence that the community will be able to meet a person's complex needs. The process takes a commitment to building relationships, overcoming barriers, and reassurance, repeated in its entirety for every prospect and family member who comes along.

CLASSIFICATION OF PROSPECTS

Prospects can be classified in terms of their urgency and desire to buy. Prospect-classification systems allow sales counselors to rank leads for effective follow-up. For example, *hot* leads, who may decide to purchase within 30 days, require more frequent contact than *warm* leads, who may be ready to purchase

in 31 to 90 days. Rarely do prospects enter the system as hot; most are upgraded from a lower classification. Other classes of leads include *active*, for those who are expected to sign in 90 to 180 days; *unclassified*, for those who may have sent in a request for information without including a phone number or who replied to a mailing but have not yet been called and classified; *inactive*, for those who may not be ready but want to remain on the community's mailing list; and *deleted*, for those who have been deleted by the sales counselor, who are deceased, or who requested deletion for any reason. This categorization allows sales counselors to spend more time working with leads who are likely to sign a residency agreement sooner, thereby maximizing productivity.

Prospects may be classified during either a telephone call or a personal visit. The sales counselor typically explores what prompted the inquiry and attempts to determine the prospect's motivations and current situation. This process establishes the level of urgency. It is the sales counselor's main job to move prospects from a lower level of urgency to a higher level.

Salespeople have been known to inactivate or prematurely delete leads who later became residents somewhere else. Because of the cost of acquiring leads, the marketing director should approve all deletions.

The classification of prospects provides a way to track the efficiency of various marketing strategies according to the level of interest that each generates. For example, a newspaper ad campaign may need to be revised if it is found to be attracting only low-interest active leads. Conversely, a direct mailing may be considered a big hit if several of the responses generated are determined to be warm or hot prospects.

THE MANAGEMENT OF LEADS

The frequency of contacting leads is the single most important controllable aspect of the sales program. Too-frequent contact risks alienating the prospect, and too-infrequent contact may leave the prospect feeling neglected or allow leads to become stale. The marketing process can involve investments of hundreds of thousands of dollars to generate targeted, qualified prospects. This money is wasted if the prospects are not appropriately contacted. Time is of the essence because the personal situations of individuals in the lead bank are changing continuously, and the individual may be dealing with your competitors as well. Prospects expect to be contacted after making an inquiry, and it can reflect poorly on the entire operation if they are neglected. Commissioned sales counselors tend primarily to work hot and warm leads and to ignore the rest of the lead bank, which can be a big mistake. Often people will inquire before they are ready, then suddenly experience a problem that necessitates immediate placement. Those families will first call the sales counselor who has kept in touch with them since their initial inquiry.

Every sales program must have a failsafe system to ensure that all leads are appropriately directed toward closing. The sales counselors must be able to manage the lead bank without losing track of any qualified leads. There are many good systems available to automate this task, but all require daily management and supervision to be effective.

Schedule all hot, warm, and active leads for regular contact. Contact hot leads weekly, warm leads three times per month, and active leads twice per month. Try to classify all unclassified leads. Individuals who send in a coupon or reply card without a phone number should receive an "unable to reach you" letter to prompt them to call. It is also possible to track leads down using the reverse directory, which lists names by address, or through a web search.

Contacts should include phone calls, personal letters, and mailings of newsletters or articles, as well as routine or scheduled direct mail contacts to the lead

Table 15.1   Sample Lead Management Analysis

Lead classification	Total leads	Contacts per month	Total personal contacts
Hot	8	4	32
Warm	32	3	96
Active	1,310	2	2,620
Unclassified	181	1	181
Inactive	1,368	0	0
Total	**2,899**	**10**	**2,929**

Productivity	Annual	Monthly	Weekly
Phone calls	17,574	1,465	366
Total hours phone time (@ 10 minutes/call)	**2,929**	**244**	**61**
Mailings and letters	17,574	1,465	366
Total hours mailing time (@ 5 minutes/letter)	**1,465**	**122**	**31**
Closing time			
Visits per sale	5		
Average hours per visit	2		
Sales budgeted	108	9	2
Total closing time (@ 10 hours/sale)	**1,080**	**90**	**23**
Total sales time required	**5,474**	**456**	**114**
Sales hours available per individual per year	1,920		

Sales time allocation		
	Percent	Hours
Selling time	85	1,632
Nonselling time	15	288
Total	**100**	**1,920**

bank. Phone calls should alternate between calls designed to close on an appointment and relationship-building calls. The approach should aim to build relationships, not just to schedule appointments, and to convey the impression that the sales counselor has a genuine interest in the individual and is not merely pestering her to visit the community. Scheduling all leads for some form of monthly contact assures the management that none is falling through the cracks.

The lead management analysis in table 15.1 bases the frequency of lead contacts on the level of urgency. All leads are contacted at least monthly to keep leads fresh and ensure that the lead bank is kept current. Mail contacts consist of event flyers, personal letters, and the monthly newsletter. For all active leads, including hot, warm, and active classifications, contacts are split evenly between phone calls and mailings. Inactive leads are routinely contacted by direct mail and perhaps telephoned quarterly to attempt to upgrade them. Any system that ensures that all leads are contacted at least monthly and appropriately directed toward closing will serve the community's objectives.

The Size of the Sales Force

The size of the sales force is a function of the size of the lead bank, the classification of the leads, the level of urgency, and the frequency of contact desired. The sales counselors categorize leads as they work with the individuals. The sales director estimates the average amount of time required for each type of contact. The next step is to calculate the number of hours per year required to make all necessary contacts. The sales director's objective is obviously to maximize the time spent selling, but some nonselling time needs to be included for each staff member. The sales director should have leads assigned to her just like the rest of the sales staff. The number of staff members required to work the lead bank is then calculated by dividing the annual hours required by the selling hours available per individual per year (see table 15.1).

Another method of calculating personnel requirements is to compare the contact frequency and time required to an average productive work week. Total monthly contact time for each lead classification is calculated and then divided among the sales counselors. This number is divided by an average of 22 working days per month to estimate the daily productivity of each person. Time requirements for each activity are factored in, and the total weekly hours needed to service the lead bank are calculated. This way, the marketing director can evaluate the overall workload. If the amount of time required by the formula exceeds 40 hours per week, then the number of full-time equivalents may need to be increased (see table 15.2).

Sales Productivity

Expectations of staff productivity should be established and managed through the lead management system. This determines the total number of personal contacts required for the entire department. Each sales counselor should be able to make at least 20 phone calls (defined as calls during which the

Table 15.2	Work Week Allocation for Sales Department

	Total		
Total contacts	2,929		
FTEs	3.5		
Monthly contacts per FTE	837		
Daily contacts per FTE	38		

Productivity per person	Monthly	Weekly	Daily
Phone calls	418	105	21
Hours required (@10 minutes/call, or 6 calls/hour)	**70**	**17**	**3**
Letters	418	105	21
Hours required (@5 minutes/letter, or 12 letters/hour)	**35**	**9**	**2**
Closing time			
Hours per sale		**6**	**1**
Total hours per week		**32.6**	**6.5**

salesperson actually reaches and talks to a prospect) and 20 mail contacts each business day. Assuming 22 average working days per month, this totals 880 contacts per month. Higher expectations may result in a pressured environment that prospects can sense. The marketing and sales director wants to create a sense of urgency among the sales staff without inducing burnout. At the same time, clearly stated productivity expectations should leave little time for activities that will not yield sales. (See the section on sales analysis for more on productivity targets.)

Contacts are equally divided between phone calls and mailings. Phone calls assume approximately 10 minutes per call; mailings assume 5 minutes per letter. Clearly, some will take more and some less, but these estimates have stood the test of time. Each sales counselor's day leaves little time for nonselling activities: three hours of phoning, two hours of mailings, and an average of one hour per day of closing time amounts to six hours of selling per day. In the previous example, each of the three sales counselors plus the sales director (part-time) will need to spend approximately 33 hours each week working the leads. The balance of the work week can be used for training, meetings, home visits, and the closing process. In short, the sales staff should be managed so that their time can be spent almost entirely on sales activities, not on paperwork or planning.

Usually a slowdown in sales results can be traced to insufficient phone productivity. If sales counselors fall short of the stated goal, the management needs to determine the cause of the problem and take appropriate action. For example, if the sales counselors are spending too much time organizing events, the management should consider reassigning the responsibility to operations staff.

Residents can be another common distraction. Having come to regard the sales staff as friends, they often visit the marketing department during the day. Although these relationships can often yield important referrals, they should not interfere with contact goals. Executive directors must protect their sales counselors' time.

It is a good idea to incorporate weekly phone-out goals into the sales counselors' incentive plans and chart their progress. In extreme cases, the marketing director might consider establishing phone quotas to ensure that all leads receive the appropriate attention.

The marketing director should organize the sales department so that all staff time is scheduled as either floor time (handling incoming visitors or phone calls) or sales time, in which the sales counselor makes phone calls, sends out mailings, schedules appointments, and conducts tours. Sales counselors should be assigned floor time on a rotating basis. The only community events they should be required to attend are marketing events.

The sales and leasing office should be open at least six and a half days per week. Weekends and holidays are times when families are together and in a position to influence the prospect's decision. It is a good idea to schedule all the sales staff for weekend duty on a rotating basis so that the office is always covered.

To allow the marketing department to spend its time on selling, operations should be responsible for planning and coordinating all major events. This can be accomplished using function sheets that fully describe the function and the associated costs of producing it. Usually the resident relations or activity department initiates the process and coordinates with the food and beverage department.

The amount of time needed for the closing process varies greatly. Some individuals will sign after only a few contacts, whereas others will require 10 or more contacts over an extended period to confirm their decision. The example in table 15.1 assumes 5 personal visits per sale at 2 hours per visit, for a total of 10 hours closing time.

Computerized Management of Leads

The decision to computerize the lead management system is usually predicated on the size of the community, occupancy, volume of inquiries, and level of detail required in analyzing results. Small and even midsized communities have effectively managed their lead banks with a card system, whereas others have chosen an integrated contact-management system with a computer on each sales counselor's desk. Several good contact-management software packages can be purchased off the shelf, some specifically designed for the senior living business, but they may have limited capacity to generate custom reports for tracking advertising results. Still other communities develop their own systems using templates in database programs.

A good program should contain two main components: lead tracking and lead analysis for both prospects and referrals. Equipped with this information, the director can quickly identify weaknesses in responses from specific marketing strategies or problems in their conversion to sales. Many of these systems have the sophistication to track residents from first inquiry throughout their residency to move-out. Components can be purchased to track care and generate billing statements to the residents or responsible parties. Some systems can further be customized to include complete financial reporting systems depending upon the company requirements.

Tracking Leads

The lead-tracking component should serve as a contact manager that automatically schedules contacts for all leads according to classification. The sales director should be able to generate a daily or weekly contact schedule that sorts each lead by classification, last contact, phone number, type of unit desired, and factors influencing the individual's decision. The lead-tracking component should also be able to generate traffic reports, such as number of walk-ins, phone-ins, returned coupons, or "be backs" (prospects who tour the property more than once). It should collect production statistics such as phone-outs, appointments made and kept, and conversion ratios by sales counselor. The system should produce reports on all move-ins, sorted by date of sale and move-in date, to track the time elapsed from first inquiry to sale and from sale to move-in.

Analyzing data over time may reveal important trends. Monitoring the number of leads by classification along with the total leads (including both new and deleted leads) can provide important clues for projecting short-term performance. For example, if the hot and warm lead classifications begin to fall, more sales need to be generated from the active classification, which may take longer to convert. If the lead bank is shrinking overall, there may be more monthly deletions than new leads, triggering a need to boost media placements.

A report that details leads or sales that were canceled or rejected, and the reason, can be useful to identify problems in the offering or weak follow-up by the sales staff or move-in coordinator. This information can also reinforce the importance of *net* sales and of follow-through. A sale is not complete until the prospect becomes a resident.

Analysis of Leads

The lead-analysis component should itemize each lead by classification and demographics and note how each was attracted to the community. For example, a lead may have originated from a coupon, a call from the website, a walk-in, or a social media inquiry. This information is usually collected and entered on a lead card by the person taking the call or meeting the prospect when he comes for a tour. It is essential to create a profile of each prospect to determine which marketing strategies are working.

The analysis should also provide an advertising summary that details the date, location, cost, size, day of week, coupon, and other details for every media placement and shows the response by prospect classification. This information enables the marketing director to evaluate the effectiveness of each ad and medium in attracting prospects. Sorting the responses from each ad by urgency classification will further help the director distinguish placements that generally yield good-quality leads from those that produce a high quantity. This way, minor adjustments can be made to one or the other. For example, the advertising summary might indicate that the quarter-column coupon "services" ad was the most productive of good-quality leads, whereas the decision-influencer ad in the local weekly newspaper produced a higher quantity of leads. Armed with these response statistics, the marketing director can begin to recognize

patterns that may deliver predictable results. Some communities employ a marketing assistant who updates the tracking database daily, entering daily sales activity logs, new leads by source and media type, and ad responses. Today most companies utilize metric and traffic tracking software such as Google Ads, which has broad tracking capabilities for evaluating your campaigns by impressions and impression share, clicks, conversions, and conversion rates. These statistics can help marketing planners understand where to maximize their online spends.

The purpose of these reporting systems is to identify the strengths and weaknesses of the combined sales and marketing efforts so that adjustments and corrections can be made each month to keep things on track and recognize any problems in sales or leasing activities.

■■■■■■ THE LEAD BANK

Communities in the fill-up phase should as a rule have approximately 20 times as many leads in their lead bank as apartments in the community. For example, a 100-unit community should have 2,000 leads. At least half of these leads should be classified as hot, warm, or active.

Communities that have reached stabilized occupancy may be able to maintain their occupancy and cover attrition with a lead bank that is 10 times the apartment count. Established communities that rely on resident and nonresident referrals may be able to get by with less. The number of referrals can fluctuate widely, so marketing directors are well advised to keep a healthy number of qualified leads in the lead bank at all times.

Trends in the size of the lead bank can indicate a need for adjustments. A continual shrinkage may indicate a poor response rate to media placements or a need for more or more-frequent placements. Shrinking lead banks can also indicate an imbalance between new leads and deleted leads. Conversely, too large a lead bank may strain staff resources. Keeping prospects waiting in the lobby for a salesperson who is overcommitted not only discourages sales but reflects poorly on the entire operation.

The marketing director should carefully evaluate the trends and composition of each lead-bank classification. Obviously, the higher the percentage of strongly motivated leads, the better. A healthy yet realistic breakdown of leads should run about 0.5 percent hot, 1.5 percent warm, 55 percent active, 10 percent unclassified, and 33 percent inactive. Too few hot leads can indicate a need to improve the quality of leads or indicate that leads are not being upgraded. Lead banks with more than 10 percent of their leads unclassified may need to reevaluate their coupon design or improve the follow-up on incoming phone calls. Lead banks with more than 50 percent of the leads designated as inactive or unclassified might indicate a need for stepped-up media placements to generate fresh leads.

A shrinking lead bank can create significant delays in sales, as new leads take some time to generate and then to convert. By the time the sales director notices that the lead bank is inadequate, it may be too late to fill vacancies as they occur.

The marketing plan establishes specific goals for the number of new leads and leases or sales required each month to meet financial projections. Other useful goals include average new walk-ins per month, average new resident-referral leads per month, and site leads originating from the sign or building from drive-by traffic. Strategies to generate leads from these types of contact need not involve significant marketing investment.

Often the differences in sales performance result from different ways of classifying and treating leads. It is not that a successful competitor necessarily has better leads, but that the sales staff is more likely to classify leads as warm, even if prospects say they are not ready. The warmer the lead status, the more frequent the contact with the prospect. The quality of contact is usually better because there is a higher expectation on the part of the sales counselor. To improve the lead split, consider the following suggestions:

- Be optimistic when initially classifying a lead. This will optimize the quantity and quality of follow-up.
- Do not automatically downgrade a lead just because the last contact with the prospect was not encouraging. Give your leads time to adjust to the idea of senior living, and make several attempts to schedule an appointment before you downgrade them.
- Implement a system whereby any inactive lead who is entered into the system and has not been contacted by phone or in person in the previous 60 days is up for grabs and can be contacted by another

sales counselor. This approach will direct attention to inactive leads and encourage sales counselors to upgrade them if there is a chance of closing.

SOURCES OF LEADS

To develop an effective marketing plan, it is necessary to identify and emphasize the strategies producing leads that ultimately convert to sales. Although sales can sometimes be difficult to attribute to a particular marketing strategy, the objective of marketing is to allocate the marketing budget according to the best conversion rate of the lead responses to sales. The inclusion of other lead sources when calculating the community's conversion rate, such as personal referrals and site leads, will inflate true marketing results.

Tracking these responses in detail will yield important information about the lead location, method of inquiry, and source. Trends in this information are then evaluated from month to month so that vulnerabilities can be identified and adjustments can be made in media planning and marketing.

The Location of Leads

The location of the lead is primarily a geographic criterion. It can be categorized by *primary market, secondary market, tertiary market, rest-of-state,* and *out-of-state.*

PRIMARY MARKET. The *primary market* is usually defined as the geographic location where 80 percent of the age- and income-qualified leads required to fill the community will be generated. This can be defined as a specified radius in miles, a zip code, or a county in the immediate vicinity of the community. Usually the boundaries of the primary market area are established relative to the size of the market in the area and their relative distance from the community. In urban areas with high concentrations of people, the community may be able to reach this 80 percent threshold within a 10-block radius of the community. A suburban community may need to expand its primary market definition to a 10- to 15-mile radius. Some rural communities have been known to define their primary market as encompassing a three-county area.

Clearly, the more concentrated the target market, the easier it is to contact leads and schedule appointments. If communities are unable to attract 80 percent of their leads from within their primary market, the marketing effort will need to be expanded to cover other, less attractive markets with consequently lower lead-to-lease conversion ratios. Most seniors prefer to move into a property near their friends and business acquaintances.

Shortages in leads generated within the primary market may also indicate that the penetration-rate analysis (see chapter 14) was flawed. In any event, the average cost per sale tends to increase with the relative distance from the property. Marketing directors should keep a close eye on the percentage of leads from the primary market and adjust the frequency and location of media placements to attract more local responses.

SECONDARY MARKET. The *secondary market* is usually defined as the geographic area outside the boundaries of the primary market but still in the general vicinity. Typically, up to 10 percent of the total lead bank should originate within this market. For example, the secondary market could include the areas beyond a five-mile radius but still within the metropolitan area reached by most major media. One community's secondary market may be a competitor's primary market. Media placements within the secondary market should be designed to improve advertising *reach* rather than *frequency* (see chapter 14). The competition will surely budget more dollars for marketing within its own primary market, and it is not usually worthwhile to attempt to match this effort. In addition, it is more difficult to schedule appointments with prospects who live farther from the community.

TERTIARY MARKET. The *tertiary market* is loosely defined in the industry. It usually involves family members who are decision influencers and who may live locally or out of state. Some marketers include rest-of-state and out-of-state markets in this category. As a rule, the proportion of interested parties (rather than prospective residents themselves) as initial contacts is approximately 5 to 10 percent for continuing care retirement communities, 25 to 50 percent for independent living communities, and 80 to 95 percent for assisted living or skilled-nursing communities. Many interested parties not only are the first to inquire on behalf of a reluctant relative but are gathering information because the relative is unable to do it.

OTHER MARKETS. The *rest-of-state (ROS)* and *out-of-state (OOS)* markets are the most costly to reach, considering their corresponding conversion rates. Communities in destination retirement locations such as Florida or Arizona may rely heavily on leads generated from these markets. These can account for up to 20 percent of new leads in some markets. But retirees usually relocate to the destination area while they are still relatively active and independent. Most out-of-state transplants enter a senior living community after living for several years in a local apartment or condominium.

Many destination senior living communities have successfully marketed before and during the summer months to "snowbirds" in colder climates. This can be done in the same manner as marketing to a secondary market, but advertising material should always include a toll-free phone number to facilitate easy response. The community may want to consider offering short-term, part-year leases to individuals or couples interested in spending the winter there. Many seniors will reserve an apartment for four to six months sight unseen. The financial benefits of these rentals need to be weighed against the drawbacks: the possibility that long-term residents may resent the temporary snowbirds, and the cost of marketing these units against the total revenue collected over the shorter stay. As a rule, the average cost per sale should not exceed two months' rent for short-term residents and three months' rent for long-term residents.

As many families become geographically dispersed, they may feel frustrated about their inability to provide sufficient assistance to an ailing parent. Therefore, many ROS and OOS inquiries are triggered by families seeking to move closer together. This is usually accomplished by the prospect's moving closer to immediate family members.

Methods of Inquiry

Methods of inquiry to senior living communities are usually categorized as *walk-in*, *phone-in*, *phone-out*, *web lead*, or *mail-in*. Prospects who inquire at the community as walk-ins eliminate the need for sales counselors to schedule an appointment. Generally speaking, walk-in conversion rates are the highest—as high as 15 percent—because the inquiries come from individuals already convinced of the advantages of senior housing. This underscores the importance of creating a positive first impression at the reception desk (see chapter 5). Walk-in traffic usually is highest shortly after the community opens. Although many visitors may be curious neighbors rather than serious prospects, they should be valued, as they represent a significant referral base. Local support and word-of-mouth advertising are vital for promotion.

Telephone inquiries are usually the result of an ad in the media or telephone directory or are prompted by a referral. Like walk-ins, these responses are also highly motivated. Many such calls are received by the receptionist, who is responsible for collecting the appropriate data to allow the sales counselors to respond. If the designated walk-in sales counselor is busy with another inquiry, the marketing director can designate another to meet with the visitor. Because these leads are usually highly motivated, they should be distributed fairly among sales counselors who are paid on commission.

Leads generated by sales phone calls can be substantial. During the call, the counselor should always ask prospects for referrals to friends and acquaintances. Many active seniors who may not be ready for the community may have friends who qualify. This inexpensive source of good-quality leads should not be overlooked.

Website leads can come from internet searches, links to your site from other sites, print media listings, or direct referral. They can be numerous, but they are often not qualified. Many people search the web for Medicaid and government-sponsored care that is not available in many senior living communities. All such leads should enter the system through email, and many can be financially qualified over the phone.

Mail-in leads can usually be traced back to a specific newspaper, magazine coupon, or direct mailing. These respondents are often only looking for information and may be seeking to avoid a sales pitch. Those who include their telephone number effectively invite a follow-up call, suggesting a higher level of motivation.

Not all leads or ultimately sales cost money to generate. Sales generated from resident and nonresident referrals and from the site itself can represent a considerable portion of the lead bank. A community situated in a good location with high visibility and good curb appeal should generate as many as 10 percent of the total leads. Curb appeal can be enhanced with attention to the landscaping, the exterior finish of the community, and neatness. Good-quality signage, offering information about the availability of apartments and directions on how to inquire, can also invite passersby into the building.

Resident and nonresident referrals can also be a valuable source of new leads. The percentage of referral leads increases with the level of care: 70 percent of leads to assisted living may come from professional referrals. Continuing care retirement communities should expect about 50 percent of their leads from referrals, primarily from satisfied, active residents. Independent living communities should expect about 30 percent: 10 percent from residents and 20 percent from nonresidents. Effective internal marketing to residents, by delivering on the promises made by the sales counselors and a commitment to service on the part of all employees, can save thousands of dollars in advertising otherwise spent to generate leads. External marketing to professionals and senior advocacy groups in the area can also be highly productive (see chapter 14).

THE SALES PROCESS

Although some prospects may recognize the inherent value of the lifestyle and convenient services or maybe planning for their future needs, few seniors research their local senior housing community simply because it looks like a nice place to live. Many inquiries are triggered by a problem: prospects may have lost a spouse, the ability to drive, or the ability to manage a household. They may be experiencing feelings of helplessness and despair. The sales counselor is likely to be dealing with a reluctant buyer whose life is in upheaval and who will grasp at any straw to avoid the decision to move.

The successful senior-housing sales counselor, then, must wear the hat of the social worker as well as the real estate and services salesperson. The traditional sales model simply will not work with this type of client. The sales process must be designed around problem-solving and trust. Many of the issues underlying the decision can be difficult for the prospect to acknowledge or discuss, and the sales counselor will need to build a relationship based on trust and patience.

Table 15.3 compares the traditional sales process with relationship selling. Both models involve information gathering, presentation, affirmation, and

Table 15.3	Traditional versus Relationship Selling		
Phases of the sales process	Traditional selling techniques	Relationship selling
Information gathering	Prospecting	Preparation
Presentation	Conversation and	Rapport building
Affirmation	fact finding	Needs assessment
Follow-through	Pitching	Proposing
	Closing and overcoming	Confirming
	objections	Assuring
	Reselling	

follow-through. In the traditional model, however, little time is spent on fact finding, and the salesperson usually concentrates her efforts on features and benefits of the product and then on overcoming objections. Often this high-pressure environment requires the process to reverse itself, and the salesperson needs to resell the features and benefits.

Contrary to popular belief, the top persuaders in the country say that the most important aspect of influence is not closing but rapport. Trust between the sales counselor and the prospect is the single most important element influencing the success or failure of a sales interview. People often buy products they do not need from salespeople they like. If they are on the edge of making a decision, a sales counselor they believe in can influence them to buy.[1] The primary aspect of persuasion is to align with someone and redirect her. This requires first earning the person's trust and confidence. The individual phases of relationship selling are described below.

Gathering Information

During the information-gathering stage, the sales counselor begins to formulate a profile of the prospect by asking key questions about the decision time frame, who will be involved in the decision process, where the person is in the search, and what prompted a visit to the community. She then uses this information to relate the community's services and amenities to the prospect's needs.

The manner in which the prospect is initially received often plays a large part in the success of the relationship-building process. The sales counselor may never be able to overcome a bad first impression. The lobby or reception area should be bright, warm, and friendly. It should have a comfortable seating area with community photo albums, newsletters, and other informational material within easy reach so that prospects can browse through them. It is a good idea to have two scrapbooks: one filled with photographs of special events at the community, and the other filled with letters, cards, and news items sent by residents, families, and community leaders commending the community or its employees for high-quality service.

The receptionist (as well as front-office personnel) should always give prospects immediate attention, trying to make them feel comfortable and relaxed. Some communities ask prospects to fill out lead cards while they wait, but this can make for a cold reception. It is better to have the sales counselor collect the information during a personal interview.

The sales counselor should lead the prospect(s) to a quiet and private area that allows uninterrupted conversation. This could be a back office, a private sitting room, or a conference room with comfortable seating.

The initial few minutes of conversation are critical. The prospect will look the salesperson over carefully to determine whether she is likely to be responsive, caring, and professional. The sales counselor must use this time to investigate a number of qualifying criteria (such as income, age, and medical condition) and to identify the prospect's needs and wants. She should also use this time to establish a friendly relationship with the prospect and to demonstrate that she is interested in finding a way to fulfill the prospect's needs rather than simply making a sale. The axiom "make a friend, then make a sale" is particularly valid in the senior living industry.

Most of all, the sales counselor will need to practice active listening. Many salespeople become so focused on what they have to say about the community that they inadvertently give the impression that they think they know what is best for the prospect. In selling, the sales counselor needs to learn as much about the prospect as possible in a short time. Here are some tips for improving listening skills:

■ Ask questions and hear the prospect out. Sometimes it is effective to use a pause to control the flow of conversation and draw out the prospect. Most salespeople feel uncomfortable with silence, but it can be a sales ally.

■ Avoid situations that may subject the conversation to interruptions, and never interrupt the prospect. This will help to keep the focus on the prospects and demonstrate a sincere interest in them. If you think of an important point while the prospect is speaking, jot it down and wait until she has finished. Ask prospects whether they mind if you take notes.

- Concentrate on the topic at hand. Listening speed is faster than talking speed, so make a conscious effort to focus on the prospect.

- Be attentive to nonverbal cues in the prospect and in yourself. Communications experts say that more than 90 percent of our messages are interpreted based on how we deliver them. A message is interpreted in this way: 7 percent is based on the words, 33 percent is based on how the words are said (pitch, tone, volume, rate of speed, and inflection), and 60 percent is based on body language. Tune in to the nonverbal cues of your prospects—posture, eye movements, speech patterns, even skin tone—and learn to mirror them, which subconsciously tells prospects that they can trust you. Look for conflicts between the prospect's words and her body language.

- Listen to all the information offered, even details that may not interest you. Skilled listeners do not discard information that could be useful later.

Experienced sales counselors use probing questions to gain insight into the prospect's needs and feelings and to keep her talking. They can also be used to help the prospect clarify her own thinking. Many prospects are unsure about what senior living communities offer and how they would fit in. The right questions can both clarify needs and create awareness. There are five types of probes: open-ended, closed-ended, operant-word, clarifying, and testing.

The *open-ended* probe is a question or statement that invites a wide-ranging response and asks for ideas, opinions, or views. They often start with "What," "Why," "Tell me about," or "What do you think of." These questions are used to open a discussion, invite the prospect to offer comprehensive responses, and give him the freedom to say what is on his mind. Such questions cannot be answered with a yes or no. For example, "Tell me what prompted your visit today."

The *closed-ended* probe is a question that limits the answer by asking for specific facts or a yes-or-no response. They often start with "Which," "Who," "When," "Where," or "How many." These questions are

useful for discovering specific details, testing understanding, directing the discussion, or asking the prospect to take a position on something. For example, "Do you think that you will be able to move in next month?"

The *operant-word* probe involves taking a key word from a prospect's previous statement and using it to create the sales counselor's next question. This method is useful for checking the sales counselor's understanding, proving that she is listening, and clarifying a prospect's needs and wants. It increases the quality of information being gathered and builds rapport. For example, if the prospect says, "One of the things I'm concerned about is security," the sales counselor may respond, "Security is important to you. What security concerns do you have?"

Clarifying a question is a type of feedback that asks the prospect for more information about a specific aspect of an earlier response. It shows that the sales counselor understands, and it prompts the prospect to provide additional information. It is also useful for refocusing the prospect's thinking. For example, "What exactly do you mean when you say that you are not ready yet?" Such a question invites the prospect to respond in more detail so that the sales counselor can tailor a response or gain some time to think.

A *testing* question asks where the prospect stands on a particular issue. It can be useful in determining the relative value of something to the prospect and in helping the sales counselor decide what topics to emphasize during the presentation. For example, "How does the continuum of care provided here match up with your wife's needs?"

The sales counselor should be polite, courteous, and respectful to prospects at all times. Even if they do not seem to appreciate a sales counselor's time and effort at the interview, when the decision-making time arrives, they will remember the help and kindness offered. This residual effect reflects favorably on the entire operation and helps set the stage for moving in.

People can spot a phony from a mile away. Senior consumers are especially knowledgeable and shrewd. If the sales counselor does not believe wholeheartedly in what she is selling, the prospect will sense it immediately. If her primary concern is in making the sale or earning an incentive, the prospect will sense that immediately too. The sales counselor's enthusiasm should be communicated in her speech, expression, and body language.

The sales counselor's appearance also plays an important part in forming the prospect's impression of the community. Dress and grooming should always be professional and tasteful, never flashy.

The sales counselor will be expected to know practically everything about the community. She should understand the limits of each service department so that she does not make promises that operations cannot fulfill. The cardinal rule is never to overpromise and underdeliver. If the sales counselor does not know the answer to a question, she should tell the prospect that she would like to consult with the appropriate person before she answers. The prospect will generally appreciate the honesty. Sales counselors should resist the temptation to try to accommodate all the prospect's wishes. They should not paint too rosy a picture. Seniors have been around a long time and do not expect things to fit their needs perfectly.

The Sales Presentation

When prospects initiate contact with a community, they have reached an important stage in their decision making and are taking a big step toward declaring their own dependence. They may be looking either for ways to enhance their current lifestyle or for ways to protect themselves from their declining ability to handle all of the pressures of daily living. Whether the prospect is seeking enhancement or protection, she is looking for someone to give her a compelling reason to make a decision.

The style of the sales presentation is as important as the content. It should be friendly, relaxed, concerned, and professional, and avoid the appearance of being canned. Use positive phrases in the current and absolute tense when describing common features. For example, "When you are living with us, your meals are always served at your table. We have a restaurant-style dining room that serves our residents their choice of entrees. We listen to our residents and design the food service around their likes and needs."

Consider where the presentation is given (the surroundings) and where it begins and ends. Avoid giving the prospect an information packet before the tour, as it could distract from the presentation of the community. Focus the prospect's attention on the messages you are attempting to communicate.

Always check the condition of the model units or other apartments before showing them. This takes only a few minutes and can save considerable embarrassment. Show an apartment only if all fixtures are in place and everything is clean and fresh. The models should be inspected and tidied daily, and all other vacant apartments should be on the weekly housekeeping cleaning schedule. The maintenance staff should be held responsible for cleaning up their own messes and should disassemble equipment only when they have parts on hand to make the repairs. If parts are not available, the fixtures or equipment should be reassembled and the marketing department notified of any apartment that is not in showable condition. The models should have the lights on, the blinds or window coverings open, and even some soft music playing.

Be aware of the possibility of interruptions during the presentation and tour. If an interruption by a resident is likely to be a positive encounter, by all means encourage it. A resident who is known to have positive views of the community can be introduced with a statement such as, "I was just telling Mrs. Cameron about our beautiful apartments. Don't you agree, Mrs. Jones?" A happy resident will agree and may even offer to show her own apartment. Such arrangements can be made in advance with residents who have nicely decorated apartments that they are proud to show off. Most occupied apartments are more homey and welcoming than the models. If the resident is known to have a negative attitude, gently but firmly refer her to another staff member and avoid any introductions or involvement with the prospect.

Customize the presentation and tour to the characteristics and needs of the prospect. Anticipate the prospect's questions after the information-gathering interview and the tour. The presentation should emphasize the areas of the community and its amenities and services that will be the most beneficial to the prospect's needs.

Leave the discussion of the costs of the program until the end of the tour, if possible. Do not bring up the subject of fees until the prospect has seen the entire community and heard about the spectrum of services and amenities. If the prospect brings up the subject earlier in the presentation, the sales counselor can respond with something like, "Well, our apartments begin at $3,600 per month and go up from there, depending on the size of the apartment you choose. The cost is relevant only when you consider the benefits of the additional services and amenities that go with it. Let me explain." Then proceed with the tour and presentation and mention an additional feature that has not been covered. If the presentation successfully builds the prospect's desire to become a part of the community, then cost will be a barrier only to those who truly cannot afford the community, an issue that should have already been determined when qualifying the prospect. When discussing rates, explain all charges the resident or responsible party can expect and when they are due. Be sure to define what services are included in the monthly fee and what other services are available at additional cost.

Many prospects may experience sticker shock when they become aware of the cost of senior living, particularly if they are living in their own home free and clear of a mortgage. Suggest that they compare what it costs them to provide all of these services for themselves. Many seniors underestimate their cost of living. Point out that the community benefits from economies of scale: all things considered, it is much more cost-efficient to provide needed services to many seniors living in a community with needs in common than for individuals to purchase similar services.

Overcoming Objections and Confirming the Sale

The best salespeople welcome objections. They provide more information and clarify the prospect's needs. Overcoming objections is part of the confirmation process. In a traditional sales approach, this is part of the closing process. In relationship selling, the sales counselor should try to identify and address the prospect's objections throughout the sales process, so that closing is less a matter of refuting objections than of confirming the decision and offering encouragement and reassurance.

Chat with your prospects before the tour to determine why they are inquiring with you and to establish a rapport. Demonstrate that you are primarily interested in finding a way to meet their needs rather than making a sale. Point out how the community's amenities match their personal interests and needs.

Throughout the tour, anticipate potential objections, selectively and patiently resolving them. Toward the end of the tour, start to close in. Ask the prospect if there is anything about the community that she may be uncomfortable with. Selling is a matter of identifying objections and then overcoming them. Try to ascertain exactly what she may be uncomfortable

with and then solve it. For example, "Mrs. Cameron, you seem uncomfortable with our reservation agreement. If it weren't for your feeling that you might be permanently committing yourself before you sell your house, do you think this type of lifestyle might make sense for you? If I could make arrangements to reserve an apartment in your name, risk-free, while you sell your home, do you think you might take us up on our offer?"

Prospects' objections can chart your course toward getting a deposit check. What follows are some sample objections and responses.

Typical Objections and Some Sample Responses

Objection: I'm not ready.
  Responses:

- Good, then it's just a matter of working on the timing, isn't it?
- I understand how you feel. But tell me, just what do you think would have to happen before you felt that you were ready? Wouldn't it be comforting to you and your family that, should such an event ever happen, you would already be in an environment where you could receive that cushion of care when you needed it?

Claiming not to be ready is a convenient way for an uninformed prospect to terminate a conversation with a salesperson. But even most serious prospects may feel the decision is premature: they want to remain where they are more than they desire to move into a senior living community.

Objection: We would have to sell the house.
  Response:

- That's right. Most of our residents have sold their homes to come here, and they will tell you it's the best decision they ever made. We can arrange a meeting for you with a competent realtor who will do a comparative market analysis on your home for no obligation. Many people are surprised at how much equity they have tied up in their homes that could be earning interest for them if they sold.

Barbara Kleger, president of Senior Living Associates, suggests, "Be patient; it takes a long time to grow old and a long time to make such a drastic decision as moving out of one's cherished home."

Objection: We have too much furniture.
Response:

- I know how you feel. Most of us spend half of our lives accumulating things and the other half giving them away. Most people find that when they start the paring-down process, it's not as painful as they thought it would be. In fact, your new spacious apartment can accommodate many of the favorite possessions you want to keep. Our move-in coordinator will be glad to assist you in determining where some of your furniture can be placed in the apartment. We assist you in every step of the move, from measuring space and furniture to helping coordinate the moving-in process.

- There are a lot of things to consider, aren't there? Our residents have all faced this issue and, as you can see, they've gained so much with all of our amenities, they don't miss their excess furniture. They decided they didn't want their possessions to stand in the way of getting what they knew was right for them. Sort of makes sense, doesn't it?

Objection: I'm too old to move now.
Response:

- That's interesting. We have many people here who are older than you. I'll bet you're not too old to get more out of life, right? This community provides you the opportunity of a secure, enjoyable, carefree lifestyle, and these could be the best years of your life. Statistics prove that people live on the average two to three years longer in a senior living community than in an apartment. There are several good reasons for this. One of them is companionship. One of the saddest things about growing older is that our friends pass away. We meet new friends, of course, but if we are not in a community setting, we don't have the ability to continually expand our friendships. Therefore, they are continually shrinking. If we stop driving in the years ahead, or our friends don't drive, or the weather is bad, we tend to spend a lot of time in our private residence. Many meals are eaten with our only companion being Vanna White. It's easy to see how one can slowly become a recluse over a period of time.

At a senior living community, companionship is always available.

Objection: I'm too young for this.
Response:

- I see. Well, interestingly, we have several people who are younger than you, and they will tell you they don't know why they waited so long. When do you think it is easier to make a change—when you're younger and have several options, or when you're older and possibly forced to make a decision under the pressure of time?

- I understand how you must feel. Retirees who have joined us here at the community support the philosophy that you should *not* wait until you need services such as health care to move to a full-service senior living community. Instead of being in the position of using the health care services and options provided for you among friends and neighbors, waiting might mean that you could find yourself in a strange nursing home several miles away from familiar surroundings. Or you might find yourself having to depend on your children or friends to take care of you, placing an undue hardship on them and taking away your independent way of life. Doesn't that make sense?

Objection: I've got too much energy for this. I'm still very active.
Response:

- Tell you what, take a look at our activities calendar, and let's assume you'll do everything that's listed. I'll bet halfway through the month you'll call time out! And just because you change your address doesn't mean you'll be less active. You'll just keep on with your fast-paced schedule without the worries of keeping up with your household.

Objection: I'm still able to take care of things around the house.
Response:

- You have done all the things to maintain your household up to this point. Although you can still do them, they are probably becoming a little more difficult with each passing year. The heavier jobs such as vacuuming, laundry, and cleaning floors and bathrooms are the kinds of things that no one likes doing. And they will become less pleasant as time goes on.

Objection: I'm just not sure.
Response:

- There's some risk involved, isn't there? And you want to be certain you do the right thing. What information would you need to be more comfortable with your decision?
- I sense that there may be something that you are uncertain about. It is the _____ [suggest possibilities like the fee, moving, apartment, etc., until you zero in]? Well, if it weren't for [the objection], do you think this lifestyle here might make sense for you? If I could [fix the objection], would you take us up on our offer?

Objection: I'm going to look around.
Response:

- Excellent. What will you be looking for?
- Good idea. We encourage all our prospects to compare what we offer and our reputation with others in the business. We can show you on our comparison chart, which details how the other communities stack up. I'm sure you will recognize how much more value you get here for your dollar.
- I understand how you feel. It's important to make the right decision about your new home. Wouldn't it be nice to be able to reserve an option for yourself while you're looking so that if you need one, you already have one picked out to fall back on? If I could show you a way to tie up a choice apartment today, risk-free, don't you think that might make good sense for you?

Objection: It's too much work.
Response:

- Could be. Anything worthwhile is worth working for, isn't it? But we can make it easier for you by doing most of the legwork of getting you situated with us. We have some excellent resources we can work with to help you with the sale of your house and your moving arrangements. By the way, will it be any less work in the future, or any easier for you at some time down the road?

Objection: I'm going to stay in my home until something happens that will make me need this.

Response:

- And then what will you do? Would you rather have a choice now or leave things to chance later? I think we all like to feel that we have control of our lives.

Objection: I don't think I can afford this.
I'm not used to spending this much on my housing.
Response:

- At first it seems high, doesn't it? I can certainly understand how you feel; a number of our residents once felt the same way you do, but when they considered everything we include in our monthly fee compared to similar expenses in their own home, they found they weren't paying any more to live here—and in some cases, less than before. Here, let me show you the value on this comparison chart and you can see for yourself.

Objection: I want to think about it.
Response:

- That's fine. Obviously, you wouldn't take your time thinking this over unless you were interested, would you?
- So, may I assume that you will give it careful consideration?
- Just to clarify my thinking, what part of this decision are you concerned about? Is it _____?
- Is there anything I have talked about that isn't clear?
- Is there anything about the community you are unsure about?
- Is it the monthly fee?
- Is it the moving problems?

Objection: I want to see it built first.
Response:

- If you were simply buying an apartment, that would be understandable. But we are not selling just bricks and mortar. We are selling a lifestyle along with a whole host of services designed to bring you peace of mind and continued independence as your everyday challenges become increasingly complex. Our program is built around the physical amenities. Your enjoyment of the community will come from the many services and intangibles it has to offer, such as activities programming, delicious meals, housekeeping, transportation services, and other things like companionship, security, and access to health care. You see, the building is only the location where all these things come together. It is secondary to the benefits of living there.

In the end, overcoming objections is a process of helping the prospect get used to the decision. Be patient. Listen for hidden meanings in their objections. Repeat the objection to clarify your understanding. Sometimes when people hear their objection repeated back to them, it sounds overstated, and they may back down. Confirm the objection by agreeing with the prospect. Do not try to argue or suggest you know better. Prospects like to have their objections acknowledged and validated. Question the intent behind the objection. Answer their concerns as best you can without being smart or glib. Confirm the answer by relating the experience of others in their situation who may have had the same objection but ultimately found that it was unwarranted. Finally, close on common ground and leave the prospect with something that you both agree on about the situation.

Overcoming objections can be a bit like handling complaints. You are seeking a positive resolution to a negative response to or drawback in your program. It may be helpful to review the checklist for handling complaints in chapter 6.

Here is a formula for handling final objections:

1. Hear it out.
2. Repeat the objection.
3. Confirm the objection.
4. Question it.
5. Answer it.
6. Confirm the answers.
7. Close.

Follow-Through

A sales counselor often spends two hours or more with a prospect, particularly if lunch or dinner is involved. It is crucial to be willing to devote the time to the meeting. A great deal of information must be covered, and if any aspect of the community is overlooked, the prospect may wrongly assume that the service or amenity is not offered. Even if the sales counselor clearly sees that the community could

meet the prospect's need well, she must still convince the prospect of that fact.

At the conclusion of the tour and presentation, the sales counselor should attempt some trial closes. This is the most difficult part of any sales presentation. Asking for the deposit risks rejection, and most of us prefer to avoid rejection at all costs. But if the presentation has clearly matched the community's offerings to the prospect's needs, then the sales counselor has prepared the prospect to consider a decision. At this point the prospect must have a clear feeling that she is not being sold something but is being offered options. Throughout the presentation, the sales counselor should be looking for common ground and making small closes on points of agreement. When the small closes have been successfully executed (the apartment selected, parking place chosen, furniture placement visualized), the decision to move ahead with the paperwork is only the next natural step. This way, the sales counselor is assuring the prospect that this lifestyle is right for her, rather than trying to convince her to sign on the dotted line.

The "feel, felt, found" answer to final obstacles is an excellent and positive way to reassure the prospect. For example, when the prospect indicates that he is hesitant to make the commitment, the sales counselor can say, "Mr. Joseph, I understand how you feel. Many of our current residents have felt the same way as you do, but what they found once they made the decision and joined the community was that they should have made the decision much earlier. Would it help with your comfort level to talk to one of our residents?" This way, the sales counselor has acknowledged the prospect's fears, assured him that they are not unique but common to many others who have already moved into the community, and assuaged the fears with the knowledge that others have overcome them and are glad they made the move. When the prospect decides to move, he chooses the community that most closely meets his individual needs and presents the fewest barriers.

Whenever possible, when the residency agreement is signed, the prospective resident's name should be passed on to operations to coordinate the move-in. This process should be handled delicately, inasmuch as the prospect will have established a relationship with the salesperson. Make it appear that you are not terminating that relationship but rather expanding it to others in the community. Many communities employ a move-in coordinator. This person is usually introduced early in the sales process, and again later after the residency agreement has been finalized, to pave the way for transition. (See chapter 16 for more on move-in coordination.) Seniors typically experience "buyer's remorse," feelings of regret or uncertainty after they have reached a decision. The move-in coordinator will need to continue to confirm the prospect's decision and offer reassurance until well after the agreement has been signed and even after the prospect moves into her apartment.

A follow-up letter should be mailed to the prospect within twenty-four hours of the initial visit. This letter serves several purposes: first, to thank the prospect for her interest for taking the time taken to tour the community; second, to prompt the prospect to recall her visit to the community; third, to show the prospect that the sales counselor is interested in helping her become a resident of the community; and, fourth and most important, to confirm the prospect's impression of the community as a positive, professionally operated place that offers the services she needs. The letter should also encourage the prospect to revisit the community or contact the sales counselor regarding any questions or concerns that were not addressed during her visit. If for some reason the prospect chooses not to move in, the follow-up letter will nevertheless leave the prospect with a favorable impression that may lead to a referral.

Some communities send a "day after" questionnaire to the prospect in a self-addressed, stamped envelope to determine how well the marketing effort was executed. This is returned to the executive director, who will discuss it with the marketing director. The questionnaire should be anonymous to elicit honest and objective answers. This feedback can be especially helpful to new sales staff members in fine-tuning their presentations.

Approximately one week after the initial prospect visit, a follow-up phone call from the sales counselor may be appropriate. During the conversation, inquire about a personal matter that the prospect may have shared during the visit and ask if he has any questions or concerns. Also ask where he is in the decision-making process. If he has decided to move into the community, schedule an appointment to coordinate the move. If he has chosen another community, tact-fully ask the reasons why. These responses can be helpful in determining the community's strengths and weaknesses in the marketplace. If the prospect indicates that he will be moving to another community, schedule another follow-up phone call approximately two weeks later to let the prospect know that you care enough to keep in touch. Many prospects may indicate alternative plans in order to delay the decision or avoid a commitment. You want to be sure that the prospect is satisfied with the decision.

On the day of the sale, the executive director should send a "thank you for choosing us" letter. This lets the prospect know that the entire community knows she will soon be coming to live there, and it emphasizes a desire to serve her. Little extras such as these letters are often the deciding factor that a prospect uses in selecting one community over another.

Wait Lists

Wait lists are useful for establishing a commitment on the part of the prospect. These can include prospects who are waiting for a specific type of unit to become available and those who plan to move to the community but may not be ready. The prospect usually submits a fully refundable deposit, which may be several hundred dollars or a percentage of the entrance fee (payment of interest on this deposit may be subject to local regulations). This deposit places the prospect's name on a wait list for a specific type of apartment. When a unit of this type becomes available, the next prospect on the list is notified and asked to sign a residency agreement within a set period (usually seven days). If the prospect does not wish to take the apartment when it is available, most communities allow her to keep her place on the list and be notified when another apartment becomes available.

The wait list prospect who is classified as "not ready" and does not wish to be called each time an apartment becomes available is treated as an inactive member. Inactive wait list prospects are contacted on a quarterly basis to assess their status and to encourage an upgrade to active status.

Prospects should be reminded that they are subject to normal rent or fee increases during their wait on the list. Other new residents might be angry to learn that someone else off the wait list was guaranteed a much lower rent.

Many communities offer additional benefits to their wait list prospects to demonstrate the value of membership and to facilitate frequent contact. Such benefits might include newsletter and event mailings, lunch or dinner at resident rates (as space permits), participation in selected resident programs and classes, or even discounts on guest apartment stays (annually limited). These benefits are designed to keep the prospect in frequent contact with the community and aware of the value associated with living in the community.

Wait lists can be a useful tool for converting a reluctant prospect. The act of making a deposit is a small close. Some prospects need to be sold in stages, and the wait list represents their first commitment. Wait lists are generally more effective as occupancy increases and the availability of specific types of apartments becomes limited. The urgency to act becomes more real because once all the available units are sold, roles reverse: the prospect waits for the community to respond, instead of the community's waiting for the prospect. In other words, during the fill-up stage, the community waits; on stabilization, the prospect waits.

Occasionally, when a specific type of apartment is not available, the prospect may elect to move into another apartment temporarily. Usually the prospect will move into a larger apartment while waiting for a smaller one. A reduction in rent can be offered on the larger apartment until the smaller one becomes available. The resident is usually asked to move into the smaller apartment within 30 days of availability or to start paying the full monthly fee on the larger apartment.

Relocation within the building can be done either by community maintenance staff or by professional movers. Some communities charge the resident for relocation costs. But if time is of the essence or if someone else is waiting for the current apartment to be vacated, the management can expedite the transfer by offering to pick up the tab. As a rule, if the building is empty, the resident pays for the relocation; if it is full, the management does.

Some companies pay commissions to sales counselors when wait list deposits are collected, but usually this payment is structured as an advance against the commission on the eventual sale. See the compensation section below.

Requests for Information

An interested party or prospect who requests information by phone should receive an information packet along with a cover letter. Requests for information should always be handled by a sales counselor to gauge how much information to give out and to attempt to qualify the caller. Most communities send out only a brochure in response to requests for information. Sending a formal letter thanking a prospect for interest in the community and issuing an invitation to visit will set the stage for a successful inquiry and sales process. He will appreciate the time and effort and will be likely to look to your community first for help with questions about senior living.

Many people call local senior living communities to gather basic information such as rates, availability of apartments, and so on before deciding which communities to visit and tour in person. Therefore, it is critical to make a good impression during the phone conversation. Sales counselors should, however, resist the temptation to give their entire presentation over the phone. Most people can remember only a small amount of information, and it is a stab in the dark for the sales counselor to try to guess what the caller wants to hear without the advantage of a personal interview.

Responses should give callers critical information while trying gently to persuade them to visit the community. After all, it is difficult to describe an entire lifestyle package in a short telephone conversation. Offer to put together an information packet and set aside some time to give the caller a tour. If the caller does not want to visit, try to get her address and phone number and then check back in a few days to see that she has received the packet. Make some suggestions on what the caller might do next and offer assurance that you are there to help her find solutions, not just to make a sale. If the community obviously will not meet her needs, then offer some suggestions for finding the most appropriate setting. This way, you are offering to perform a service rather than pitching a sales presentation.

Many inquiries come from interested parties—family members, usually the children, of the prospect who have already recognized a need. They are typically motivated by either feelings of guilt stemming from a geographical or work-driven inability to care for their parents or serious concerns about the safety of their living alone. Many family members visit one or more senior living communities and choose one they would like to see their parents move into. The next step is to approach them with the idea of considering such a move.

For many, this is a difficult step because of the role reversal that occurs. It is not easy for a child to become the caregiver, offering advice or even taking charge. No one wants to push and doing so would likely meet resistance anyway. The prospect needs to recognize the importance of the decision and the fact that moving to a senior living community does not mean a loss of independence. She should be encouraged to visit the community with the parent and have lunch. Many communities have guest apartments and can arrange for a trial visit or weekend stay, which gives the prospect an opportunity to experience the lifestyle and talk to a few people who live there. Often, residents living in a community have a way of selling the place themselves.

SALES ANALYSIS

Often the causes of a failing community can be traced to flawed marketing strategies or to productivity issues in the sales department. Sales analysis is the detailed study of sales statistics to evaluate performance. It can equip the management to adjust marketing tactics and allocate sales efforts effectively. As sales directors identify weak areas in their sales department, individually and overall, they can develop short- or long-term incentives to focus the sales counselors' attention appropriately.

Marketing departments can collect data in a variety of ways, using traffic reports, summaries of prospect lead cards, computer activity reports, and the personal logs of the sales counselors. This information can be compiled by a marketing assistant or secretary, the marketing or sales director, the executive director, or even the night concierge. As discussed earlier, it may be advisable to have one employee personally responsible for maintaining the computerized lead bank, marketing responses, and sales statistics. This approach produces more-consistent data entry and greater proficiency in customizing reports.

Analyzing sales performance statistics is an absolute necessity. Although each community or market is unique, evaluation of the results against industry standards enables the sales director to quantify the relative strengths and areas of vulnerability of the sales counselors.

Phone-outs

The telephone is the single most effective method of reaching the lead bank. It can be used to build relationships, initiate the sales process, coordinate appointments, prompt action, and solve problems. The average sales counselor should complete approximately 20 phone-outs per day. To be counted, a phone-out must reach the intended lead and have at least a minimal exchange of information: either the caller or the recipient must gain some new information as a result of the call. The number of calls to each lead is established by a tickler system, or contact management software, and urgency classification. This schedule can be overridden by the sales counselor as appropriate: he may defer a call if the client is out of town, sick, or awaiting news from a physician, for instance. If the sales counselor is not averaging at least 10 personal contacts per day, then something is wrong, and the sales director needs to address it. An excellent book on how to "reach out and touch someone," *The Phone Book*, by Richard Zarro and Peter Blum, is a good resource for improving the effectiveness of telephone communication.[2]

In addition to reaching the leads by phone, expectations should be established for the conversion of phone calls to sales appointments. The call-conversion rate is the percentage of calls to the lead bank and from phone-ins combined that result in appointments. For calls to new leads, this conversion ratio is a good measure of the quality of new leads responding to a specific marketing strategy. The call-conversion rate for new, good-quality leads should be approximately 20 percent: that is, one in five calls to new leads should result in an appointment. For follow-up leads, the call-conversion rate should be about 5 to 10 percent. The average sales counselor should therefore be able to set up at least one appointment per day from calls from his own leads.

The objective of personally contacting individuals in the lead bank is, of course, to set up appointments and build relationships. After appointments are set, they must be kept. Occasionally, a prospect will agree to an appointment to get the caller off the phone, and then fail to show. The appointments-kept statistic is a measure of the quality and motivation of leads as well as sales skill at booking appointments. Transportation to the project is often difficult for the prospect to arrange, so the more difficult the logistical obstacles, the more serious the client. Experienced salespeople generally have a much higher appointments-kept percentage, often close to 100 percent. They know the value of their time and are not inclined to waste it on reluctant prospects and tire kickers. Because it is relatively rare to make a sale on the first appointment (except for skilled nursing or assisted living), the appointment-to-move-in conversion rate for new leads is meaningless. But the appointment-conversion rate for follow-up or repeat appointments is a good measure of prospect motivation and sales ability. The rate of sales from single follow-up appointments should approach 25 percent. At the very least, the sales counselor should secure a wait list deposit. Caution should be exercised, however, because the deposit can at times provide a haven for "not-ready" clients.

With sales-activity expectations established, it is possible to make sales forecasts. For example, if a sales counselor is making 20 phone-outs per day with an average call-appointment conversion rate of 10 percent, she should be scheduling approximately 2 appointments each day, or 10 per week (and certainly at least 1 appointment per day). With an appointment-to-sale conversion rate of 10 percent on 10 appointments per week, an average sales counselor should be able to close approximately 1 sale each week, or 4 per month (although site-specific results will vary).

The greater the number of follow-up appointments for a single prospect, the less productive the sales counselor becomes. In fact, after five or six successive appointments without a sale, the sales director should become involved to help determine the sales strategy. Some people simply like to come to the events or enjoy the free lunch.

The appointment-conversion rate usually increases with the level of care. Assisted living prospects are usually more need-driven and have a higher urgency level than do congregate prospects or those interested in continuing-care retirement communities. Finally, it can be helpful to keep track of appointment-conversion rates to the wait list, particularly if wait list deposits qualify for commission rewards, as this arrangement may reduce the sales counselors' motivation to complete the sale.

Mail-outs

In contrast to phone calls, which are often considered annoying interruptions in our day, most of us look forward to opening the day's mail. We usually look for personal notes and letters and open those first. Most seniors enjoy receiving mail and will respond with a phone call thanking you for the personal touch.

Top sales counselors send out hundreds of personal letters and mailings each month. Most sales directors set a target of at least 20 mail-outs for each sales counselor daily. Bulk mailings of event flyers, newsletters, and seminar and other announcements should be excluded from this count. The letters can include "tried to reach you" letters to unclassified mail-in leads, "day after the tour" letters, notes or cards expressing sympathy for illness or bereavement, responses to requests for information, phone call follow-ups, letters passing on industry news or press releases, and the like. One dementia care community developed a card that on the outside simply said, "Gratitude is the heart's memory," with the inside left blank for a personal note. It's a nice touch that links the dementia care concept with the overall purpose of the card, which was to thank the person for touring. Handwritten envelopes, notes, and cards have a much bigger impact than computer-generated letters. Some communities mail small gifts and cookies to their active prospects to remind them gently of the caring atmosphere that the community offers.

Seniors are often inundated by telemarketers because many of them are home all day. It is difficult to avoid being seen as just another pushy salesperson trying to trick them into buying something that they may not need. Telemarketers rarely, however, take the time to send a personal note; those who do can quickly cut through the barrage of advertising rubbish and get their message across. There is nothing like a personal note to communicate the sentiment that "I care about you, and I'm not just in this for the sale."

The expectations of conversion rates from the various types of contact are discussed in the "Sources of Leads" section above.

Number of Contacts

The average ratio of contacts to sales is a good measure of the quality of the leads and the sales counselors' closing skills. The lower the ratio, the higher the productivity of the sales counselor. Selling senior living, as we have seen, involves the development of a rapport between the sales counselor and the prospect. The more quickly trust is established, the sooner the prospect will be converted to a resident. Training sales counselors in methods of advanced communications and relationship building can accelerate this process and decrease the average number of contacts to sale and days to sale. In fact, these two statistics can be used to evaluate the effectiveness of such training.

Another measure of the quality and motivation of the lead bank is the percentage of sales that are generated within the first 30 days. These are essentially hot leads at first contact. Many prospects interested in assisted living or skilled nursing fall into this category. A congregate community that is priced competitively and has a good reputation in the community should expect to generate at least 30 percent of its sales within 30 days. This number should climb toward 50 percent for the more need-driven assisted living prospects.

Table 15.4 details typical sales performance targets for three types of community. These are guidelines for an average community in a fill-up stage. Actual targets and relative performance will of course vary according to local conditions and the owners' expectations.

COMPENSATION

The compensation package for the sales counselors can be structured to energize the sales effort and target weaknesses in the program. The single biggest cause of failed projects has been the inability to meet occupancy projections. Operators have now reached a better understanding of the marketplace through more sophisticated feasibility studies. If the community is priced right and has a good location, adequate demand, and a service package that demonstrates value, then the only missing element is sales. Even the best offering requires motivated and savvy people to promote it.

Often, the management will scrutinize a $500 commission check payable to a successful sales counselor but sign off with barely a second glance on a $1,500 advertising invoice that produced only five leads. Yet investing in the sales team may produce higher returns than paying advertising fees. It is more productive to offer cash incentives to sales staff to work *current* leads, many of whom may have al-

Table 15.4   **Sales Performance Targets**

Performance category	Congregate	CCRC	Assisted living
Lead-lease conversion rate	7%	4%	10%
Average phone-outs per day per person	15–20	15–20	15–20
Average mail-outs per day per person	20	20	20
Call-appointment conversion rate (new leads)	20%	15%	30%
Call-appointment conversion rate (follow-up leads)	5%–10%	5%–10%	10%–15%
Appointment-sale conversion rate (follow-up leads)	10%	5%–10%	10%–15%
Percentage of appointments kept	95	95	95
Appointment-to-wait-list-deposit conversion rate	10%	10%	5%
Percentage of sales with interested party as initial contact	25–50	5–10	80–95
Percentage of sales from referral sources	10	5	20
Walk-in-to-sale conversion rate	10%	7%	15%
Phone-in-to-sale conversion rate	8%	5%	12%
Phone-out-to-sale conversion rate	5%	5%	7%
Mail-in-to-sale conversion rate	3%	2.5%–5%	5%
Referral-to-sale conversion rate	12%	7%–10%	15%
Average number of contacts to sale	10	10	3–5
Average number of days to sale	100	120	60
Average number of days from sale to move-in	60	90	45
Percentage of sales generated within 30 days	30	20	50

ready visited the community, than to spend additional advertising dollars to attract additional leads who may not even be qualified. It is always better to work the lead bank that you have already bought and paid for. The trick is then to put your money where your mouth is and convince the sales counselors that the old leads are likely to produce sales.

A good compensation plan should be designed to reward and motivate. To do this, it must meet several requirements:

■ It must provide a living wage in the form of a secure income. Sales counselors who are worried about money do not concentrate on doing their jobs well. Relationship building takes time, and to be successful at building rapport with the prospect, you must avoid giving the impression that your sales staff is financially pressured to make sales.

- The plan must not be divisive. It should offer a mix of individual rewards and team incentives that encourages the sales counselors to work well together. For example, individuals can earn commissions on personal sales, and the team can earn incentives based on collective goals, such as total sales or total appointments scheduled, phone-outs, or conversion rates for the whole department.

- The plan must be fair and realistic, and not penalize sales counselors for factors beyond their control. If the community is not competitively priced, no incentive plan will suffice to increase sales. Performance goals must be within reach and the rewards worth striving for.

- The compensation plan must be easy for the sales counselors to understand, and they must be able to calculate their own earnings. Complex compensation formulas can be used as long as the sales director explains them thoroughly, with several examples. The ability to calculate potential earnings in advance allows sales counselors the opportunity to set their own financial and performance targets and work toward them.

- The plan should reward incremental improvements in performance. This way, there is always an incentive to do more, even if the sales counselors are already having a good month.

- The plan should be designed around the objectives of the sales and marketing department. It should align with the expectations of each sales counselor, the sales director, and the executive director and the community's budgeted occupancy forecasts.

The typical compensation plan has several components: a fixed salary to provide income stability; variable elements such as commissions, bonuses, and incentives; and fringe elements such as vacation and sick benefits, insurance, and disability coverage. Straight salary plans, while providing the management considerable control over the sales staff, also have weaknesses. Without financial incentives, the sales counselor is not motivated to maximize his or her earning potential. Straight commission plans pay based on performance but afford the sales director little control over the sales staff. Most companies use a combination of the two. The proportions of each element will vary, but for inexperienced salespeople the split between salary and commissions often works out to be about 50/50 or less. As their performance improves, so does the level of commissions relative to their base salary. The income of top sales counselors consistently producing six or seven sales per month is typically split 20/80 between salary and commissions.

Often an adjustment to the structure of the sales compensation plan is sufficient to jump-start a sales department. For example, a community with a team commission structure that divided each sales commission equally among the sales staff, regardless of who made the sale, was consistently producing about 3 or 4 sales per month and about a 50/50 split between salary and commission income for the counselors. When the commission structure was redesigned to provide individual commissions along with team incentives, the sales counselors were quick to understand the benefits of increasing their productivity. Within three months, the sales department had tripled the average sales to 12 per month, and, because of the increase in productivity, the average cost per sale was cut in half! Although the team approach was simple to administer, it offered no reward to the counselor who made the sale. In fact, many productive sales counselors were reluctant to work harder if they had to share their hard-earned commissions with other sales counselors who were satisfied with selling only 1 or 2 units per month. In effect, the team approach resulted in the productive sales counselors carrying the nonproductive ones. The sales compensation plan should be designed to motivate and reward top producers, not subsidize poor performance.

The base salary level should be determined through a wage survey of the local competitors, and it must be competitive to attract new recruits. If the base salary is low and the sale price of the units (even if well commissioned) is too high, the applicant will realize that the earning potential may be limited. The management must consider the experience and potential productivity of the applicants and set base salaries accordingly. Some companies operating multiple communities base their sales compensation plans on a formal evaluation of the entire company. Such a plan, however, may not be competitive across all regions of the country and may not address the specific performance requirements of each community. It is better to design a compensation plan that has a basic salary and commission shell and to customize incentive programs for each site, within budgetary guidelines.

Most companies in the industry use a sliding scale for commissions, so that each additional sale in a given period, such as a month, is worth more in commissions. The weakness of this system is that it encourages sales counselors to cluster their sales within one sales period: for example, they may have a "good" month every other month to maximize their commission payment per sale.

Payment time frames for these commissions also vary by company. Forty-four percent of the companies surveyed paid the commissions when the resident moved in, whereas 33 percent paid half at the point of sale and half at move-in. Other companies (12%) used variations of this approach, such as 40 percent payment at point of sale and 60 percent at move-in, to emphasize to the sales counselors the importance of follow-through to ensure a prompt move-in. This is understandable, as the revenue from the sale is generated only after the resident has moved in.

Commission plans vary greatly among companies. Fifty percent pay commissions on the basis of the number of move-ins per month, whereas 33 percent pay on the basis of the number of sales per month. Again, the emphasis was clearly placed on move-ins, which generate the revenue to offset the commissions paid. Thus some companies used the commission structure to focus the attention of the sales staff on issues critical to the communities. Companies willing to be flexible and creative with commission structures can respond effectively to changing community needs. Some companies will individually price every unit in the building based upon what may be unique about that apartment. This way they can create a premium pricing based upon view, proximity to the elevator, unit features, or configuration. Marketing counselors can say, "I understand your mother likes to watch the sunrise or wants a garden view. We only have two units left with garden views, so if you leave a deposit today, you can reserve one and have right of first refusal if another family wants it." Management can then offer sales counselors a share of the upside from the premium pricing. For example, if the salesperson was able to get $100 more

per month for that particular unit, management can increase the commission on that unit to give the salesperson the first month's premium on that unit as an added incentive. Management then earns the additional $100 per month in revenue for the remainder of the lease.

Companies that employ a move-in coordinator are often split on paying them commissions: half do, and half do not. Many companies have no such position, perhaps because their high occupancy rates rendered it unnecessary. Generally, move-in coordinators are employed during the fill-up stage to facilitate a smooth transition into the community after the sale and free up the sales counselors' time.

The majority of companies do not pay wait list commissions. Communities with a high level of turnover can use wait list commissions to ensure a safe number of prospective new residents on the wait list. But this practice can also give the not-ready prospect a means of avoiding a firm commitment.

For canceled sales or a new resident who moved out voluntarily after a short period of time (less than 90 days), most companies charge back the commission paid to the account of the sales counselor. The rationale is that a canceled sale or rapid move-out (which may indicate an inappropriate placement) does not constitute a completed sale. Moreover, the commission is ultimately funded from the resident's monthly fee, which is not forthcoming if the resident cancels or leaves.

The majority of companies pay marketing or sales directors overrides on the sales generated by their staff. These payments are in addition to the commissions they receive on sales that they personally make. Some companies pay overrides to marketing assistants on each sale to encourage them to focus on customers.

In addition to the commission plan, many companies use sales incentives. Some companies use special bonuses to reward both the executive director and the marketing director for a rapid fill-up of newly opened communities. Reaching an occupancy threshold of 75 percent within the first 90 days could result in a $10,000 bonus, split between the executive director and the marketing director. Reaching 95 percent in 90 days could lead to a $15,000 additional incentive.

The total levels of compensation vary considerably. This wide range reflects both the variety in compensation plans commonly used in the industry and the differing abilities of the sales staffs.

In addition to a compensation plan, many companies offer other forms of incentive. Some organize team-oriented monthly sales contests using a theme and prizes. A $25 Amazon gift card might be a prize for making the fourth sale of the month, a $50 department-store gift certificate for the sixth sale, $100 theater tickets for the tenth sale, and a $300 cash bonus for a dozen sales in one month. The point of such prizes is to provide incentives to improve performance incrementally and to sustain enthusiasm among sales counselors. Recognition dinners, additional training, motivational books and audiobooks, weekends away, and pats on the back are all effective forms of motivation. Creative sales directors who identify a weakness in the sales program can develop inexpensive and fun contests to refocus their staff. Sales staff members are by nature competitive, and many will invest extra hours selling to reach designated award levels.

Many companies have a top-producers' club. These are common in real estate offices as well. Most programs define specific performance levels, with associated awards. A sales counselor who averages four sales per month could qualify for the minimum package, which might include $50 retroactive commission payments, a crystal trophy, and an award package with a letter from the president and perhaps a gift bearing the company logo. For five or six sales per month, the award package and trophy might be more impressive. It is amazing how effective these programs can be. Salespeople crave recognition, and programs like these enable them to attain a high profile in the company while keeping them constantly aware of their performance statistics.

TRAINING

Sales training can decrease the number of contacts required before close. This change can dramatically increase productivity. If the average number of contacts before close can be reduced, through training and skills practice, from 20 to 10, you have effectively doubled the productivity of each sales counselor.

Considerable opportunity exists for improving sales through training. In many communities, the training of new and experienced salespeople, beyond an introduction to the service package, financial options, and office paper flow, receives little attention

or financial support. In this relationship-oriented business, improvements in performance generated by training existing employees exceed improvements resulting from employee recruitment or replacement. So why don't we do more of it?

Perhaps the answer to this question is that people tend to gravitate toward the activities that they do best and avoid those that require them to step outside their comfort zone. Most marketing directors arrive at their position by demonstrating success in selling. This process typically involves expertise in one-on-one situations. Training is also a selling exercise, however: the trainer is selling a thought process and ideas or techniques. The difference is that training generally involves speaking before groups or leading a discussion. Training is a new ball game for the marketing director, and he may fear that it will cause him unnecessary stress and even, if it is not well received, hurt his credibility as a supervisor. Yet marketing directors who are successful at defining training needs and building effective training programs can inspire confidence, raise morale, add variety to the daily routine, and experience professional growth.

The typical employee-development model begins with setting expectations, then moves on to determining needs, training to fill needs, giving feedback on performance, and coaching for career growth. It can be broken down into four major components: the needs assessment, the training methods, the format, and the evaluation of results.[3]

Needs Assessment

The marketing director must first evaluate the training needs and the vulnerabilities of the entire department, and then of each individual. Training sessions should be separated into two main components: initial training and continuous training. Initial sales training programs typically have a broad scope and are intended to orient new employees or transferred employees to the community. Categories for initial training could include the following:

■ Understanding the market
■ Basic gerontology
■ Competitive analysis and market share
■ Departmental policies and procedures
■ Management of leads
■ Community image

- Service package
- Showing the community
- Inventory and pricing
- Limits of authority
- Record keeping
- Orientation to other departments and their services

Continuous sales training programs may concentrate on specific aspects of the job in which experienced sales counselors may have deficiencies, or they may introduce new concepts. Categories for continuous training could include topics such as the following:

- Relationship building
- Closing techniques
- Improving telephone productivity
- Advanced communication skills
- Neurolinguistic programming
- Personality and temperament testing
- Information gathering and probing
- Affirmation and imprinting
- Overcoming objections
- Handling difficult people
- Dealing with conflict
- Time management
- Marketing planning
- Community outreach
- Public relations
- Motivation and self-esteem

The objective of the training plan is to eliminate weaknesses that directly affect performance and to create learning environments that enhance it. It's a good idea to have all sales counselors rate their own skills in each area to identify any patterns in the group, and then use the results to develop a specific plan.

Experienced salespeople can be invited to assist in training new recruits. This way new employees can gain an appreciation for the skills of their coworkers, which can build team cohesiveness and cooperation.

Training Methods

The marketing director has several training methods at his disposal: group lectures, personal conferences, demonstrations, role-playing or skills practice, case studies, impromptu discussions, games, on-the-job training, and programmed training. The method should be tailored to the material. Some content is applicable to the entire group, such as new policies, company direction, and skill development. Other content, such as improving call-conversion rates, may be of a more personal nature and better imparted one on one.

LECTURES. Professional trainers generally consider lectures the least effective training method. The format establishes a passive rather than active mode of participation. Lectures emphasize teaching, not learning. Studies have shown that the average retention of material disseminated at a lecture can be less than 10 percent. Even with the use of visual aids, trainee absorption can be disappointingly low. People learn best when they are active participants and have a role to play in the process. Brief lectures can be useful, however, to introduce new material, summarize major topics, communicate company philosophy, and provide an orientation to the industry, the market, and the residents.

PERSONAL CONFERENCES. The personal conference is often the most effective training method. Personal meetings demand the participants' complete attention. Instruction can be customized to the needs of the trainee, and the trainer can offer constructive advice and specific suggestions privately, avoiding embarrassment. The conference can be structured or unstructured, formal or informal, depending on the content and context.

DEMONSTRATIONS. Demonstrations are indispensable in training. When training new sales counselors, the marketing director needs to demonstrate the best methods of showing the community. Demonstrating to the trainee how to focus a prospect's attention by using the techniques on the trainee herself is the best method of getting your point across. Demonstration is also a useful technique for teaching hands-on skills, such as using the computer system and operating apartment appliances, HVAC equipment, and door locks.

ROLE-PLAYING. Role-playing involves having trainees act out parts in specific scenarios. These situations can be either problematic or designed to create awareness. Generally speaking, role-playing is an effective method for training employees to handle challenging situations, such as managing difficult people or learning closing techniques. In addition, role-playing provides experienced sales personnel the opportunity to test responses out on the management and to clarify company policy. Role-playing, sometimes referred to as skills practice, can be fun and stimulating even for experienced salespeople, who may welcome the opportunity to display their sales talents to the group. At the same time, each participant learns to accept criticism openly from others as the group realizes that sound suggestions benefit everyone.

CASE STUDIES. Case studies can be an efficient training method when sales staff time is at a premium. Using this method, the marketing director, executive director, or senior sales counselor presents a problematic and potentially complex selling situation. Controversial issues such as smoking, medical screening, family conflicts, or the application of the Fair Housing Amendments Act can be presented for discussion by the group. The case description should be concise but include all relevant facts and information. The group should then discuss the problem, clarify the facts, suggest possible solutions, and choose one. The point of the discussion is not so much to reach a consensus as it is for the group to grasp the complexity of the issue and to understand the process for resolution. Case studies can also explore problems and outcomes experienced by other operators in the business to learn from their mistakes.

IMPROMPTU DISCUSSIONS. Impromptu discussions can be conducted during weekly sales meetings to explore specific problems or learn new techniques. For example, the sales department should have a weekly "hots" meeting to enable each sales counselor to discuss the current status of the best leads. During these meetings, each sales counselor discusses her top 10 or 15 current prospects, describing their personal situation, motivation, obstacles, timing, and likelihood of closing. The sales staff can offer suggestions on how to bring the prospects to closure and discuss any obstacles to setting a move-in date. The "hots" meeting is an excellent opportunity for the sales staff to share excitement about pending closes and estimate the likelihood of reaching month-end targets.

As the marketing director becomes aware of any problematic trends in sales activity, he or she can use an impromptu discussion to raise the issues and introduce potential solutions. Discussions can also be facilitated by the executive director or other department head to educate the salespeople about other departments and job functions. In addition, they can be used to keep the sales staff informed about move-outs or potential problems with operations in the community so that they can steer prospects around them or be prepared to overcome potential objections. Impromptu discussions are an excellent forum in which to disseminate information about the availability of inventory, pricing structure, or policy changes. They afford the opportunity for immediate feedback from sales counselors who are in constant contact with prospects and market trends.

GAMES. Games are another method of training that can be fun and productive in large groups. Television quiz games such as *Jeopardy* or *Wheel of Fortune* can be adapted to highlight important information about the community and its services. Employees from one or several departments can participate. Generally, the larger the group, the less structured and formal the occasion. These events work well to break down barriers between sales and operations while celebrating the accomplishments of each.

Games can also be used to familiarize employees with the management's problem-solving process. There is an excellent YouTube training video entitled *Sales Process for Assisted Living* with tips on how to conduct a winning sales presentation.[4]

ON-THE-JOB TRAINING. On-the-job training provides supervised practice. There is simply no more effective method to learn a job or communicate expectations. It is a progressive sequence of tell, show, do, and review. Most marketing directors employ some version of this method to train new sales employees. The supervisor usually first introduces a new employee to the organizational structure of the department and the finer points of selling the community and its service package. Shadowing new employees on mock tours or during presentations then provides a good opportunity to rehearse methods of overcoming prospects' objections and to discuss possible responses to vulnerabilities in the community's service package, pricing structure, amenities, or location. Even experienced salespeople occasionally need to practice and hone their skills when selling an unfamiliar community.

On-the-job training should be conducted by the marketing director and other senior sales counselors, each with an organized agenda. Many experienced sales counselors who are paid on a commission basis may be reluctant to assist with this training, as it takes them away from sales activities. This problem can easily be remedied by paying bonuses or overrides on the trainee's sales. There is no better role model than someone who is already successful.

Each of the training methods above is relatively inexpensive and, if properly deployed, can cover the vast majority of a department's training needs. The only resources they require are research, planning, creativity, organization skills, and time management. Other methods of training may require a somewhat larger financial outlay, but the expenditure may be justified when tackling a particularly stubborn problem, imparting a lot of new information rapidly, or setting especially ambitious departmental goals.

PROGRAMMED LEARNING. Programmed learning involves the delivery of instructional material in seminar format or broken down into lesson plans or units. Programmed learning or training by consultants is generally the most expensive and least targeted of all training methods at the marketing director's disposal. Still, it has some advantages. These programs are usually developed by professional trainers or consultants and are marketed as a package or in individual components. They have the advantages of introducing fresh ideas into the training curriculum and conveying the impression that employees are receiving something of value. Many employees believe that these "professional" programs have inherent value and are a demonstration of the company's commitment to investing in its employees. Whether or how well the expenditure translates into incrementally higher productivity is difficult to measure. But such programs may produce improvements in employee morale and loyalty, and many good packages are available for a minimal investment.

How to Conduct Training

Training can be conducted by a variety of facilitators and instructors, depending on the material content. Initial training and orientation are usually conducted by the marketing director or direct supervisor. Continuous sales training can draw on the resources of other successful salespeople, marketing directors, and top sales producers from other company properties (that are at stabilized occupancy), company executives, or outside consultants.

The starting point for a successful training program is to train the trainers. Effective training requires more refined and sophisticated influencing skills than those needed to sell the community. With training, you are selling intangible techniques and ideas rather than products and services. Not all experienced and successful salespeople are naturally good trainers. In fact, most sales counselors tend to be results-oriented and can become frustrated with the time it takes for their training efforts to yield results. Moreover, the mechanics of teaching and learning alone do not guarantee the success of train-the-trainer programs. It helps to have a well-planned and well-organized curriculum to assist the trainer in his or her delivery.

Initial sales training should be scheduled at the time of hiring. Continuous sales training should be conducted informally, daily and weekly, as needed, and formally at least monthly. If it does not happen at least monthly, then it is not continuous! The marketing director can develop a training plan based on a departmental needs assessment. It can then be delivered during monthly meetings, with weekly follow-up modules to keep concepts fresh. Regular review and practice will improve retention.

Training manuals, workbooks, and video and audio materials can be developed or purchased for a minimal investment per employee. The best programs include statements of objectives, summaries or outlines of the main concepts, related reading materials, orienting questions, and case studies.

Evaluation of Training

Sales training programs can represent the investment of considerable time, effort, and expense. Although the management hopes to improve morale and gain a sense of goodwill in the process, it is primarily interested in seeing a return on its investment in the form of improved performance. The relationship between training and results can take many months to become evident. The management can devise various methods for analyzing productivity, such as phone-out-to-appointment or call-conversion ratios, but relating results back to training is rarely conclusive.

The best method for evaluating any training program is to compare individuals' track records before and after the training. It is also useful to mystery-shop your sales counselors (see chapter 14). Although some sales counselors are naturals at the job, most benefit from training. For a relatively small investment, training can keep the sales team fresh, sharpen their skills, and clarify the manager's expectations.

Managers who create a clear vision for their department, define a set of expectations and standards to support that vision, build consensus among their staff, and create a sense of urgency in a positively charged environment will position their community for success. There are no shortcuts.

NOTES

1. A. Robbins, *The Magic of Rapport* (La Jolla, CA: Robbins International, 1986).

2. R. A. Zarro and P. Blum, *The Phone Book: Breakthrough Phone Skills for Fun, Profit, and Enlightenment* (Barrytown, NY: Station Hill, 1989).

3. R. R. Still, E. W. Cundiff, and N. Govoni, *Sales Management: Decisions, Strategies, and Cases* (Englewood Cliffs, NJ: Prentice Hall, 1991), 341.

4. Pearce, Benjamin. The Winning Sales Presentation: Senior Living Communities, YouTube, https://www.youtube.com/watch?v=UwuQz7AExIA.

Coordinating the Move

16

Moving can be an overwhelming experience for people of any age. For seniors, it is especially emotional, for often they are moving from homes in which they have lived for many years, raised families, and created precious memories. The prospect of having to shed decades' worth of possessions can lead them to postpone moving to a senior living community, even though their lives are likely to be enriched by the move.

The services a community offers to coordinate the move are an invaluable part of the sales process. (See exhibit 16.1 for a checklist for coordinating a smooth move.) Knowing that a capable professional will be on hand to help them eases the doubts and fears in prospects' minds and can shorten the time between lease signing and move-in.

Communities that have an average of eight or more move-ins per month should consider hiring a move-in coordinator, especially during the fill-up stage. Even larger, mature communities with 300 units and 20 percent annual turnover will need to coordinate approximately five move-ins and five move-outs each month. Managing these moves can involve a serious commitment of time. Using sales staff to perform this function wastes time that could otherwise be committed to keeping the apartments fully occupied.

The volume of monthly turnover at the community will determine the allocation of staffing hours to the coordination of moves. Move-in coordinators can also assist with community outreach and networking, activities, resident orientation, driving, concierge backup, and even night management during slow periods. Some moving coordinators also assist with family issues and help the resident deal with health care professionals. As a community reaches full occupancy, a full-time moving coordinator may no longer be necessary, and the marketing assistant can be trained to perform these functions. The feasibility of this arrangement will of course depend on the size of the community and the amount of turnover.

Some communities structure the move-in coordinator's compensation package to provide incentives for accelerating the move-in date. In one community, the move-in coordinator accelerated the move-in time frames to produce 1,000 additional revenue days for her community, resulting in an additional $65,000 in revenue annually.

The move-in coordinator should introduce him/herself to as many prospects as possible at community tours, marketing functions, or resident programs. Depending on a prospect's needs and concerns, a marketing representative may choose to involve the move-in coordinator in the sales process even before a lease or residency agreement has been signed. At this stage, the move-in coordinator's role is to calm the prospect's fears by explaining what assistance can be offered during each stage of the move and what to expect on move-in day.

Throughout the process of assisting a resident, the coordinator should keep in mind the primary objective: expediting the move. During the fill-up stage of a community, sales counselors are typically flexible on scheduling the move-in date. The longer the delay, however, the less likely the sale will result in a move-in. Move-in time frames allowing longer than 60 days do not create any sense of urgency in the prospect to move in, and actual dates become meaningless. The prospect should be encouraged to pick out a particular unit and be prepared to pay rent on that unit if someone else becomes interested in it, or else run the risk of losing his choice of unit.

■■■■ THE INITIAL CONTACT AND HOME VISIT

Once a prospect signs a lease, the move-in coordinator should call the prospect within three days and schedule a home visit. For out-of-state prospects for whom a home visit is not feasible, the initial phone call to the prospect takes on even greater importance. During the telephone conversation, the coordinator should do the following:

- Reemphasize the features of the community that led the prospect to sign a lease.
- Acknowledge and minimize any concerns the prospect has about moving.
- Listen for any subtle changes in attitude (is the prospect getting cold feet?).
- Look for opportunities to shorten move-in time.

The home visit is the best opportunity to establish credibility with the prospect and earn his or her trust, but preparation is paramount. A briefing with the sales counselor will enable the coordinator to learn as much as possible about the prospect before the visit. Because a prospect is likely to feel more comfortable and in control at home, questions and concerns about all aspects of the community—not just the move—are likely to surface during the home visit. The prospect will constantly be evaluating the move-in coordinator's confidence about, and knowledge of, the community. The coordinator's main objective at this stage is to *remove barriers to getting things done*, saying "I can take care of that for you" or "This is what we need to do now," rather than "This is what you need to do."

Presenting the welcome package. Presenting a personalized welcome package at the home visit can be especially effective. All of the following items should be included in a welcome package, although discussing every item may prove overwhelming for the prospect.

- A welcome letter personalized with the prospect's new address, including a list of the items with which you can assist during the move (see exhibit 16.2)
- Several blank floor plans for the apartment style the prospect has selected
- Pictures of the view from the prospect's apartment (for long-distance moves)
- A list of goods and services available in the prospect's new neighborhood (e.g., banks, dry cleaners, 24-hour pharmacies, markets, florists, places of worship)
- Local utility companies' phone numbers for canceling or transferring service
- Local newspapers' phone numbers for transferring subscriptions
- Change-of-address cards to send to the prospect's current post office branch and contacts
- A list of reputable Realtors and moving-and-storage companies—at least four of each
- A list of local charitable organizations that accept donations of furniture and household items
- A list of antique appraisers, tag-sale managers, decorators, resale shops, upholsterers, drapers, and so on
- Several community postcards so that the prospect can spread the good news about the move to friends and acquaintances
- A current resident newsletter and events calendar

The resident newsletter can serve as an icebreaker during a home visit. Because it highlights exciting aspects of the community, it can help you determine which programs the prospect will find most interesting. Come equipped, too, with a floor plan of the common areas, a tape measure, and some imagination. Gently walk the prospect through the downsizing process. Ask questions about furniture, wall hangings, and personal possessions. Identify the items the prospect absolutely will not part with and work around the rest. Sometimes it will be necessary to ease the prospect's mind about the downsizing with comments such as "It seems as though we spend the first half of our lives accumulating possessions and the last half giving them away. Once you start the paring-down process, it won't seem as big an obstacle."

Exhibit 16.1   Moving Checklists

Master Checklist

Resident's name: _____

Apartment number: _____

_____ Review the client's special needs with marketing representative.

_____ Make initial contact with the client.

_____ Make sure the resident's application paperwork is complete and approved.

_____ Confirm the resident's plans for sale of house or notice to vacate rental property.

_____ Schedule home visit to measure furniture and develop floor plan.

_____ Confirm the resident's plans for selecting and hiring a mover.

_____ Confirm the resident's plans for sale, disposal, or storage of unneeded items.

_____ Help the resident with change-of-address procedures for utility companies, magazine and newspaper subscriptions, post office, etc.

_____ For dementia care residents, check that all clothing, glasses, and assistive devices have been marked with the resident's name.

_____ Inspect apartment, arrange for any needed repairs, and prepare it for the resident's arrival.

_____ Contact appropriate community staff to prepare for the resident's arrival.

_____ Visit the new resident and schedule an orientation date.

Move-in Checklist

Resident's name: _____

Apartment number: _____

30 Days Before Move-in

_____ Sit in on lease signing to meet with and establish a personal relationship with the resident. Deliver and discuss resident handbook.

_____ Schedule a home visit to counsel the resident and discuss the move-in process. Establish a move-in time frame. Provide moving company referrals.

_____ Be present in the resident's home when moving company estimates are given.

_____ Arrange with several real estate companies (if appropriate) to do a free comparative market analysis of the resident's home and make listing presentations.

_____ Make personal phone contact weekly to answer questions or concerns. Keep the resident updated on any maintenance requested on apartment, such as painting or wallpapering.

_____ Be sure all forms required for residency (e.g., application for residency, medical form) are submitted and that the resident's file is approved by the executive director prior to move-in.

Two Weeks (Minimum) Before Move-in

_____ Inspect the apartment. Notify appropriate departments (housekeeping, maintenance, dining room) in writing of the resident's arrival.

_____ Notify the resident relations staff so that they can prepare welcome information and an orientation for the new resident.

_____ Confirm that telephone service (and any other utilities) will be transferred on the date of the move.

_____ Notify the community's postal carrier of the new resident's name and apartment number.

(continued)

Exhibit 16.1 Moving Checklists *(continued)*

_____ Mail change-of-address cards to the local postmaster.

_____ Call the moving company and confirm the move.

_____ Include the new resident in the community resident directory.

_____ Order a name tag for the new resident. This will help existing residents get to know the new resident and will also help the new resident begin to feel like part of the community.

Two Days Before Move-in

_____ Inspect apartment: check all light fixtures, activate appliances, set clock on stove, etc.

_____ Assemble a move-in package and display the contents in the kitchen of the apartment: kitchen treats and amenities basket, resident newsletter and activities calendar, complimentary meal tickets, resident directory, telephone directory, chamber of commerce information (for out-of-state moves), cable television information, and a welcome card signed by the staff. Post transportation schedule and dining room hours on refrigerator.

_____ Involve welcome committee or arrange for a resident with similar interests or hobbies to escort the new resident to dinner on move-in day.

_____ Write maintenance ticket for television connection.

Moving Day

_____ Provide two folding chairs for the apartment.

_____ Check to see that a welcome snack or fruit basket and beverages have been placed in refrigerator by the housekeeping staff. Provide coffee and tea for the resident and family.

_____ Place a welcome plant on a shelf outside the resident's door, or have a member of the welcome committee deliver it personally.

_____ Turn on heat or air conditioning if appropriate.

_____ Notify concierge staff of the resident's name, estimated time of arrival, apartment number, and telephone number.

_____ Check the resident's mailbox and remove any mail for previous resident.

_____ Greet the new resident, escort her to the apartment, issue keys, have her sign the new-resident form, and get her situated.

_____ Offer lunch certificates to the resident and family or friends who are helping with the move.

_____ Greet movers, show them to the apartment, and restate any appropriate policies (responsibility for damage, elevator availability and lock-off, refuse disposal, time constraints).

_____ Reconfirm the new resident's dinner escort.

_____ Install telephones and confirm that telephone service is connected.

_____ Stay with the new resident until after the bed is made up, bath linens have been unpacked, apartment has sufficient lighting in place, traffic paths have been cleared, alarm clock and telephone are placed by the bed, necessary medications and toiletries have been unpacked, the television has been connected, the emergency response system has been tested, and the new resident feels secure.

_____ If the new resident seems overwhelmed, offer room service on the first night at the community.

Soon After Move-in

_____ Review the resident handbook with the new resident, including policies and procedures, a map of the community areas, and the community's organizational chart.

_____ Schedule appointments for all department heads to visit the new resident and discuss the services available through their respective departments. (These meetings should take place within one week of move-in.)

Department	Contact	Date
Resident relations	_____	_____
Dining room	_____	_____
Kitchen/chef	_____	_____
Maintenance	_____	_____
Housekeeping	_____	_____
Programming	_____	_____

_____ With the new resident's permission, send a notice to all residents with some general information about the new resident.

_____ With the resident's permission, post a photo of the new resident near resident mailboxes, along with a welcome sign.

_____ Post a photo of the new resident in the employee cafeteria so that employees will begin to associate the new resident's face with his name.

_____ Schedule two hours to help the new resident get acclimated to her apartment, unpack, hang pictures, and so forth. Some general comforting will be in order.

_____ Schedule resident orientation.

If the new resident must stay in a guest room while waiting for furnishings to be delivered, no charge should be assessed. Rent and meal allowances, however, should begin immediately.

What to look for. During the home visit, as the prospect begins mentally to adjust to community living, recording observations about her concerns will aid the operations staff in easing the transition into the community. Get a feel for the prospect's temperament: is she a worrier, detail-oriented, indecisive, attached to possessions? Try to gauge the level of assistance the she will require and then provide it without being asked. Anticipating a prospect's needs is as crucial as being able to fulfill them.

Take note of the prospect's surroundings during a home visit. Does the house have stairs that have become an obstacle? Is yard maintenance a problem? Are there medical appliances in the house? Ask questions and make comments about the difficulties of home ownership: "It must be tiring to climb those stairs all the time," or "How do you manage to take care of that big yard?" Avoid talking about how desirable the home is other than to say that it should sell easily.

Reinforcing the sale. The sale is never complete until the resident moves into the community. It is especially important to reassure the prospect during the home visit that he has made the right decision. Pay special attention to the way he frames questions, and accentuate the positive in your answers. For example, if the prospect asks, "How will I ever fit all of my dishes in that kitchen?" emphasize the dining services offered at the community, including the use of the private dining room for special family gatherings. Take inventory of the kitchen and make suggestions for selecting a few pots and pans: chances are the prospect won't be cooking as much at the community. Perhaps half of the family heirloom china could be available for use and display and the rest could be stored or passed on to family members. Use an upbeat tone when making suggestions.

Wrapping up the visit. Always close the visit with a date for follow-up, whether it is with a phone call or an additional home visit. Then follow up with a phone call the next day to thank the prospect for his time and to reiterate your availability to assist.

Reporting back to the community. After the visit, brief the sales representative who will assist the marketing department in expediting the move-in. Then set up a calendar that brings the prospect up to move-in day, with milestones along the way. Alert the marketing staff if you sense any hesitation on the part of the prospect, so that they can follow up with the additional attention needed to ensure the sale.

Sharing observations on the home visit with other department heads will help them get to know the prospect before the move-in. If a new resident has a hearing impairment, employees can make her feel more welcome by speaking directly to her in a clear, distinct manner, so that she can read their lips. If a new resident is visually impaired, the dining room servers should be prepared to describe the menu items to him in a noncondescending way. It also helps to know if a new resident is recently widowed and still grieving. If employees know that a new resident loves volunteer work, they can suggest projects in which she could get involved. Any insight that can be offered from the home visit will help the entire staff to smooth the new resident's transition into the community.

■■■■■ PREPARING A WELCOME PACKAGE AND COMPILING A LIST OF AREA RESOURCES

All the resident's possessions require some type of action, whether they are to be packed and moved, updated or altered in some way, donated to a charity, given to family, or sold. Limit your involvement in this process to offering advice and resources. Becoming involved in giving possessions away runs the risk of offending a family member who may have wanted a particular item. Stay neutral as family possessions are distributed. *Do not* accept any of the prospect's belongings as a gift without the approval of all family members. To do so could constitute a conflict of interest and could expose the community to legal liability.

Keep an up-to-date card file or database of resources for various types of services, filed or tagged by both company name and type of service. For instance, filing an art dealer under both "Jones, Frank; art dealer—consignment (will pick up)," and "Art dealer, Frank Jones—consignment (will pick up)" saves you having to remember the vendor's name.

■ *Area services.* The most efficient way to compile this information is through referrals. Current residents who know the area will be happy to share their consumer experiences, good and bad. Next, turn to the telephone directory or a local senior services directory and look under subjects such as

tailors, banks, pharmacies, and places of worship, as well as services targeted specifically to seniors, such as hearing-aid replacement and service.

Verify business hours and charges. Are senior discounts available? Is the store open 24 hours a day? Is it located within walking distance? Is it accessible to wheelchairs? Does the merchant deliver to the community?

■ *Realtors.* Gather the names of the largest, most reputable real estate firms in town. Larger firms have more resources at their disposal and offer the broadest possible exposure to the marketplace through the multiple listing service, newspaper and television ads, open houses, and office tours. Provide at least four companies' names. If the marketing department has a Realtor referral program, get the names of Realtors who have referred prospects in the past or who work well with seniors. The local multiple listing service usually keeps statistics of sales volume and average home sales prices by real estate office or broker. With a little digging, you can find the most productive Realtors in the community. The faster they sell the prospects' homes, the shorter the move-in time.

■ *Estate auctioneers.* The auction has been the traditional method for disposing of an estate. Professionals who specialize in these sales—which can be called tag sales, estate sales, garage sales, house sales, patio sales, or yard sales—can arrange for the complete or partial liquidation of residents' belongings. After appraising the belongings to establish their fair market value, they coordinate, advertise, and conduct the sale. Average proceeds from a sale range from $8,000 to $15,000, but they can be as high as $75,000.

When contacting estate-sales professionals, be sure to inquire about their charges, which are usually a percentage of the total sale (usually 30 percent or less, depending on the valuation amount). Also inquire about their preference for the location of the auction or sale. If they prefer to hold it in the prospect's home, the prospect may have to move out beforehand. Here are some suggested questions:

■ Will the owner receive a clear financial agreement specifying the commission charged?

Exhibit 16.2   Sample Information for New Residents

Move-in Coordination Services

The community's move-in coordinator will be glad to assist with the following tasks and to answer any other questions you may have about your move:

- Organizing the details of your move
- Providing information about moving, packing, storage, and furniture rental companies
- Coordinating the logistics of your move with the moving company
- Assisting with the planning and organizing of garage sales or tag sales
- Assisting with furniture measurement and placement
- Helping with the selection and placement of household items
- Transferring telephone service or ordering new service
- Handling details at the US Post Office, such as change-of-address forms
- Transferring newspaper and magazine subscriptions
- Conducting apartment and community orientation

CHANGE-OF-ADDRESS FORMS

Enclosed in this packet you will find a change-of-address form to be sent to your local post office branch. The form has been filled out and needs only your signature in order to effect the change.

If you like, you can request that your mail be sent to the community beginning a few days before you move. Please send this form to the post office as soon as your move-in date has been confirmed.

Once you send in your change-of-address form, you will receive a moving kit from the post office. It will contain change-of-address notification cards that you can use to inform all correspondents of your new address.

Your mail will be forwarded to the community by the post office for six months, beginning on the date specified on your change-of-address card; therefore, it is very important to send out the notification cards promptly. If you would like assistance filling out the cards, please bring them by on your next visit, or I will come to your home and help you fill them out.

It is recommended that you inform the Social Security Administration in writing of your new address.

Your new address will be:

_____

_____

_____

Your address including apartment number

_____

_____

_____

- When and where will the sale be advertised?
- How will you handle the traffic flow inside the residence to minimize theft and breakage?
- Will the owner receive an inventory of the property before sale? (This is essential.)
- When will the final accounting be due to the estate or owner? (The interval is usually between 15 and 30 days.)

When deciding between a tag sale and an auction, owners should keep in mind that prices in a well-run tag sale are established by the knowledgeable professional, whereas prices in an auction are established by the audience.

- *Antique dealers.* Valuable or unusual items can be sold most profitably through antique dealers. Call around and secure the name of contacts in at least three businesses on whom you can rely when a prospect wants to have something appraised. Encourage the prospect to compare offers.

■ *Refurbishers.* Some personal treasures are in better shape than others. Restorers and refurbishers can breathe new life into sentimental items so that prospects can keep familiar things around them. Find a local draper who can turn draperies into valances or other styles of window treatment that are currently popular, a carpenter who can fix or restore an old table, an electrician who can rewire an old lamp, and a frame shop that can update the look of family photos or artwork.

■ *Charitable organizations.* Many charitable organizations gratefully accept donations of household items and clothing. If your community has an affiliation with a local hospital or nursing home, either group may be able to pass along some names to you. Some churches and synagogues have resale shops. The key is to work with two or three reputable organizations that will pick up the merchandise (either from the prospect's current residence or from the community) and provide receipts for tax deductions to the donors. Prospects can then select organizations from the list that you have compiled. Find out if there are items that these organizations will not accept, so that the prospect can make other arrangements to dispose of such items.

■ *Libraries.* The local public library is usually happy to accept used books from prospects. Call to find out how to make such donations. Senior centers, nursing homes, and some university libraries also look for donations of used books. Most used bookstores will pay cash or give the prospect credit toward future purchases at the store.

■ *Garage sales.* Garage sales represent big business for your local newspaper's classified section. Call the paper and inquire about any special rates it may have for advertising garage sales: some papers even give out garage sale kits with signs, price stickers, and inventory sheets. Also ask for several ad-copy forms so that you can assist the prospect in preparing an ad.

■ *Storage units.* The best way to research local storage-unit companies is to visit them personally so that you can see exactly what each company has to offer, decide whether it will meet a prospect's storage needs, and obtain rate schedules.

■ *Vintage clothing and consignment shops.* Many prospects own vintage clothing, and shops specializing in such goods have increased in popularity in recent years. Call them and find out what types of clothing and accessories they will accept and whether they will pay for them. Consignment shops offer to sell items for the prospect in exchange for a percentage of the sale price. A third option for prospects is to place a classified ad in the local paper in the clothing section.

■ *Post office.* Ask the local post office branch for several change-of-address forms and stamps-by-mail order forms and distribute them to prospects.

All potential resources must be screened thoroughly before they are recommended to prospects. And because not all businesses conduct their affairs consistently well, it is crucial to evaluate resident satisfaction with the services that were recommended. When a resident uses a service or purchases goods based on the community's referrals, find out whether she was satisfied with the service and the price and would recommend the service to someone else.

UNDERSTANDING THE HOME SALE MARKET

To meet the goal of reducing time and obstacles to move-in, it is helpful for the move-in coordinator to understand the process of selling a home. This knowledge will equip move-in coordinators to advise prospects on the marketability of their homes and provide counsel to those whose homes may be slow to sell.

The listing. Most people selling a home use the services of a residential Realtor. Although a Realtor's sales commission may be as high as 8 percent (the percentage decreases as the price of the home increases), the Realtor has the expertise and access to professional resources to market the home effectively. The multiple-listing service publishes a listing and description of every home on the market for sale by professional Realtors. This listing gives the home much more exposure than could be achieved by an owner trying to sell the home himself. Listings are sorted according to price and location and distributed to every real estate agent in the area.

Several top Realtors should be asked to prepare a listing presentation, which usually includes a comparative market analysis, a detailed analysis of value based on comparable home sales in the area. It includes the essential elements of a home appraisal and recommends a listing price and a sales strategy. If the homeowner is not satisfied with the suggested sales price, it may be advisable to have the home valued by a certified Appraisal Institute appraiser. The homeowner should evaluate each Realtor's presentation not only on the basis of the recommended price but also on the Realtor's track record and projected length of time to sell.

Once the owner has selected a Realtor, a listing agreement is usually signed to establish the parameters for selling the home and the fees charged. Such an agreement is normally made for a minimum of six months. Shorter agreements usually command more attention from the real estate agent. Commonly, the listing agreement may be terminated by the seller before its expiration date without obligation if she is dissatisfied with the listing agent's progress in selling the home.

The best agent for selling a home is not necessarily the busiest or the most successful agent in town. Agents who are already managing more than 10 listings will have little time to devote to each. If the listings are not worked aggressively, they quickly become stale, and clients may be well advised to terminate the listing agreement and hire another Realtor.

Price. The single biggest factor affecting the length of time to sell the property is the price. When the home is priced above its market value, fewer prospective buyers want to see the home. When it is priced below market value, interest increases. The key is to match the list price with the selling goal. If the seller wants a quick sale, then the home should be priced competitively. For example, in any given market, a home priced at fair market value will attract about 60 percent of the prospective buyers looking to purchase. At 5 percent below market, the home will attract 80 percent, and at 10 percent below, it will attract 90 percent of the prospective buyers. Conversely, if the home is priced at 5 percent above market value, it will attract only 30 percent of the prospective buyers, and at 10 percent above, it will attract virtually no one. If a home is overpriced, fewer salespeople will show it, fewer prospects will respond to ads, and the seller may risk losing buyers who might be willing to negotiate.

Homes for sale receive the most attention from buyers during the second to the fifth weeks they are listed. After the fifth week, if no offer has been made, the activity level declines sharply. Therefore, it is critical that the home be priced accurately during the first five weeks. If no offers are made during this period, something is wrong, and the price should be reevaluated.

The sales process. On listing the home, the listing office will erect at its expense a "for sale" sign on the property and announce the new listing to its office Realtors during their weekly meeting. All agents of the listing office preview new listings of the office each week. The listing Realtor will hold a broker's open house to allow agents from other real estate companies to view the home before the general public does. This event is held midweek (usually on a Wednesday or Thursday), with refreshments offered to entice agents to view the home. Usually, other agents will come to see the home if they have a current client in that price range—or if the food is good. The agent who sells the home usually receives half of the commission. The listing agent will receive the entire commission if he sells the home himself, but this rarely happens: obviously, the more exposure the home receives through other agents, the quicker the sale. Each time a home is visited or shown, the law requires the visiting agent to leave her business card. Therefore, the more cards and the more showings, the more likely it is that an offer will follow. Too few cards may indicate that a listing is too expensive, poorly marketed, or undesirable for some other reason.

In addition to brokers' open houses, the agent should hold twice-monthly public open houses on Sundays to allow passersby and neighbors to view it. A desirable home with good curb appeal in a good location should attract between 50 and 100 prospects on a sunny day. These open houses should be advertised in the Sunday paper, along with a photo. Some larger real estate firms advertise Sunday open homes on television.

Once a buyer has expressed the intention to purchase the home, an *earnest money agreement* is usually signed and a nominal deposit (1–5% of the purchase price) is paid to the seller. This agreement outlines the proposed price and method of payment. After negotiation, the agreement is followed by a *purchase and sale agreement* for cash sales, or a *real estate contract* if the seller is offering to finance all or a portion of the sales price. Once the purchase agreement or contract has been signed, the deposit is usually increased to 10 percent of the purchase price.

The real estate agent should continue to market the home and solicit backup offers in case the sale falls through. This happens quite often, owing to the buyer's inability to consummate the deal or failure to perform on a contingency. A contingency is a clause in a contract that protects the buyer against unforeseen difficulties in closing. For example, the sale may be contingent on the sale of the buyer's existing home, on the buyer's ability to secure acceptable financing, or on an engineer's inspection and approval. If any of these should fail, the deal is usually off: all deposits are returned, and the seller and the buyer have no further obligations to one another. Depending on the nature of the contingencies, some sales may be tenuous at best.

Escrow and closing. After contingencies have been cleared, the transaction is turned over to an attorney or escrow agent for closing. During this time, the buyer selects a title insurance company and applies for a loan to finance the purchase. The mortgage broker conducts research on the buyer to determine creditworthiness and submits the loan application to the company's underwriting committee for approval. If the loan is rejected or some problem is discovered during the title search, or if a structural engineer discovers an irreconcilable problem with the property, the deal can dissolve.

The point of this description of the pitfalls of real estate sales is to emphasize the importance of continuing to market the home. The move-in coordinator needs to be in constant contact with the prospect to ensure that the sale moves forward so that the move into the community can be made without delay. If the home is not shown on a regular basis, then the reasons need to be investigated and dealt with. The problem is usually price. The seller may need further counseling or advice on the opportunity costs associated with holding a home on the market too long. In fact, delays caused by unrealistic price expectations could render the home less marketable. Realtors look for a good deal for their clients and will avoid overpriced homes. The coordinator should be very cautious, however, of urging the owner to settle for too low a price: a sales price resulting in lower-than-expected net after-tax proceeds may affect the prospect's ability to qualify financially for the community.

During the sale of the home, the move-in coordinator should periodically ask the prospect about the frequency of showings and other sales activity. If activity is slow, it could delay the eventual move-in. On receipt of a bona fide offer, it may be helpful to advise the prospect of the importance of backup offers, especially if the sales agreement or contract contains contingencies.

WORKING WITH MOVING COMPANIES

The primary goal when contacting movers should be to find several who understand senior living communities and their prospects' special needs. The first step is to set up screening interviews with reputable, long-established companies that can provide references and that hire only full-time workers, as opposed to seasonal part-timers. Emphasizing the expectation of good service will help establish a positive working relationship with the movers from the start. Inquire about professionalism. Do the employees wear uniforms? Are they friendly and patient enough to deal with seniors? Perhaps a crew can be assigned to work exclusively at your community during fill-up months so that a strong rapport can be developed. Offering prospects a list of three or four local and two long-distance movers from which to choose is sufficient.

Understanding rates. How are rates established? Are the mover's rates competitive? Why do some movers charge more than others? Will the mover provide a guaranteed estimate, meaning that the final charge cannot exceed the estimate? Some companies will offer a low estimate in order to get the job, then charge more on delivery. Sometimes an extra charge is assessed because the items being moved weigh more than the estimator thought they would. Ask if the mover will drop off goods at a local charity free of charge if the resident has items to donate.

Getting competitive bids. Explain to each moving company that at least two competitive bids will be solicited on all moves.

Securing insurance. All movers must have documentation proving that they are insured and bonded by the state. Inquire about insurance for moving specialty items—pianos, works of art, and the like—and request that a representative of the moving company thoroughly explain the insurance coverage to the prospect. Keep copies of the companies' documentation on file.

Sharing information. Evaluate each company according to the type of move for which it is best suited. For example, if Mrs. Jones cannot do any packing or unpacking, recommending the company with the most efficient packers and unpackers will save her time, money, and stress. If everything is left in boxes on the day of her move, she will be overwhelmed with the clutter, and it will take longer for her to get settled. If Mr. Smith prefers to pack his own belongings, perhaps a less costly moving company is sufficient for his needs.

Long-distance moves. Long-distance moves require extra time and attention. First, it is essential that the movers guarantee the delivery date. The new resident will need to stay in a guest apartment or hotel until her belongings arrive. The sooner delivery can be arranged, the sooner the new resident can settle in and make the community her home.

Long-distance movers frequently give a two- to three-day window for delivery. Many are reluctant to guarantee a delivery date, but this point is negotiable. Insist on it. If the company wants the business, its representatives will be flexible.

Several factors determine the date of delivery: the size of the load, the route it will take, and the number of shipments in the truck. If a resident has a large load that will fill a truck, the delivery date will be based on the time it takes to travel straight to the community. If it is a relatively small load, as is usually the case, other loads will be collected to fill the truck. The delivery date in that case will depend on where the load is in line for removal from the truck.

Long-distance movers typically arrive first thing in the morning and want to unload as soon as possible, so plan to be available and have the loading dock clear by 7:00 a.m. Coordinate the delivery schedule with the new resident. If he is not an early riser, suggest a wake-up call.

Residents will be new not only to the community but also to the surrounding area. If possible, arrange to have a resident volunteer with similar marital status and interests show the new resident around the neighborhood. A driver could be assigned to spend a few minutes driving the new resident around the area and pointing out things of interest. The information in the welcome package will go a long way toward making new residents feel more at home.

SCHEDULING MOVE-INS

Because most long-distance movers arrive in the morning for delivery and unpacking, in high-rise communities it is necessary to schedule the freight elevator to avoid conflicts with other deliveries or move-outs. Schedule no more than two move-ins or move-outs per day. Movers can make a building look shabby after only a few move-ins if they think they do not have to be careful: explain to them that their company will be held responsible for any damage they do to facility walls, corners, or carpeting. It is usually advisable to ensure that a maintenance employee is on site during all move-ins to hook up appliances and see that everything runs smoothly after the resident moves in.

Communicating with Other Departments

Moving in can be smooth only when all departments are involved and committed to doing their part. The move-in coordinator is responsible for coordinating their efforts.

On a weekly basis, prepare a list of who will be arriving during the upcoming week and distribute it to all the staff. This information will help the staff become familiar with names and apartment numbers. Residents also take an interest in the arrival of new residents.

MAINTENANCE. Completing a maintenance request update on a weekly basis will keep the maintenance department informed as to who is moving into which apartment, when new residents are moving in, and what type of assistance will be required from the maintenance department (for instance, installing grab bars or hanging fixtures). Incorporate into the maintenance request list any deliveries, decorating, or customizing to be done to the apartment. The maintenance department should be informed as soon as an apartment is leased, regardless of the move-in date (within reason). This gives them a chance to schedule apartment work conveniently, avoiding a crunch if the move-in date changes. Distribute this list to the housekeeping supervisor as well.

HOUSEKEEPING. Because residents often bring a few personal items to the apartment before the official move-in date, the apartment should be cleaned and presentable a few days ahead of time. If a new resident is moving in on Tuesday, the apartment should be ready no later than the previous Friday. Let maintenance and housekeeping know when they need to have their work completed. To avoid wasting effort, request that housekeeping clean the apartment after painting is complete, or that additional closet organizers be installed after any wallpapering is done but before closet doors are rehung.

DINING ROOM. If the dining room schedules multiple seatings, let the dining room manager know which seating the new resident has selected. Request certificates for lunch and dinner on moving day, and specify whether other residents or family will be dining with the new resident that day. Discuss any special dietary concerns.

ORIENTING NEW RESIDENTS

Moving can be an unsettling experience, and new residents will need sympathetic assistance in adjusting to the community. Even though new residents may have toured the community several times before move-in, they will appreciate having important information repeated. There is a big difference for residents between going on an escorted sales tour of the building and having to find their own way around once they have moved in. In the case of long-distance moves, orientation may be a resident's first introduction to the community. Either way, orientation for every resident should include all of the items on an orientation checklist. Exhibit 16.3 shows a sample orientation checklist.

Emergency Information

Complete a multiple-copy emergency medical face sheet (see description in chapter 6 and exhibit 6.4) before move-in. One copy should be kept at the concierge desk and another in the personal care or assisted living center, if applicable. In an emergency, this face sheet will allow the concierge or other responding staff to relay pertinent information to emergency medical personnel. Another copy of the emergency medical face sheet should go into the resident's file: for quick reference, attach it to the front inside cover of the file. Finally, a copy should be accessible in the resident's apartment.

Update the emergency medical card as needed to reflect changes in residents' doctors, medications, allergies, family phone numbers, and so on. Distribute memos requesting that residents update their cards twice a year.

All consideration must be given to the residents' privacy. Only the executive director or department heads should notify family members of a resident's emergency or illness.

MANAGING MOVE-OUTS

Moving a resident out of the community should be given as much care as moving a new resident in. The move-out is likely to be more traumatic than the move-in, so be considerate of the resident or family and offer to help organize the move. On the death of a resident, the family should be asked if they would like to have the move-out coordinated and the apartment cleaned.

Residents are responsible for removing all furniture, food, and personal belongings from the apartment. The apartment should be left in "broom-clean" condition. Small picture holes and marks on the wall constitute normal wear and tear and should be repaired when the apartment is being repainted.

Residents should be held responsible for removing all garbage to the outside bins, as other residents may not be able to get to the garbage rooms if they are cluttered with moving debris. The housekeeping department should be on call to provide assistance if the resident wishes to have the garbage removed for a small fee. In addition, the maintenance department should be notified in advance to assist with any furniture breakdown that the movers will not provide.

No fees should be prorated on move-out. Most states will allow more than a 30-day move-out time, but some states require that the apartment be vacated 5 days before the lease expires to allow the landlord to return the apartment to rentable condition. This means that the resident may need to move out on the 26th of the month for the apartment to be available on the first day of the next month. If the community maintains a waiting list, the new lessee should start paying rent as soon as the apartment is in move-in condition, if possible. In other words, move-ins should not be prorated, in order to minimize the possible loss of revenue on the unit. If the lessee is not willing to take the apartment when it becomes available, it may go to the next person in line.

The security deposit should not be considered the last month's rent. On move-out, the resident services director or maintenance personnel should inspect the apartment for any damages. Normal wear and tear is not considered damage. Chargeable damages usually

---

Exhibit 16.3   Sample Resident Orientation Checklist

Resident: _____

Apartment number: _____

COMMUNITY AREAS
Tour all common areas and refer to the types of activities that occur in each.
_____ Concierge desk and the services coordinated there (transportation, parcel deliveries, maintenance requests, program sign-up, etc.)
_____ Administrative offices and functions performed there (billing, etc.)
_____ Department heads' offices (reiterate who handles what)
_____ Dining areas (select seating time)
_____ Mail area (explain use of in-house mailboxes)
_____ Commissary (hours, information on volunteering)
_____ Beauty shop (hours, services provided)
_____ Library (policies for use)
_____ Art studio (describe classes, activities)
_____ Health club (hours, classes, use of equipment)

ALSO DISCUSS THE FOLLOWING:
_____ How to sign up for events
_____ How to sign up for and use transportation
_____ How to make lunch and dinner reservations for guests
_____ How to arrange for room service

RESIDENT'S APARTMENT
Apartment orientation should take place just before the move or on moving day itself and should cover the following:
_____ How to lock and unlock the door properly
_____ Location of light switches and corresponding sockets
_____ How to set and reset electrical outlets
_____ How to operate the climate control system
_____ Explanation of circuit breaker box
_____ Explanation of emergency generator
_____ How to work kitchen range, timer, overhead hood (fan and light)
_____ Refrigerator setting and icemaker operation

_____ Garbage disposal
_____ Bathtub stopper
_____ How to open, close, and lock windows
_____ How to operate window blinds
_____ Use of emergency assistance pull cords
_____ How to open mailbox
_____ Garbage collection
_____ Laundry facilities

---

include damage to carpeting less than five years old, damage to window coverings that belong to the building, and damage to wallpaper. Any room that has been painted a color other than white should be returned to its original color. Any structural changes to the apartment must be undone to return it to its origi-nal condition unless the executive director approved the changes in writing. The resident can undertake to have the damages repaired herself if the executive director approves this arrangement in advance. The security deposit should be returned within 30 days of the move-out, unless otherwise specified by state law.

The renovation of vacated apartments should be given priority above all maintenance work orders except emergencies so that the unit can be returned to move-in condition within 48 hours of move-out. The maintenance department should anticipate the need to order parts or fixtures for the unit. Painting and repair work should be scheduled in advance of the lease ending date. Obtain permission from the resident or responsible party to enter the apartment for this purpose before the lease expiration date. The vacant apartment should be thoroughly cleaned and left in showable condition immediately after the maintenance work is finished. With the resident's or family's permission, apartments should be made available to the marketing department so that they can be shown before the residents have vacated them.

As the community nears full occupancy, the ability to manage the final few units proactively can make a big difference to the bottom line. For example, the difference in cash value of 95 percent occupancy and 100 percent occupancy in a 100-unit project, at an average rate of $4,000 per month, is $240,000 per year. At a 10 percent capitalization rate, this can add $2,400,000 in value to the property. The incremental expenses associated with these additional units are minimal at this occupancy level. In addition, marketing should evaluate the current market rent for each vacated apartment as it becomes available, and at least semiannually for all units in the community. The vacated unit should be repriced at market rate, not at the rate the previous tenant was paying.

The resident services coordinator or the executive director should make a follow-up call to the resident or family to confirm receipt of the security deposit, to offer the community's best wishes, and to ask for an evaluation of their experience at the community.

IV

Providing and Tracking Care

Assessments and Interventions

17

Across the continuum of senior care there has been a disconnect between the varied interests and agenda of families, medical professionals, mental health specialists, and senior living communities, whose responsibility it is to deliver the care needed by the residents. Many professionals with a vested interest in the resident's well-being share certain common frustrations relating to the accurate diagnosis and prescribed most effective treatment for their patients.

Common challenges of medical professionals:

- Physicians have a limited period of time during their appointment to accurately and comprehensively screen, diagnose, and prescribe effective treatments for their patients.
- Patients are often accompanied to their appointments by family or caregivers with very limited knowledge or experience with the patient and are unable to comprehensively communicate to the physician patient history, behavior, psychosocial and/or nutritional status.
- Physicians are often contacted repeatedly by caregivers or senior living professionals seeking solutions to behavioral problems or care delivery challenges, which reflect a lack of understanding and/or training on how to work successfully with dementia patients and provide a quality environment where they can thrive.

Common challenges of dementia caregivers:

- **Behaviors.** Many people suffering from dementia are often in denial and have an altered state of reality. While they try to desperately hold on to their former self, they sometimes act out in frustration. Often this "behavior" is treated with anti-anxiety medications, leaving them in a stupor and despondent.
- **Engagement.** We need to understand a person not only as someone who suffers from illness but also as someone who inhabits healthy parts and personality that remain even though it seems to be hidden by illness. People with dementia are like everyone else—they attach personal meanings to their activities. Keeping people actively engaged makes them easier to supervise and builds quality of life.
- **Depression.** Depressed residents often do not have positive outcomes and are greater risk of discharge to nursing homes and death. Chronic depression can lead to loss of appetite and weight loss, lethargy, and a host of other premature health complications. The body follows the mind, and depression often leads to catastrophic health failure.
- **Balance and stability.** People with dementia are less aware of the potential consequences of a fall and are less guarded in their mobility efforts. People who are sedentary and allow their muscles

to atrophy have a high risk of falling. Proper nutrition can also help reduce the risk of falling. Seniors who are undernourished are often unsteady on their feet and can even feel dizzy when they stand up. Inadequate nutrition can also lead to a number of other health failures and diseases that further destabilize the body. Medicines affect gait and balance for most adults. It may be possible to reduce the number of medications used, particularly tranquilizers, sleeping pills, and antianxiety drugs.

■ **Care refusal.** People with dementia often become paranoid as they struggle with experiencing continued losses and fear losing control over decisions regarding their lifestyle. This can cause them to become suspicious regarding their medications and refuse treatment. This is combined with a tendency for them to become tactilely defensive during attempts by staff to provide direct care that is often of an intimate nature.

■ **Wandering or exit seeking.** Many residents with dementia also experience anxiety disorder. This is typically manifested in the afternoons and often referred to as "sundowning." Residents who walk or wheel about unrestricted become a threat to engage in conflict with other residents or may leave the facility unattended without the knowledge of the facility staff due to their state of confusion.

Managing care needs within a resident population starts with gathering information about their functional status then monitoring trends in those functionalities and implementing interventions at the right time to fully support the residents' changing needs. Once these changes are identified, if caught early and treated, staff can avoid further deterioration and resident risk. The better job that staff can do at identifying and arresting risks, the fewer surprises for the family and physician and the better quality of life for the resident. The steps below can help providers create their own system for monitoring, identifying trends, implementing interventions, and communicating with interested parties in this regard:

1. Create a protocol for communicating with medical professionals.
2. Utilize medically accepted standardized tools to assess, track, and measure metrics in order to provide the primary care physician meaningful data

to empower them to make an accurate diagnosis and prescribe effective treatments.
3. Screen residents using medically accredited assessments to determine care plan needs.
4. Create specific and person-centered interventions for each resident according to their needs and functional status.
5. Create best practices programming and provide a system for enrichment of residents that will keep them engaged, interested, and entertained, while exercising many different areas of the brain (music, reminiscence, social, brain fitness, eye-hand coordination, memory games, household, cognitive, psychosocial, craft art, and sensory).
6. Create tools that collect data and analyze metrics so that changes in condition, functional status, cognition, and happiness can be measured and managed.
7. Provide staff with dementia training or certification enabling them to learn dementia-specific techniques for communicating with and managing behaviors common in persons afflicted with Alzheimer's disease or related dementias.

With OBRA (Omnibus Budget Reconciliation Act) guidelines, HCFA (Health Care Financing Administration), in some cases JCAHO (Joint Commission on Accreditation for Hospitals Organization), state regulators, and CARF (Certification Administration for Rehabilitation Facilities), the care delivery programs of skilled nursing and senior living communities are being scrutinized more than ever. This trend can be expected to proceed down the continuum of care as regulators look to assisted living communities as a more cost-effective setting in which to deliver care.

Further, primary care physicians, geriatricians, psychotherapists, social workers, and hospital discharge planners, whose responsibility it is to make informed recommendations to families as to their senior living options, have been reluctant to do so or to partner with a particular provider. This is because most providers do not or cannot meet their expectations regarding consistent care delivery with measurable outcomes that support the interests of the referring professionals in a sophisticated and reliable manner.

ASSESSMENTS

There is ample research in the field of geriatrics that has produced accredited studies detailing measurable

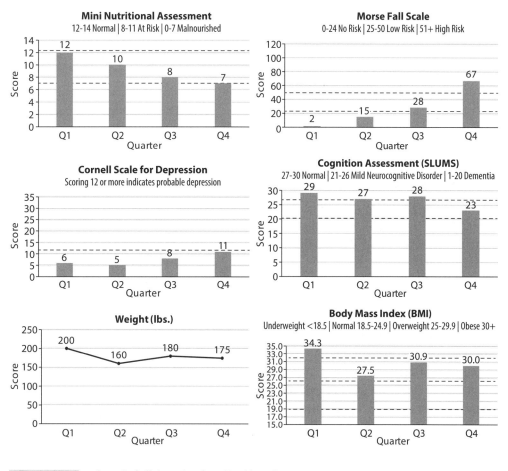

Figure 17.1   Sample Collaborative Care Dashboard

outcomes from assessment tools designed to quantify characteristics of persons in the areas of depression, cognition, nutrition, behavior, and even happiness. Using these tools to create baseline assessments and measure changes in condition will enable providers and primary care professionals to measure and understand the disease progression and determine the best course of treatment for these residents that will enable them to achieve the highest possible functional status and quality of life. See figure 17.1, Sample Collaborative Care Dashboard, for an example quarterly report that tracks the functional status against the baselines for each assessment.

These assessments are in addition to mandatory assessments for admission, routine care, and changes in condition required by applicable state regulations.
Assessment tools:

■ The Mini-Mental State Examination (MMSE) or Folstein test is a 30-point questionnaire that is used

extensively in clinical and research settings to measure cognitive impairment. It is commonly used in medicine and allied health to screen for dementia. It is also used to estimate the severity and progression of cognitive impairment and to follow the course of cognitive changes in an individual over time, thus making it an effective way to document an individual's response to treatment.

■ The Geriatric Depression Scale (GDS) is a 30-item self-report assessment used to identify depression in the elderly. In the GDS, questions are answered "yes" or "no." A five-category response set is not utilized, in order to ensure that the scale is simple enough to be used when testing ill or moderately cognitively impaired individuals, for whom a more complex set of answers may be confusing or lead to inaccurate recording of responses.

■ The Cornell Scale for Depression in Dementia (CSDD) is a way to screen for symptoms of depression in someone who has dementia. Unlike other scales and screens for depression, the CSDD takes into account additional signs of depression that might not be clearly verbalized by a person. For example, if your loved one or patient has Alzheimer's disease, vascular dementia, or another kind of cognitive impairment, he might not consistently be able to accurately express his feelings. The Cornell Scale measures observations and physical signs that could indicate depression.

■ The Morse Fall Scale (MFS) is a rapid and simple method of assessing a patient's likelihood of falling. A large majority of nurses (82.9%) rate the scale as "quick and easy to use," and 54 percent estimated that it took less than three minutes to rate a patient. It consists of six variables that are quick and easy to score, and it has been shown to have predictive validity and interrater reliability. The MFS is used widely in acute care settings, both in the hospital and in long-term care inpatient settings.

■ The Comprehensive Geriatric Assessment (CGA) is a multidimensional, multidisciplinary assessment designed to evaluate an older person's functional ability, physical health, cognition and mental health, and socioenvironmental circumstances. It is usually initiated when the physician identifies a potential problem. Specific elements of physical health that are evaluated include nutrition, vision, hearing, fecal and urinary continence, and balance. The CGA aids in the diagnosis of medical conditions, development of treatment and follow-up plans, coordination of management of care, and evaluation of long-term care needs and optimal placement. The CGA differs from a standard medical evaluation by including nonmedical domains; by emphasizing functional capacity and quality of life; and, often, by incorporating a multidisciplinary team. It usually yields a more complete and relevant list of medical problems, functional problems, and psychosocial issues.

■ The Mini Nutritional Assessment is an effective, easily administered tool designed to identify older adults who have or are at risk for developing malnutrition. It consists of 18 questions and can be completed in about 15 minutes. A short form, containing the first 6 questions, can be used for screening.

■ Saint Louis University Mental Status Examination (SLUMS) is a method of screening for Alzheimer's and other kinds of dementia. It was designed as an alternative screening test to the widely used Mini-

Mental State Examination (MMSE). The idea was that the MMSE is not as effective at identifying people with very early Alzheimer's symptoms. Sometimes referred to as mild cognitive impairment (MCI) or mild neurocognitive disorder (MNCD), these symptoms occur as people progress from normal aging to early Alzheimer's.

Implementation

Residents should be assessed at the following intervals:

■ Initial assessment upon application and 30 days post-admission
■ Quarterly following admission
■ Upon readmission after rehabilitation or hospitalization
■ Upon significant observable change in condition or behavior
■ Upon significant injury or fall
■ At physician request
■ Upon significant weight loss from normal body weight
■ Upon determination of a significant decrease or increase in a tracked metric
■ Upon director of nursing recommendation

Changes in Condition

A significant change in condition is one or more of the following:

■ Deterioration in two or more activities of daily living (ADL) services
■ Change in ability to walk or transfer
■ Change in ability to use one's hands to grasp small objects
■ Deterioration in behavior or mood to the point where daily problems arise or relationships have become problematic
■ No response by the resident to the treatment for an identified problem
■ Threat to life such as stroke, heart condition, or metastatic cancer
■ Emergence of a pressure ulcer at stage two, which is superficial ulcer presenting an abrasion, blister, or shallow crater, or higher
■ A new diagnosis of a condition likely to affect the resident's physical, mental, or psychosocial well-

being, such as an initial diagnosis of Alzheimer's disease or diabetes

- New onset of impaired decision-making
- Continence to incontinence or indwelling catheter
- Resident's condition indicates that there may be a need to use a restraint and there is no current restraint order for the resident
- Serious fall with injury
- Two incident reports on same resident within 45 days or less
- Behavior change with effect on others
- Unintentional significant weight loss (>2% decrease in baseline body weight in one month, >5% decrease in three months, or >10% in six months) in persons older than 65 years is associated with increased morbidity and mortality. In this population, unintentional weight loss can lead to functional decline in activities of daily living, increased infections, pressure ulcers, and failure to respond to medical treatments.
- Improved behavior, mood, or functional health status to the extent that the established plan of care no longer matches what is needed

Quarterly Assessment for Collaborative Care Dashboard (CCD)

The following process is recommended for follow-up on changes in condition:

Change in condition = Assessment → Care plan → Interventions → Verify implementation

The purpose behind this process is to properly identify any changes in functioning through the use of a comprehensive assessment; then amend the resident's care plan to include interventions needed to maintain resident health and safety; then verify the actual interventions are being routinely and consistently implemented. The nursing department should then ensure that the additional costs (if any) associated with the additional interventions are captured through the level of care billing process.

Should a significant change in condition occur, the resident's physician (or other appropriate licensed health professional such as mental health professional, nurse practitioner, physician assistant) should be notified and an assessment should be done within 10 days. If the change in condition poses an immediate

risk to the resident, the physician or appropriate licensed health professional should be notified immediately and in writing. A new or revised individual written care plan (ICP) should be developed for each resident in conjunction with the resident assessment. The ICP will normally specify the needs of the resident, including activities of daily living for which the resident requires assistance:

- What assistance, how much, who will provide the assistance, how often, and when
- Requirements and arrangements for visits by or to physicians or authorized health care providers (such as therapists or specialists)
- Advance directives or health care power of attorney
- Recreational and social activities that are suitable, desirable, and important to the well-being of the resident
- Nutritional needs

State regulations will specify precisely what is required in the resident's individualized care plan. The ICP delineates the responsibilities of the facility in meeting the needs of the resident, including provisions to monitor the care and effectiveness of the facility in meeting those needs. Included are specific goal-related objectives based on the needs of the resident as identified during the assessment phase, including adjunct support service needs, other special needs, and methods for achieving objectives and meeting needs in measurable terms with expected achievement dates.

Comprehensive Assessment Tools

The use of comprehensive assessment tools in senior living has historically been very limited and confined mostly to regulatory requirements. Management of the care of assisted living residents has been structured around maintenance of dignity, cleanliness, and nutritional support. But the typical assisted living resident profile has changed dramatically over time. The typical assisted living resident is an 84-year-old female who will statistically live there for 22 months. Forty percent of the residents will be dependent on assistance in three or more activities of daily living (ADLs); 82 percent of the residents will be taking at least one prescription medication, and

29 percent will be taking five or more medications. In the US, seniors account for 40 percent of all prescription medications although they comprise only 15 percent of the population. One-third will have a serious injury-related fall after the age of 65, and one-half will fall after the age of 80.

These statistics paint a vivid picture of an aging population with increasingly medically complex health care challenges who are currently living in an environment that was originally designed to accommodate patients whose needs were less dense. Therefore, to properly serve this population, staff and management need to understand and respond to assisted living as an environment for treatment as well as housing and support services.

Specific challenges to expect:

- Physician skepticism regarding the enhanced care delivery at assisted living communities
- Staff resistance of measurement and care delivery expectations
- Scheduling time to create, evaluate, and communicate assessment results

Possible solutions:

Problem	Solution
Physician participation	Communicate program, discuss advantages, follow up
Creating care metrics	Create assessment and care metrics toolbox for staff use
Staff skill sets	Provide free online training to certify staff
Staff participation	Communicate rationale, solicit ideas and gain support

Solutions

Seniors naturally undergoing their aging process need coordinated support from families, their friends, the community, their physician and therapists, and in their living environment. These support services are often offered piecemeal or haphazardly due to the residential nature of their environment. Even when the patient is living in a homelike setting, they still may need complex professional services to attain the highest possible failure-free functional status. Even though they have a disease, it doesn't mean they become the disease. As professionals in

senior living, it is incumbent upon operators to seek out and coordinate the appropriate array of services and engagement that they need delivered to them right in their home.

Specifics:

- **Attentive personal care.** From proper nutrition, hydration, and medication management to compassionate assistance with activities of daily life, the needs of the residents are central to each care pathway. Once a personalized path of care is created, the staff can work daily to strengthen their abilities and promote independence.
- **Person-centered care.** Staff assess and collect data on each resident's functional status so that metrics can be shared with primary care physicians, therapists, dieticians, activity professionals, social workers, hospitalists, and others who together weave the fabric of care surrounding each resident. Person-centered care focuses both on the quality of life and the quality of care with the ultimate goal of optimizing individual well-being. Person-centered care realigns the traditional model of care away from what may be best for all to what is best for the individual.
- **Positive social engagement.** The emphasis should be placed on making personal connections. Staff members visit each resident multiple times per day, and make it a point to facilitate connections among residents with similar interests. Outings to foster connections with the surrounding community can also be offered.
- **Sensory enrichment.** Promote a full and rich quality of life for residents who are confined for their own safety or functional status that incorporates multifaceted engagement that they have been accustomed to throughout their life prior to dementia diagnosis.
- **Physician collaboration.** Physicians are programmed to seek positive outcomes. They are not interested in simply keeping their patients safe and supported, they want to see them flourish. They become frustrated with the erratic and high turnover world of assisted living whose efforts to deliver the care they prescribe may at times be inconsistent. People define quality as the difference between what they expect and what they get. This is no different for medical professionals. They

want to see their treatment efforts rewarded by the positive outcomes that can only be delivered by trained, competent, facility-based staff who provide them with solutions rather than problems to solve. The more they receive in terms of good news and consistent reporting about their patients, the more patients they will refer.

Benefits of Frequent Assessments

Overall the goal is to support the residents by collaborating with community professional resources to provide the highest quality of life possible. The aim is to support quality of life beyond building a secure and safe environment. There is a need for metrics and assessments that measure quality of life parameters that are important to monitor status changes so that timely interventions can be implemented to possibly arrest decline. Information that brings a better understanding of functional status, and tracking changes observed in baselines can empower medical professionals and facility staff to steer their care efforts and supportive treatments to respond rather than react to the ever-changing lifestyle challenges the residents may face. See table 17.1, which summarizes the benefits of tracking person-centered outcomes to all interested parties.

Further, families who can see how the assessment scores change over time can have a better appreciation of how the disease is progressing in their loved one and be better prepared to understand how caregivers will respond to their increasing needs.

Table 17.1   Benefit Summary for Tracking Outcomes

Benefits	Meaning
Physician support	Partnering with personal care physician for better outcomes
Resident support	Better quality of life, longer stays, can accommodate medically challenged cases
Family support	Reassure families that they have the best care possible
Staff support and retention	Provide options for career enhancement and quality of care identity not available elsewhere
Marketing implications	Redirect and improve the flow of professional referrals who seek measurable outcomes for their patients

■ INTERVENTIONS

Upon completion of at least two quarters of assessment, a trend can be observed from the differences in the scores. It will be important to moderate the risk of negative trends by intervening with a menu of alternatives for each. These will include nutritional interventions, falls prevention, depression mitigation, and cognitive support interventions.

Nutritional Interventions

Seniors have a special relationship with food. Each phase of the aging process presents different nutritional challenges. Although good nutrition is not a treatment for memory loss, it does improve quality of life dramatically. Good nutrition helps to combat infections, depression, skin breakdown, pneumonia, confusion, as well as risks for falls and urinary tract infections. Here are some of the changing nutritional needs presented with the three general progressive phases of Alzheimer's disease (AD).

In phase one, loss and confusion typically fuel depression, which causes changes in appetite. Weight changes may occur. People with AD may anxiously eat nonstop, or they may forget to eat altogether. They may forget how to shop for food or how to prepare a meal. They may forget how to use kitchen equipment, like a microwave or toaster, and become frustrated.

The increased activity, agitation, and wandering that are prominent in phase two increase residents' energy needs. Active residents in this phase may require an extra 1,600 calories per day just to maintain their body weight. Getting those extra calories may be challenging if the resident loses interest in food. Swallowing difficulties, inability to recognize or distinguish foods, tasting difficulties, shortened attention span, physical changes like tremors or apraxia and the inability to cope with the stimulation at the meal site all work against a confused resident.

In phase three, people with AD are usually confined to a wheelchair. Typically, they forget how much food to put in their mouths or how to swallow. Most people in phase three need to be fed. In order to ensure the maximum nutritional intake, caregivers should take their time, offering cues, coaxing, and proper positioning. Appropriate food consistency is essential, as there is a risk for choking. Having the main meal at midday helps too, because that is typically when the resident is at his sharpest.

Alternatives for nutritional intervention:

Have foods available at all times.

Include the resident in choices, preparation, and cleanup.

Encourage hydration at least six times per day.

Have portable/finger foods available for residents who wander, have limited attention spans, have difficulty using utensils, and/or would benefit from six meals per day. (Examples of finger foods: hard-boiled eggs, bananas, baby carrots, orange sections, graham crackers with peanut butter, cookies, cheese, chicken nuggets, etc.)

Offer smaller portions of food frequently throughout the day.

Offer favorite foods, with a preference on nutrients. (If a resident likes both brown and white rice, serve the nutrient-rich brown rice.)

"Bulk up" snacks with peanut butter, cheese, and margarine. Use dry milk in sauces and soups. Add ice cream and chocolate syrup to milkshakes and desserts. Sprinkle sugar over everything (unless a no-concentrated-sweets diet is needed).

Choose dinnerware for special needs: large handles on mugs and bowls to increase steadiness; plates with a lip to help get food on a spoon or fork; solid-colored dishes to highlight food and minimize confusion; contrasting linen colors to make food easy to see.

Move the plate a quarter-turn to compensate for vision problems.

Use dark table linens so spills won't show up easily. Use aprons, not bibs, at mealtimes if necessary.

Consider a swallowing evaluation for residents who are observed doing the following: pocketing of food, coughing or choking after meals or liquids, frequent throat clearing, drooling, gurgling voice quality, effortful chewing, complaining of pain while swallowing, watery eyes or running nose while eating, reflux, prolongation of meals. Implement diet modifications, positioning and swallowing techniques, and modify food consistencies.

Positioning techniques:

Keep the resident's head and upper trunk as upright as possible with head at midline; the head should be slightly forward in relation to the neck and shoulders.

The hips and small of the back should be centered at the back of the chair.

Arms should be resting on the table to facilitate proper shoulder posture.

Keep resident's feet flat, adjust the table height, and have the resident sit close up to the table.

Serving and food preparation techniques:

Talk to the resident, tell her who you are and what you will be doing.

Speak slowly and clearly, feed slowly while alternating foods.

Don't startle the resident with the feeding utensil.

Feed small amounts of food at a time, alternating sides of the mouth.

Offer sips of liquid often, and tell the resident when you are done to put closure on the activity.

Nutritional strategies:

Remove or substantially modify dietary restrictions.

Encourage the use of flavor enhancers.

Encourage more frequent small meals.

Offer liquid nutritional supplements for use between (not with) meals.

Improve protein intake by adding meat, peanut butter, or protein powder.

Treat depression with antidepressants that do not aggravate nutritional problems.

Remove or replace medications that may have anorexia-producing side effects.

Staff interventions:

Ensure that residents are equipped with all the necessary sensory aids (dentures, hearing aid, glasses).

Ensure the resident is seated upright at 90 degrees, preferably out of bed in the dining room in a chair (residents eating in the dining room are much less likely to have low intake).

Remove or minimize unpleasant sights, sounds, and smells.

Pharmacological nutritional intervention:

Megestrol acetate is a synthetic derivative of the female hormone progesterone. It can promote increased appetite and is very tolerated. The medication is designed to increase food intake, BMI, albumin, prealbumin, hemoglobin, and lymphocyte count. This will require a physician order.

Falls Interventions

Ninety-five percent of the more than 300,000 hip fractures in the US each year are the result of a fall.[1] The remaining 10 percent of hip fractures occur spontaneously due to low bone density or osteoporosis. Spontaneous fractures can then precipitate the fall. Women have two to three times as many hip fractures as men, and white post-menopausal women have a one in seven chance of a hip fracture during their lifetime. The hip fracture rate increases at age 50, doubling every five to six years. More than one-third of adults aged 65 and older fall each year.

Alternatives for Falls Intervention

Physical measures: Using a recliner or rocking chairs. Seating adaptations such as a wedge cushion. Lowering bed or removing bedframe to put mattress on the floor. Teaching residents to dangle their legs before rising from bed, Commode/urinal at bedside. Assistive devices such as quad canes and walkers. Call bell within reach. Monitor blood sugar and oxygen levels. Check for presence of infections (URI or UTI). Anti-tippers for wheelchairs, self-releasing Velcro lap belt. Fall mats at bedside. Orthostatic blood pressure (BP) and pulse (P) monitoring. Reposition resident routinely in high visibility areas. Discuss with physician discontinuing or decreasing doses of medications associated with cognition changes, hypnotic or sedative effects (sleeping medications), bradycardia, hypotensive episodes, or sensory changes. Consider medications for pain relief. Review of current medications that may destabilize gait and balance (such as benzodiazapines). Also consider identifying high-risk residents for falls using a color-coded bracelet, falling star sticker or similar tag and relocating them to rooms near the nursing station.

Environmental measures: Anti-rollback device on wheelchair. Remove wheelchair foot supports when not in transport. Remove visual barriers, clear pathways, remove clutter that can fall and pose a hazard (magazines are very slippery on the floor). Brakes on beds, bed in low position. Repositioning for comfort. Personal items within reach. Assess seating. Brake extenders for wheelchair. Walker/cane tips in good condition. Assess siderail use. Bed/chair alarms. Pressure sensor alarm. Reminder signs to alert staff to residents at risk. Nonskid strips on floor. Remove wheels from overbed tables. Consider motion detection night lights to illuminate pathway to bathroom. Nonskid socks while in bed. Properly fitting footwear and nonskid shoes. Clothing that does not interfere with or restrict movement. Create and manage a toileting schedule. Room monitor. Spills and wet spots should be mopped up as soon as they happen.[2]

Psychosocial measures: Active listening. Behavioral strategies. Sensory stimulation. Increased surveillance. Mental health evaluation.

Activity measures: Structured daily routines. Physical exercises, evening exercises. Buddy system to monitor, PT/OT and pharmacy consultations. Music therapy. Restorative ambulation. Frequent toileting post-opioid pain medication and constipation relief measures combined with a proactive bowel and bladder training program.

Behavioral Interventions

The primary goal in behavioral interventions is to first recognize and attempt to prevent bad behaviors. Employees need to be taught to recognize subtle changes in residents' condition. Employee longevity enables the staff to gain an intimate knowledge of their residents' personal habits and characteristics, much as a parent would recognize a subtle change in their child. This enables them to spot problems quickly as they arise. Many health problems, when detected early, can be managed by a physician, enabling residents to continue to function independently and live in more comfort.

To assist with this, a behavior card system that is individualized and updated constantly can prove to be an invaluable communication tool. Similar to dining cards that indicate residents' food preferences, behavior cards are posted in staff-only areas where they can be referenced when issues begin to arise. These behavior cards will list specific individual behaviors commonly exhibited by residents, as well as individualized interventions that have worked in the past to prevent or deescalate potential behavior deterioration. It is important that all staff share their insights so that proactive actions and interventions can be deployed to reduce or eliminate challenging behaviors before they start. Frequent physician visits on behaviorally changed and medically at-risk residents should also be done on an as-needed basis.

Alternatives for Behavioral Intervention

In a recent study, researchers found that many behaviors are triggered by often undiagnosed pain or other medical conditions. These results indicate a strong need to properly assess residents for behaviors. Seek interventions for those suffering who are undiagnosed and corrective actions for those who may respond favorably to them. Identifying these at-risk residents and advising attending physicians and family members may help operators to avert unnecessary mental health triggered discharges, while improving the quality of life for each individual.

Physical factors: Medication interactions, multiple medications, side-effects of psychotropics, diuretics or antianxiety medications. Check for infections such as upper respiratory, urinary tract, fever, blood tests. Dehydration and constipation can also cause changes in mental status, pain and discomfort triggering behavioral episodes. Monitor personal comfort by checking for pain, hunger, thirst, constipation, full bladder, fatigue, infections, and skin irritations. Check for bowel sounds, abdominal distention and impaction. Check for signs of dehydration, including skin elasticity, temporal wasting, and urine color. Sleep deprivation is a well-known trigger of behavioral issues. Evaluate sleep and wake patterns. Bedtime routines should be ritual. Limit stimulants in the afternoon such as caffeine. Avoid hypnotic medications and other stimulating drugs. Engage in deep gentle exercise. Avoid napping.

Psychosocial factors: Assess resident for delusions, hallucinations, and depression. Assess aggressive behaviors and attempt to determine triggers. Assess psychoactive medications. Provide cognitive therapy and failure-free activities, focus on remaining abilities, not losses.

Evaluate staff approach (calm, flexible, guiding and not controlling). Avoid being confrontational or arguing about facts. Redirect the person's attention. Try to remain flexible, patient, and supportive by responding to the emotion, not the behavior. Validate feelings. Consider breaking down large tasks into smaller ones (task segmentation). Nonverbal approaches can include therapeutic touch, aromatherapy, approaching patient on equal or lower level, also adjusting approach to deescalate—attitude is contagious. Also consider music therapy, distraction therapy (redirection), recreational engagement, exercise, and remotivation.

Environmental factors: Assess physical surroundings. Evaluate roommate, nighttime activities, staff interactions, interpersonal preferences. Evaluate the environment for sensory overload, furnishings, room personalization. Create a calm environment by avoiding noise, glare, insecure space, and too much background distraction. Relocate the person away from other residents and attempt to deescalate them one-on-one.

Staff factors: Street clothes to be less threatening. Decrease staff turnover. Resident chooses caregiver. Permanent assignments rather than rotating caregivers. Consistent scheduling to create and maintain routines.[3]

Use the four-step approach "I Can Respond Professionally" (ICRP) = Identify, Calm (or Control), Resolve, Prevent. Identify the problem from the resident's point of view. Empathize and put yourself in their place and understand their triggers. For many residents, a challenging behavior is often their only way of communicating a need or unpleasant feeling. Calm the situation by using reassuring, nonthreatening body language. In order to calm an escalating situation, staff must also remain calm. Staff should ask themselves, "Am I the best person to handle this, or does the resident respond better to someone else?" Residents with dementia can be redirected and distracted. Offering them something pleasurable, such as a snack or a stuffed animal, or asking them to help you with something can calm the situation. Once the problem has been identified, take steps to resolve it by modifying the environment. Bring the resident to a less stimulating area. Separate the resident from another resident who may have been the trigger. Resolve hunger or thirst. Toilet, clean, or change the resident. Offer reassurance and speak softly to the resident to distract them and prompt them to listen to you. If there is a possibility that the resident is experiencing pain, it should be reported to management. The final element in the four-step process is Prevent. Staff can do this by looking for patterns that may indicate an "episode" is coming. Many residents have experiences that will trigger a behavioral pattern. These triggers might be recognized by one employee but totally unknown to another. Communication between staff regarding potential triggers and what may have worked in the past to avoid or redirect the resident is good person-centered care and can help staff anticipate issues and respond before the resident has a chance to escalate.

Common Behavioral Challenges

Agitation is a broad term that refers to a variety of verbal, vocal, or physical behaviors that appear distressing to the person and are considered inappropriate or unusual or disruptive to others. Common behaviors observed in a person experiencing agitation include restlessness, complaining, repetitive statements or repetitive movements, and constant request for attention.

Response to agitation. Consider integrating them into a small group or one-on-one activity. Try calming music, reduce level of stimulation, brief hand massage with essential oil. Feeling agitated is a very uncomfortable feeling for the resident, and their response to this may make them combative or put them at risk for falls or self-injuries.

Aggressive behaviors are actions that are threatening or harmful and can be physical in nature (hitting, kicking, biting, grabbing people or things, throwing things) or verbal (screaming, cursing, or making threats). Aggressive behaviors may be the result of a person having unmet needs and not being able to express them to staff, too much sensory stimulation, or frustration related to reliance on memory.

Response to aggressive behaviors. Explain to the person step by step in a calm voice that you understand and are there to help. Remove any other residents or staff in the immediate area who may be in danger or contributing negatively. Be mindful of your body language and voice. Keep a pleasant face, a calm voice, and a nondefensive posture. Approach an aggressive person from the side, not from the front. Attempt to initiate a time-out to deescalate the situation. Slowly assess for unmet needs and attempt to meet the resident's need with caution and in a safe manner.

Resisting care, sometimes referred to as combative with care, is a common behavior that is different from agitation or aggression. A person who is resisting care may pull away, attempt to leave, or become agitated or aggressive while expressing resistance to care. Resistance toward care usually occurs during hands-on care activities such as mealtimes, bathing, toileting, or administering medications. The resistance may be occurring because the person does not understand the care activity or why it is important or because they are afraid or uncomfortable with how the activity is occurring.

Responses to resisting care. Assume a nonthreatening posture by smiling and speaking in a pleasant tone of voice. Keep arms open and not crossed. Conduct care at the resident's eye level and from the side. Do not stand over the resident. Slow down the care, and make sure you are communicating clearly and explaining the task in a step-by-step process as you do it. Attempt to redirect the resident's focus away from themselves and try focusing on something or someone else. Give them a job to do while you perform the care. Encourage them to do as much for themselves as they can. Put objects necessary for the task within their field of vision so they are more easily located and remove objects that are unnecessary or distracting. If the resident is agitated, consider reapproaching them at a later time when they are quieter or distracted. Also consider having the care done by someone else. Consider whether the activity may be uncomfortable and painful or consider pain treatment before the activity.

Repetitive behavior refers to mannerisms, questions, or behaviors that a person frequently repeats. Repetitive behaviors are thought to occur because of changes in the brain due to dementia as well as the resident's reaction to those changes, which may include anxiety, fear, and a sense of loss of control. Repetitive questions may occur because the resident has dementia and cannot recall the answer they recently received, or because it is something that is important to them and the caregiver can't remember.

Responses to repetitive behaviors. Maintain consistent routines. Give the resident your full attention and pay attention to what he or she repeats. If a specific object triggers repetitive questions or statements, consider removing the object. Ignore behaviors that are not harmful. If tapping or clapping is especially annoying, try a hand warmer or a squeeze ball to occupy the person. If the person frequently forgets the day, consider having calendars visible and accessible. Whiteboards may be helpful for addressing repetitive questions. This board may include information about frequent questions the resident asks along with the appropriate answer. Index cards can be used in a similar way and may be kept in the resident's pocket or wallet, with the question on one side and the answer on the other side. Focusing on the emotion of the question may help you identify a more appropriate response.

Sexually inappropriate behaviors include socially unacceptable behaviors toward self in public or inappropriate behaviors directed at others, such as sexually explicit comments and inappropriate touching. Behaviors that are considered sexually inappropriate may be related to the human need for intimacy, although it may also be triggered by something in the environment such as a suggestive television program or another resident or staff person.

Responses to sexually inappropriate behaviors. Remain calm and professional and gently yet firmly redirect the behavior by telling the person it is inappropriate and unacceptable. Let the resident know how their behavior affects you and others. Try to redirect the behavior through the use of food, drink, activity, or alternate conversation. Distract the resident through activities that have been meaningful for them and involves the use of the resident's hand, such as exercise or folding towels. Provide stuffed animals to the resident for grasping and fondling. To help prevent disrobing and masturbation, choose clothing for the resident that opens in the back. Identify and try to eliminate triggers for the behavior.[4]

Disruptive vocalizations are any verbal noises, such as screaming, yelling, nonsense talking, or cursing, that are generally considered unusual, inappropriate, or upsetting to others. Disruptive vocalizations may be the result of a resident having unmet needs and not being able to express them to staff or may be due to too much or too little sensory stimulation.

Responses to disruptive vocalizations. Listen to what the resident is saying and see if you can identify any concrete needs or requests in the vocalization. Assess for unmet needs, such as the presence of pain, hunger or thirst, hot or cold body temperature, or need to go to the bathroom, and attempt to meet that resident's needs. Try to redirect the resident. One way to do this nay be to engage them in one-on-one social interaction or individual or small group activities. Playing white noise or nature sounds in a relaxing environment may be helpful. Taking the disruptive resident for a walk outside or away from the group of people can help to deescalate.

Apathetic or withdrawn residents may be experiencing a loss of interest or motivation. Behaviors that may reflect being withdrawn or apathetic might include sitting alone in one's room, avoiding contact with others, and making limited eye contact with other residents or staff.

Responses for apathy or withdrawn behaviors. Sensory stimulation may be helpful and can involve stimulating hearing, sight, or touch. Some ways to do this might include playing music, looking through visually stimulated things such as pictures from holiday cards, and touching or holding a stuffed animal. Involving the resident in cooking or baking activities can help stimulate a sense of smell and be a good time to talk and reminisce with the resident as their memory allows. Aromatherapy might be tried if someone on staff is trained in the correct implementation of this approach. Aromatherapy can benefit stress-related problems and promote a positive state of energy, health and well-being. Essential oils are some of the oldest and most powerful therapeutic agents known.[5] There is ample research to demonstrate the human response to essential oils. Some oils such as Peppermint, Rosemary, Jasmine, Lemongrass and Grapefruit stimulate and have an uplifting effect on the body. Others such as Lavender, Rose, Geranium, Sandalwood and Ylang-Ylang have a relaxing or sedating effect on the body. For many, simply sitting outdoors for a short period of time can offer valuable sensory stimulation.[6]

Wandering or pacing is sometimes referred to as "aimless" walking. This can also refer to restlessness or excessive moving around during the day or evening. While the behavior of wandering appears pointless to the outside viewer, it often has a purpose for the resident with dementia. Common reasons a resident with dementia wanders are to increase exercise, reduce boredom, reduce anxiety or confusion about where one is, attempt to return to a similar place or resident, exit seek or search for a specific location or familiar person.

Responses for wandering behavior. Make sure the area that the resident wanders in is safe for them. Create "rest stations" with benches and additional engaging stimuli such as pictures, scents, recorded sounds, wall art or an activity board in the hallways or wandering areas that provide opportunities for tactile stimulation. Wandering and pacing can be indicative of discomfort, so check for pain, hunger, thirst, constipation, full bladder, fatigue, infections, and skin irritation. If the resident is exit-seeking (trying to leave the unit or constantly looking for doors or exits), they may be bored or may be expressing interest in returning home or going outdoors. Disguising doorways with murals or wall hangings might reduce cues to exits. Schedule outdoor time or off-unit walks in other secure parts of the building for someone who is frequently exit-seeking, if such areas exist. If the resident seems to be looking for personal items, consider producing duplicates for them, such as a wallet, purse, or keys, and make them readily available. Many people identify these items with independence.[7]

Finally, while you sometimes cannot control the behavior of another resident, you can always control your response to it. Always share your successful findings with other staff and interested parties so that everyone who interacts with the behaviorally challenged individual is equipped with techniques that have been proven effective with that resident.

Alternatives for Depression Intervention

Treatment for depression depends upon its cause and severity and, to some extent, on personal preference. In mild or moderate depression, psychotherapy is often the most appropriate treatment. But incapacitating depression may require medication for a limited time along with psychotherapy. In combined treatments, medication can relieve physical symptoms quickly, while psychotherapy enables the patient to learn more effective ways of handling his/her problems.

- **Personal measures.** Mild exercise. Music therapy. Pet therapy. Gardening or other hobbies. Social engagement. Volunteerism. Intergenerational ac-

tivities. Reminiscing with family members or other residents. Social interventions to help with isolation and loneliness (group outings, regular visits from volunteers, participation in a support group). Humor. Maintaining a healthy diet. Religious or spiritual groups. Continuous engagement in stimulating activities. Craft programs.

- **Medical measures.** Treatment of underlying medical conditions. Antidepressants, hormone replacement therapy, changes in prescription dosages or considering alternate medications without side effects. Antidepressant medication can help some people feel better by controlling certain symptoms. This can be helpful in mobilizing people who survive the repair of a broken hip but lose the will to get out of bed. It should be noted that antidepressants can potentially lead to falls as they are sedating and can cause a sudden drop in blood pressure when a person stands up. Also, selective serotonin reuptake inhibitors (SSRI) drugs can create dependency and may lead to self-destructive thoughts.

- **Psychotherapy and counseling measures.** Supportive counseling includes religious and peer counseling. It can help ease the pain of loneliness and address the hopelessness of depression. Both peer counseling and pastoral counseling usually are provided without cost. Cognitive behavioral therapy (CBT) helps people distinguish between problems that can and cannot be resolved and develop better coping skills. Interpersonal psychotherapy can assist in resolving personal or relationship conflicts. Somatic or trauma psychotherapy with a professional can help bring about resolution of traumatic experiences.

- **Why it is important to treat.** The body often follows the mind, and depression substantially increases the likelihood of death from physical illnesses. Depression can increase impairment from a mental disorder and impede its improvement, while psychological treatment frequently improves the treatment success rate for a variety of medical conditions. Untreated depression can interfere with a patient's ability to follow the necessary treatment regimen or participate in a rehabilitation program. According to a study conducted by the RAND Institute, depressed elderly patients use six times more prescription medications and spend four times more in total health care dollars than their nondepressed counterparts. Seniors who are vulnerable for depression experience more comorbidities and run a higher risk of catastrophic health failure.

Cognitive Interventions

Cognitive interventions must be blended with a perspective that allows the caregiver to understand a person not only as someone who suffers from illness or unhealthy conditions, but also as someone who inhabits healthy parts and personality that remains even though it seems to be hidden by illness. For staff and families, engaging the person behind the impairment will allow everyone to feel good about participating with the residents in the activity experience and improve in the likelihood that the therapy will be effective (see chapter 8).

Everyone benefits from better information. Equipped with baseline data and measurable metrics to evaluate changes, we can better understand the residents' needs and changes in their health progression. Everyone can partner together to weave a tapestry of care to surround the resident in health and happiness.

Specifications and Tools

Mini-Mental State Examination
  https://cgatoolkit.ca/Uploads/ContentDocuments
    /MMSE.pdf

Cornell Scale for Depression in Dementia
  https://cgatoolkit.ca/Uploads/ContentDocuments
    /cornell_scale_depression.pdf

Morse Fall Scale
  http://networkofcare.org/library/Morse%20Fall%20
    Scale.pdf

Comprehensive Geriatric Assessment
  https://www.bgs.org.uk/sites/default/files/content
    /resources/files/2019-02-08/BGS%20Toolkit%20
    -%20FINAL%20FOR%20WEB_0.pdf

Mini Nutritional Assessment
  https://www.mna-elderly.com/sites/default/files
    /2021-10/mna-mini-english.pdf

Saint Louis University Mental Status Examination (SLUMS)
  http://www.memorylosstest.com/dl/slums
    -english.pdf

Geriatric Depression Scale
  https://geriatrictoolkit.missouri.edu/cog/GDS
    _SHORT_FORM.PDF

Body Mass Index
  https://www.nhlbi.nih.gov/health/educational
    /lose_wt/BMI/bmicalc.htm

NOTES

1. J. Parkkari, P. Kannus, M. Palvanen, A. Natri, J. Vainio, H. Aho, I. Vuori, and M. Järvinen. "Majority of Hip Fractures Occur as a Result of a Fall and Impact on the Greater Trochanter of the Femur: A Prospective Controlled Hip Fracture Study with 206 Consecutive Patients," *Calcified Tissue International* 65 (1999):183–187.

2. *CNA Fall Pocket Guide: Risk and Defensibility—Fall Risk Assessment and Prevention* (November 2016), 17.

3. Karen D. Doll, "Addressing Problem Behaviors in Long Term Care: Interventions for Communication, De-escalation and Prevention for Cognitively Impaired Residents," YouTube video, October 2021, https://www.youtube.com/watch?v=NiJFoZjAtug.

4. Nursing Home Toolkit: Promoting Positive Behavioral Health, http://nursinghometoolkit.com/sexrelated.html.

5. *Essential Oils Desk Reference,* 3rd ed. (Orem, UT: Essential Science Publishing, 2004).

6. Nursing Home Toolkit, http://nursinghometoolkit.com /apathy.html.

7. Nursing Home Toolkit.

Personal Care

18

The introduction of personal care to the senior living community or the development of a freestanding assisted living community can be attractive to seniors looking for cost-effective alternatives to home health care or a nursing home. As a rule, the cost of assisted living is about two-thirds that of equivalent care in a skilled nursing facility. The economies of scale of delivering personal care in a multiple-family residential environment such as an assisted living community, as compared to purchasing home health services delivered in a resident's home, are driving the current boom in assisted living.

According to Consumer Affairs, there are more than 810,000 people who reside in assisted living facilities at an average cost of $4,500 per month. The demand for assisted living will continue to accelerate as the baby boomers require services. The population of adults older than 85 will double by 2036 and triple by 2049, and 70 percent of these people will require assisted living services during their lifetime.[1] About 71 percent of the residents are women, and 71 percent of those have some memory impairment. The average age of residents is now 84 and residents stay an average of 22 months. Most are discharged to a nursing home (46%) or to a hospital (12%), which could lead to readmission. Fewer discharges (24%) are due to death.

As people live longer, their personal care needs increase. Figure 18.1 illustrates the average personal care needs for people 85 or older in the general population. Fifty-seven percent of this population require some assistance with activities of daily living (ADLs) or instrumental activities of daily living (IADLs). Thirty-five percent need assistance with one or more ADLs.

Levels of care for residents in assisted living communities are considerably higher than those in the general population. These residents have clearly identified the need for assisted living and have higher personal care needs than those living at home with family or other support. Figure 18.2 illustrates the need for assistance among residents in assisted living communities. The greatest need for assistance is in bathing and medication reminders, followed by dressing and escort services.

The most common disease states encountered in the assisted living setting are arthritis (42.6%), dementia or emotional illness (33%), hypertension (28.1%), asthma or other pulmonary disease (11.5%), and diabetes (10.6%). The assisted living residents in the study averaged 2.9 diagnoses per resident. The most commonly used medications are cardiac drugs and diuretics (48.6%), CNS medications (46.3%), and laxatives or cathartics (17.2%). Thirty-five percent of residents had four to seven prescription records, and 19 percent had eight or more.

The methods of delivering personal care vary among providers, as does staffing. Typically, 6 hours

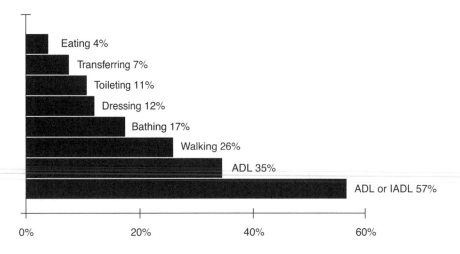

Figure 18.1   The Need for Assistance in the Population 85 and Older

Source: Data from US Department of Health and Human Services, Agency for Health Care Policy and Research, *Functional Status of the Noninstitutionalized Elderly: Estimates of ADL and IADL Difficulties*, Publication No. PDS-90-3462, June 1990.

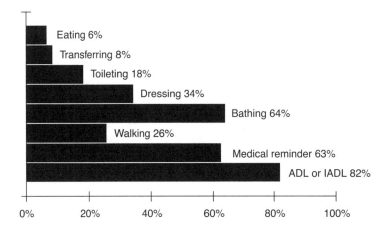

Figure 18.2   The Need for Assistance among Residents of Assisted Living Communities

Source: Data from Coopers and Lybrand, Assisted Living Federation of America (ALFA), acuity study within assisted living communities.

per day of home health services cost as much as a monthly service package that includes 24-hour staffing and 45 minutes per day of personal care services. Clearly, for those seniors who have extensive needs and can afford it, assisted living can be cost-effective while providing the added benefits of companionship and 24-hour emergency service.

The decision to move into an assisted living community is generally made by adult children seeking an affordable alternative to placing a loved one in a nursing home. The advantages of a private residential unit and the noninstitutional, homelike environment can help ease feelings of guilt common to families considering institutionalization.

METHODS OF DELIVERING SERVICES

As the assisted living business has grown and matured, service delivery and billing methods have evolved. Assisted living originally developed as a way for congregate or independent living communities to maintain their occupancy by enabling existing residents to age in place. Over time, those residents required additional services. Some communities met this challenge by introducing home health agencies, some discharged these residents to a higher level of care, and others designated a section of their independent community for personal care or assisted living. In the continuing care retirement community, the progression was a planned one, and a full continuum of care, including assisted living and skilled nursing, was offered. Many new operators faced with significant staff shortages are now looking to develop communities where residents contract for their own personal care services with outside agencies. This is a growing trend as the costs of staffing these communities balanced against the residents' ability to pay more negatively impacts operating margins.

Subsequently, developers recognized that prospects were becoming more aware of the limitations of traditional congregate communities and began developing properties with both independent living apartments and a separate assisted living component. This option, of course, was popular with seniors who were interested in having access to services if they needed them but did not want to live with infirm elderly people. Conversions of hotel properties, multiple-family dwellings, and nursing facilities to assisted living, and of nursing facilities to subacute and rehabilitation facilities, have been tried, with mixed results. The elderly will always be attracted to assisted living communities that allow seniors access to health care services in a residential setting while avoiding admission to a nursing home.

Assisted living communities employ a variety of methods to deliver the care residents require. The following discussion describes the four main methods and identifies their advantages and disadvantages.[2]

Home Health Care Agencies

With the home health option, the community developer or management provides the basic service package, such as meal service, housekeeping, maintenance, laundry, activities, and transportation, and subcontracts with a Medicare-certified home health care agency to deliver personal care. This arrangement gives residents of the community access to personal care services using their collective purchasing power. Home health agencies benefit because they can deliver a wide array of services, many of which are reimbursed by Medicare, without the expense and inconvenience of traveling to individuals' homes. Hospice care, which is largely palliative care for the terminally ill and is reimbursed by Medicare, has become increasingly popular for assisted living residents who qualify. The program not only provides nursing supervision but also covers the cost of medications.

The home health option enables the community to deliver a higher level of care than would be possible under assisted living regulations in most states. Because the operator is not directly providing the care, they are not required to become licensed as assisted living and subject to regulations. It can provide relief to residents who are experiencing financial pressure as their health care needs increase. The community can benefit from reduced turnover, stabilization of the assisted living population, control of the continuity of care, and differential billing structures to account for differing care needs.

Subcontracting for health care services with a single provider is attractive to owners looking to minimize their overhead to defray expensive nursing costs, particularly during the fill-up period, when the continual changes in occupancy make it difficult for the management to optimize staffing. By contracting with a single Medicare-certified home health agency, the management can provide residents with needed care while avoiding the risks of several different home health agencies delivering services to its residents with little or no control over the quality of these services. Should a medication error or resident abuse occur at the hands of a home health staff member, the community may be exposed to legal liability, and its reputation will suffer even though it is not directly responsible for the incident. In one assisted living community, no fewer than 15 home health agencies were delivering services to residents, making the community vulnerable to problems with control and quality assurance.

Operators must be careful to conform to federal regulations. Medicare and Medicaid antikickback provisions contained in U.S.C. 1320 a-7b(b), section 1128B of the Social Security Act, are enforced by the Office of the Inspector General. Because of the broad scope of the federal antikickback laws, the secretary of Health and Human Services issued regulations on July 29, 1991, commonly known as the "Safe Harbor" regulations (*Federal Register* 56 F.2d Reg.35951), which clarify the applicability of the federal regulations. It is critical to document the arrangement with the independent contractor through the use of a "safe harbor" agreement to protect against any possible infringement of the Social Security Act.

The home health arrangement must be kept totally separate from services provided by the owners and management of the business. First, there can be no duplication of services that the facility is obligated to provide under the existing contract. The contract can, however, be modified to exclude those services so long as the home health agency provides for residents who do not qualify for Medicare. Medicare also does not allow any inducement to residents for the provision of Medicare-reimbursable services. Therefore, the community must not gain financially or receive any services in exchange for or as a condition of the subcontract. An arrangement in which the community is delivering personal care services with its own staff, in conjunction with a preferred home health agency that manages the program through nursing staff provided to the community at no cost, may be violating federal regulations by receiving services in exchange for providing access.

Further, providers cannot legally deny any Medicare beneficiary the freedom to choose among health care providers. The agreement must therefore be a nonexclusive arrangement in which the certified agency may engage other contractors to provide similar services or allow other certified home health agencies to provide its services. The provider must at all times refrain from recommending or referring residents to any single agency. Because the owner or manager is not providing personal care services, the residents are free to choose whichever provider they wish. Most, if not all, will choose the main contracted agency in any case, out of convenience and because they may already know its staff. Finally, the owners and management of the community cannot receive any payments from the agency. This stipulation takes into account the volume or value of any referrals or business generated between the parties for which the payment may be made in whole or in part by Medicare or a state-funded health program. The owners and management should also avoid creating a supplemental staffing company, consisting, for example, of a nurse and home health aide, and billing the agency for their services. Medicare views this practice as an abuse of the system and considers it an inducement for referrals. But the occasional use of specific subcontracting services is permissible. The community can provide office space for a Medicare home health agency as long as it charges the agency a reasonable and customary rent.

Differential Service Levels

Personal care services usually include bathing, dressing, escort to meals or tray delivery, medication reminders, additional housekeeping, personal laundry, dementia care, orientation and cuing, grooming, scheduled toileting, and safety checks. Under the service level program, different levels of services are provided. On admission, residents' needs are assessed, and a personal care service plan is created. (Many states require an assessment by a medical professional before admission and periodically thereafter to evaluate the appropriateness of placement.) Premiums for ascending levels of service are usually based on additional time required per day, translated to a monthly rate. For example, a community that includes 45 minutes per day of personal care in the basic service package may charge an additional $210 per month for an intermediate level that provides up to 60 minutes per day ($28.00 per hour × 0.25 hours = $7.00 per 15-minute increment × 30 days per month = $210.00). Additional 15-minute increments are charged at the same rate. Any significant change in a resident's status that requires a permanent increase in care, or a significant increase in care on a short-term basis, triggers a review of the service plan with the resident and family.

Although this type of system works fine for residents who usually require 45 minutes or less per day of personal care, as a resident's needs increase, it can be difficult to convince them or their family that they need to move up to the next level of service and incur the additional expense. Residents and families who have been accustomed to one rate on move-in can see their monthly service fees climb by as much as $2,000 per month as the resident's care requirements increase. In addition, a service-plan review that coincides with lease renewal and the usual rent increase can be a tough sell.

Staffing the service level option can bring challenges because it is difficult to quantify the amount of service delivered to the residents. Personal care aides are constantly being pulled in different directions to serve residents on demand. The management will find that some basic-level residents require more care on an intermittent basis, while higher service level residents may demand special attention because they pay more.

Point System (ADL Guide)

In the point system, the resident's needs are assessed and assigned a numerical score. For each ADL, the amount of assistance required is rated on a scale of 1 to 5. For example, a resident's need for assistance in bathing and dressing might be assessed on the following scale:

1 point: Independent in bathing and dressing.

2 points: Requires assistance only in transferring into and out of bath; can bathe self.

3 points: Requires assistance in bathing and dressing but does most of the work.

4 points: Requires considerable assistance with bathing and dressing.

5 points: Completely dependent on staff for bathing and dressing.

The final score is derived by adding the points from each category of service, then dividing by the number of categories, usually 10. The higher the score, the higher the monthly fee. Levels of 4 or 5 can demonstrate a need for nursing home care and trigger discharge planning.

Assessments are conducted on admission and periodically thereafter. If the personal care director waits until an obvious reassessment is needed, chances are that the personal care aides are already providing more service than the resident is paying for. Consequently, significant amounts of care are given away, and the facility is always understaffed.

Like the service level option, the point system leaves room for interpretation. Residents and family may contend that the assessment may vary from one week to the next depending on how the resident is feeling. The management needs to perform regular assessments for every resident and resell the increase in fee structure many times throughout the lease term. In addition, the time required to perform ADLs can vary widely among residents. One resident may require 20 minutes to bathe and get dressed for breakfast, while another may need 45 minutes to accomplish the same task with assistance. There is no way to directly correlate the nursing time needed for each resident with the amount charged for services.

Actual Care Provided

Under the actual care option, residents are allocated a daily amount of care (say, 45 minutes) in their service fee, and additional time required is billed in arrears. On admission, a resident is assessed, and a personal service care plan is developed. The service plan measures the amount of personal care the resident needs in a seven-day period, usually Sunday through Saturday. The plan itemizes each ADL for which the resident requires assistance.

An initial time study, performed by the personal care aides assigned to the resident, serves as the foundation of the service plan. The total number of minutes of care required is added up; if the total for the week exceeds 315 minutes per week (45 minutes per day for seven days), the excess is billed to the resident's account, and this becomes the amount of additional care regularly provided and charged for. The time study is repeated under one or more of the following conditions: (1) the resident returns from the hospital after a short stay, (2) the resident's physician significantly alters the resident's medications or treatment, (3) the resident's overall personal care needs increase or decrease, or (4) the resident experiences a cognitive decline. A care conference is then called among the personal care director, personal care aides, family, and physician to update the service plan. Usually, personal care aides account for every minute of their day during the time study, so that all interactions between personal care aides and their residents are documented. (This process can also be used to monitor employee performance.)

Another time study is completed during the first week on the revised service plan. The total time that exceeds the allotment in the service fee is then billed separately—for example, at 50 cents per minute ($30 per hour). This system benefits residents and families because it allows for the fact that a resident may need more care on some days than on others. The resident is charged only for the care that exceeds 315 minutes per week even if he or she needs extra time on a given day.

On completion of the time study, a weekly schedule is prepared that documents the time needed to deliver each service to the resident. This should be reviewed by the management and then discussed with the family or resident, along with the associated additional fees. If the resident or family objects to the additional cost, the management can ask them which services should be deleted from the plan and explain the implications of such actions.

The actual care system allows the management to recover the cost for the actual time of service delivered rather than impose a flat fee, as in the service levels option. On completion of all time studies, the management also has an accurate tally of the total staff hours required to deliver services to the resident. This can be an effective tool for measuring overall staffing needs.

Each personal care aide is assigned specific residents and has a set daily schedule. The schedule includes the time of service, apartment number, resident name, assignment detail (with check-off boxes), and minutes allocated to perform the service. The aide's entire day is fully scheduled, and he or she is expected to complete all assignments before clocking out. Under this system, it is common to reach 80 percent efficiency (meaning almost all staff time is billable to the residents) in the delivery of services. Schedules do have some flexibility to allow for unscheduled service and personal attention. Also, the night shift does not provide a significant amount of personal care so those employee hours are not subject to additional pricing. Some companies use software to develop the personal service plan, schedule care for each resident, assign a staff person to the resident and track each interaction using a bar code scanner, generate a billing statement, personal information sheet, medication record, and report of need. Programs such as these can also be used to optimize staffing and manage the overall profitability of the ancillary care delivery system.

■■■■■ QUALITY ASSURANCE

Quality assurance must be an integral part of the management and culture of a senior living community. The long-term success of the community depends on its reputation for problem solving and consistent delivery of good-quality care and service.

In contrast to skilled nursing, in which quality assurance can be managed through traditional physicians' rounds, the assisted living environment is more challenging. In a community where residents live in private apartments, the management must demand effective communication by the personal care aides of changes in residents' conditions and needs and be prepared to act on that information.

The management should not wait until it hears of a problem from the resident's physician or family member to address quality assurance. Personal care service plans for each resident should be developed and periodically evaluated to ensure that the appropriate level of care is planned for and consistently delivered.

Supervision of the care plan by a senior caregiver or licensed practical nurse (LPN) can help ensure that services are in fact delivered. This individual can also be available for emergency response and to answer aides' questions about their residents' needs and problems. Residents who are identified as at high risk can be visited regularly throughout the day.

Periodic care-plan reviews for each resident can also serve as quality-assurance tools. Each service should be evaluated in terms of timing, frequency, duration, and resident response. Reviews should be done at least every six months, or sooner if changes in the resident's needs or condition are observed. From an operations perspective, the review helps detect whether aides have been coaxed into providing more care than a resident's plan provides for. Residents have a habit of asking for small amounts of extra care that staff may be reluctant to refuse. As a resident's health declines incrementally over time, these requests become more frequent, contributing to higher costs. Reviewing personal care plans frequently will ensure that the cost to deliver this additional care can be identified and recovered from the resident.

Quality assurance is even more challenging in assisted living communities with special care units, such as those for residents with dementia. In later stages of the disease, residents lose the ability to communicate health complications and pain. Common disorders such as urinary tract infection can go undiagnosed until they become serious enough to require hospitalization.

State regulators have promulgated extensive regulations in assisted living and monitor care delivery on an annual or more frequent basis. Table 18.1 summarizes many of the most common deficiencies found by surveyors during their on-site investigations.

■■■■■ STAFFING

There are three basic ways to categorize personal care staff assignments: universal worker, rotation, and pri-

Table 18.1 Most Common Survey Deficiencies

- Background checks on staff or volunteers not being done prior to hire.
- Pills being removed from original container (loose pills) and/or pharmacy review not being done.
- Medication management: Audits show order, but medication is not in cart and there is no note saying it is on back order. If there is an order, it must be in the facility or noted why not.
- Notes of observation of resident not being conducted at least monthly, or if a condition or incident occurred requiring more frequent documentation, that was not being done and documented.
- Inservice training not being delivered by a properly certified person performing training, or documentation not signed by the person trained, or conducted prior to resident contact or absence of annual basic training
- TB testing must have annual risk assessment documented.
- Menus not being planned and written at least one week in advance and posted in a public place.
- Food and food storage: At least one week's supply of nonperishable staple foods and two days' supply of perishable foods not being maintained.
- Failure to implement and monitor interventions subsequent to a change in resident condition or accident.
- Resident physical examinations: physical not completed within 30 days prior to admission and at least annually after admission or change in condition by licensed physician. Exam lacking any of the following: appropriateness of placement, medication ordered, self-administration status, identification of special needs, including needs that must be delivered by a nurse.
- Water supply and hygiene—domestic hot water temperature outside the range of 100–120 degrees in faucets that are accessible by residents.
- Failure to safeguard and secure stored medications. Expired medications comingled with current meds.
- Medications refrigerated outside the range of 36 to 46 degrees, thermometers missing.
- Facility and grounds not clean and free of vermin and offensive odors. Equipment not clean and disinfected. Chemicals not safely stored and secured.
- Outside areas unkept with presence of weeds, rubbish, overgrown landscaping, and potential breeding grounds for vermin.
- Controlled substances: Narcotics without their own control sheet (date, time, resident's name, signature of who administered it and who ordered it). After each shift change: no audit that narcotics were properly administered, documented, errors and omissions indicated, addressed and corrected.
- Resident care services: Render care services, follow orders by physician or authorized health care provider, take precautions for residents with special conditions, assist with ADLS as needed and appropriate.
- Medication administration record review: Required at each shift change, lack of documented review of the MAR, outgoing and incoming staff without corrections made.
- Maintenance: All equipment and building equipment in less than operating condition and in good repair,—light bulbs, faucets, etc.
- Care plan: Lack of ICP development within seven days of occupancy with signature of resident or responsible party, and administrator or designee. Failure to revise semiannually or if resident has had a change in condition.
- Administration of medications: Failure to be administered by the same staff member that prepared them, no earlier than one hour prior to administration. Failure to properly recorded *when rendered*. Failure to ensure that physician ordered medication is available and properly managed. Failure to document that employee has successfully completed medication management training if they are administering medications.

mary care. All three systems are commonly used in assisted living communities but are rarely mixed.

Universal Worker

In a typical assisted living community, services such as bathing and grooming, meals, housekeeping, and activity programs need to be provided every day. The traditional operation accomplishes these tasks through departmentalization. For example, the housekeeping department cleans the community, the food and beverage department prepares and serves the meals, the activity department organizes leisure activities and events, and the nursing department delivers the personal care. Each service is generally supervised by a separate department head. Because staff members are trained or experienced in only one type of service, there is little crossover or communication between departments. Consequently, the entire service package becomes compartmentalized, and department heads may become territorial and bureaucratic. The more the residents' needs are passed from one department to the next, the higher the risk of a communication breakdown that will cause a problem for the resident.

Under the universal-worker concept, which has become popular among providers, employees are hired as care managers and are cross-trained in several departments. Because they are conditioned to accept responsibility for all of a resident's needs, there is little "buck passing" on service requests. An employee may be hired as a personal care aide, for instance, and then cross-trained as a housekeeper or server in the dining areas. He might spend the first four hours of his shift bathing and dressing residents and then move to cleaning apartments or assisting in activities. In assisted living–based dementia care units, the care manager usually handles all of the care needs of the residents to whom she or he is assigned. Facility management or department heads act as facilitators and trainers. The system is designed to make everyone in the operation accountable for meeting the residents' needs, whatever they may be. Some technical skills, such as maintenance, cooking, and bookkeeping, do not lend themselves to cross-training, but the majority of services that are delivered to the residents in a community can be performed by universal workers.

Clearly, it is easier to set up a new community under this structure than to break down the compartmentalized paradigm in an established community. The universal-worker idea is often met with resistance from established employees who believe the management wants them to work harder for the same pay. Moreover, people are by nature resistant to change. Some operators have restructured their compensation plans to overcome this objection. They hire for attitude, then train for skill: employees are hired in one specialty and then, as they learn and pass competency tests in each new discipline, their base compensation is increased. For example, a personal care aide may be hired at $12 per hour, then cross-trained in housekeeping for an additional 25 cents per hour, then as a server for 25 cents more or a dishwasher for 15 cents more. As employees learn and grow in their positions, they become more flexible and consequently more valuable, and they are motivated by a sense of accomplishment and reward.

Typical assisted living community requires approximately 0.49 full-time equivalents (FTEs) per resident. Under the universal-worker concept, some op-erators suggest, this figure could drop to 0.356. One operator suggests that segregating job functions can reduce productivity by as much as 40 percent. In the competitive assisted living environment, it is no wonder that operators are embracing the universal-worker concept. It works well in many stand-alone dementia care communities, especially in smaller homes where separate departments are not practical. (See chapter 19 for more on staffing of dementia care units.)

The drawbacks of the universal-worker concept are in quality assurance and employee support. Service to the residents can become inconsistent when employees skilled at performing one job are learning another. The staff can become frustrated, feeling that they are doing many different tasks without being given a chance to excel at any of them. The management must respond to this frustration with continuing skill testing and retraining to develop proficiency and by continually reinforcing the merits of the concept to staff, residents, and family members.

ROTATIONAL SYSTEM

In the rotational system, staff are assigned to specific tasks, but they work with different residents in rotation. Many operators rotate housekeepers and personal care aides. While rotating staff may have a number of advantages, residents who are served by the same employee every day (as explained below) can benefit from the relationship that develops and the unique needs of the resident's care can be learned. See chapter 11 for more information on staffing patterns.

PRIMARY CARE ASSIGNMENTS

Also known as modular nursing, the primary care system assigns specific personal care aides to specific residents. The daily personal care needs for several residents are scheduled and assigned to one personal care aide on each of three shifts. This approach allocates responsibility for the delivery of care to the smallest number of employees. Residents prefer this system because the delivery of personal care is an intimate business. It requires a considerable amount of trust and is best accomplished through the development of personal relationships between the resident and the caregiver.

People who are attracted to the personal care business are usually compassionate. They are motivated by their ability to improve the lives of the residents they serve and often become attached to their residents, as the residents do to them. As a mutually supportive relationship develops, the resident generally receives the best care the aide is capable of giving.

Personal care aides who work with the same residents each day become intimately aware of each resident's condition and overall health. They can detect minor changes in a resident's health, activity level, and even bathroom habits, much as they would at home with their own children. They can alert the management and families to changes so that problems can be recognized and treated immediately. This is the essence of good-quality care: it is not about people delivering purchased services to residents in a consistent manner, but about people caring about their residents personally and taking responsibility for their health and happiness because they want to. Families feel more connected to personal care aides whom they know, and are better able to support them when residents exhibit difficult behaviors. They are also more likely to trust the management of the community if they come to know and trust the aides.

When staff members are rotated, even the best-intentioned caregivers have no baseline from which to evaluate the present condition of the residents. They can go on only what they can see today and what their instincts, training, and experience have taught them. It is nearly impossible to recognize the often-subtle changes that can signal big problems. More important, it is not easy for the residents to constantly remind their ever-changing caregivers about their specific needs for assistance. This system is disturbing to the residents and their families.

CALCULATING STAFFING REQUIREMENTS

There are several ways to calculate staffing requirements in the personal care department. Staffing can be calculated based on the number of minutes of daily care included in the residents' monthly fees, on coverage in the building throughout the day, on actual care scheduled in each resident's care plan, or on ratios of caregivers to residents.

Scheduling residents for personal care is an important consideration. If aides' tasks are not carefully scheduled at the beginning of the day, problems will snowball. Residents who cannot finish bathing and dressing before the dining room closes will order room

service—and will, of course, blame the management for not attending to them in time, in an effort to have the room-service charge waived. At the same time, personal care aides will be found in the kitchen waiting for trays that were already ordered, which creates a bottleneck in the kitchen and delays service to the residents who did make it to the dining room (and are now complaining about slow service). As the personal care aides are forced to wait, still more residents waiting for help in their rooms will miss breakfast. This cycle of poor service can be avoided or minimized by encouraging some residents to rise earlier for their bathing and dressing assistance and by limiting the number of morning baths. The residents' expectations must be managed so that everyone can be assisted without adding staff. Baths can be scheduled after dinner, before residents go to bed, so that the next morning they need assistance only with dressing.

Creative scheduling can often improve service to the residents *and* reduce the cost of delivering that service. For most residents, there are 14 to 16 hours available in which to schedule their care. Although some care must be scheduled at certain times during the day, typically around mealtimes, some of the heavier tasks can be distributed throughout the day and evening. The use of part-time personal care aides (job share with housekeepers or dietary staff with personal care assistant (PCA) training) during the morning rush, between 6:00 and 10:00 a.m., can also help defray the costs and improve care. Some operators run an 11:00 p.m. to 9:00 a.m. shift (10 hours per day, four days per week) so that they have two aides available to help during the morning rush. This adds four hours to the night shift but eliminates two four-hour morning shifts, for a net savings of four hours per day. Teach the staff to be flexible so that the community can deliver the best possible care with the resources available. Often it is a matter of learning to adapt an established routine to new requirements. In the long run, the residents will receive better care and be more satisfied.

Staff should also support and enhance the residents' ability to care for themselves. Many residents can learn to be more independent in some tasks and less dependent on the personal care aide. Aides might start or complete difficult tasks for the residents and encourage them to do the parts in the middle. This approach builds strength and self-confidence in the residents while easing the burden on the staff. Residents respond well to encouragement and to recognition for small victories over the effects of aging.

The care plan should also encourage family involvement. Families who are willing and interested can perform small services routinely. Such efforts can reinforce family bonds and generate a sense of teamwork between families and the staff. Moreover, if the family is directly involved in the resident's care, they are on hand to observe problems that may develop and can be involved in the solution or more easily accept the cost of additional care.

Flexible scheduling can be used to increase the efficiency of care delivery; some directors may also be tempted to use it to accommodate employees with personal scheduling problems such as childcare or transportation difficulties. Such accommodations, however, almost always result in higher costs to the operation. It is crucial in this low-margin operating environment to match the employee to the job requirements, not the job to the employee's requirements.

To monitor labor costs, it is also vital to make sure that the hours on the staff schedule tally with the assignment sheets for individual residents, which should also agree with the department's staffing budget. If the level of care increases, the staffing level can be increased accordingly, provided that the additional cost to deliver that care can be recovered through additional billing. The executive director should audit timecards weekly or bimonthly to control the inevitable cost creep.

There has been much debate about the most efficient number of units in an assisted living community. If there are too few, the overhead in supervision cannot be fully amortized by the residents' fees; if there are too many, quality control requires prohibitively complex supervision. Because of the relative seclusion of assisted living residents in private apartments, as the number of units increases, it becomes increasingly difficult to keep track of their individual care needs. Moreover, communities with more than 100 units tend to have residents aging in place. As their needs increase, so does the need for additional supervision; the turnover rate increases as the average length of stay decreases, costing more marketing dollars to refill the units. In a competitive environment, this trend can lead to financial difficulty. A stand-alone assisted living community should not exceed 80 units for maximal efficiency, unless there is a special care unit associated with it on the same site. Nursing supervision and other staffing can be shared by both units.

A nurse supervisor (a registered nurse [RN] or LPN) can reasonably be responsible for approximately 60 assisted living residents in one building. This work includes care planning, supervision, scheduling assignments, monitoring medication, dealing with families and physicians, emergency response, and some direct care. Larger units require additional supervision, depending on the overall level of need and cognitive impairment. For maximum coverage, schedule the LPN to work from 1:00 to 9:00 p.m. daily and from 10:00 a.m. to 6:00 p.m. weekends. Schedule the RN personal care director from 8:00 a.m. to 5:00 p.m. daily. This way, there is nurse coverage most days from 8:00 a.m. to 9:00 p.m., when the residents are most active and when families are most likely to visit. It is also a good idea to schedule the activity director to be available at lunch and dinner, when extra hands are needed to move residents safely to and from the dining room.

Most state regulations establish minimum caregiving staffing levels. The number and qualifications of staff members or direct care workers is normally determined by the number and condition of the residents. Typically, regulations call for there to be sufficient staff members to provide supervision, direct care, and basic services in a safe manner for all residents. Some states further go on to define staff minimums for peak and nonpeak hours. For example, for assisted living this ratio can be 1:15 during peak hours and 1:25 for nonpeak. In practice these minimums are adjusted for resident acuity and cognitive ability that impacts the residents' ability to assist or complete activities of daily living on their own. When determining the level of acuity for residents, the industry typically looks at the level of assistance they require with their activities of daily living and/ or their Mini-Mental State Examination cognitive score. The three main levels of acuity can be defined as follows: Low acuity = assistance with <3 ADLs and/or a MMSE score >19; Medium acuity = assistance with 3–5 ADLs and/or MMSE score of 11–19; High acuity = assistance with >5 ADLs and/or MMSE of <10. In terms of staffing minimums, while most state require "adequate staffing to meet the needs of the residents," in practice the specific needs of your resident population will determine the staffing you need for coverage.

	Assist with ADLs	MMSE Score
Low	<3	>19
Medium	3-5	11-19
High	>5	<10

Industry norms ratios are generally 1:15 (from 7:00 to 3:00 and 3:00 to 11:00) and 1:25 at night for assisted living residents. For memory care, those ratios are normally 1:7 ratios throughout the day and night. A facility with 1:20 throughout the day would need to have low acuity patients (requiring 54 minutes of personal care per day or less). Heavy care residents would require approximately a 1:11 ratio of staffing. When determining staffing efficiency for direct patient care, one needs to calculate time spent with the residents versus nonresident activities. So out of an 8-hour shift, the personal care assistant has two 15-minute breaks, a 30-minute lunch break, and approximately 10 minutes per hour of nonresident duties (charting, travel time, communications, training, dealing with urgent needs). This totals 2.3 hours per day nondirect duties, leaving 5.7 hours per day direct patient care. So 5.7 of 8 hours is approximately 70 percent efficient in round numbers.

The following is an example of what the staffing would look like for a 60-unit assisted living facility at 93 percent occupancy (56 residents) for low, medium, and high acuity:

Low Acuity = 77 minutes PRD @ 70% efficiency— 54 minutes PRD

56	Persons	Daily	Weekly	FTE	Ratio
7:00-3:00	3.5	28	196	4.9	16
3:00-11:00	3.5	28	196	4.9	16
11:00-7:00	2	16	112	2.8	28
		72	504	12.6	

Medium Acuity = 90 minutes PRD @ 70% Efficiency—63 minutes PRD

56	Persons	Daily	Weekly	FTE	Ratio
7:00-3:00	4	32	224	5.6	14
3:00-11:00	4	32	224	5.6	14
11:00-7:00	2.5	20	140	3.5	22.4
		84	588	14.7	

High Acuity = 111 minutes PRD @ 70% efficiency—78 minutes PRD

56	Persons	Daily	Weekly	FTE	Ratio
7:00-3:00	5	40	280	7	11.2
3:00-11:00	5	40	280	7	11.2
11:00-7:00	3	24	168	4.2	18.6
		104	728	18.2	

Typically, assisted living communities have a mix of low, medium, and high acuity residents that is constantly changing as residents age in place. The best way to accurately calculate staffing requirements is by tracking care delivered directly to each resident. This can be accomplished manually by assigning personal care aides to specific residents and recording each encounter. There are also cloud-based software programs such as PointClickCare that can use barcode technology to track and manage data from every encounter with any resident. These programs can also create service plans, keep patient records, perform medication management, and capture additional care delivered for accurate billing. Reports can be customized to produce an accurate picture of where staff time is currently allocated and determine how much actual time each resident is using—even the efficiency of the staff delivering the care. This way families can see progression in the needs of their loved ones and understand how that translates to additional hours and cost to provide that care.

ELECTRONIC RECORD-KEEPING

The benefits of using electronic health records (EHR) touch every area of operations in the health care continuum of care: relationships with family members, physicians, long-term care providers, therapists, specialists, resident engagement, employee satisfaction and turnover, compliance, operational efficiency, and operational cost. EHRs are the future of health care, including assisted living, because they provide critical data that can help coordinate care between residents and all providers in the health care ecosystem. They improve access to medical information for doctors, nurses, patients, and long-term care residents and restrict information access via passwords and biometric scanners.

While both EHR and EMR are commonly used terms, the term EHR (electronic health records) is now referenced more frequently. This is likely due to the

Centers for Medicare and Medicaid Services (CMS), as well as the Office of the National Coordinator for Health Information (ONC) preference for the term. When speaking of health care reform, CMS always uses the terminology "meaningful use of an EHR." The ONC exclusively uses the terms EHR and "electronic health records," explaining that the word "health" is more encompassing than the word "medical." The term "medical records" implies clinician records for diagnosis and treatment, while the term "health records" more broadly denotes anything related to the general condition of the body. A personal health record (PHR) is just that: personal. It is those parts of the EMR/EHR that an individual person "owns" and controls.

It is important to distinguish EHR and EMR, both parts of long-term care software as well. The EMR, or electronic medical record, refers to everything you'd find in a paper chart, such as medical history, diagnoses, medications, immunization dates, and allergies. While EMRs work well within a practice, they're limited because they don't easily travel outside the practice. In fact, the patient's medical record might even have to be printed out and mailed for another provider to see it.

An EHR or electronic health record is a digital record of health information. It contains all the information you'd find in a paper chart but a lot more. An EHR may include past medical history, vital signs, progress notes, diagnoses, medications, immunization dates, allergies, health care directives, lab data, and imaging reports. It can also contain other relevant information, such as insurance information, demographic data, and even data imported from personal wellness devices.[3]

The EMR is a digital version of the paper chart used by facility nurses, but an EHR goes further by providing a more expansive view of a long-term care resident's health and medical history. A fully functional EHR system goes beyond basic functionalities such as clinical notes and documentation.

The EHR software systems can perform some key functions in assisted living facilities, including documentation, storage, and retrieval of patient and resident e-documents, such as electronic medical records, minimum data sets, care plans, e-prescribing, admission/discharge/transfer records, physician orders, medication administration and refill requests, finan-cial records, incident reports, referrals, and many other continuity of care modules that are readily accessible and easy to use.

There can also be calendar modules that enhance communication with families about the resident, which can be particularly useful for memory care patients, who might report no activities despite having had a full day. When family members can confirm a digital check-in, they're less likely to confront nursing staff with demands about why their loved one isn't doing more.

Some of the best EHR vendors provide interoperable software, allowing not only for interfacility communication but also information exchange with other EHR systems. The power of an EHR lies not only in the data it contains, but how the data are shared. Health information becomes instantly accessible to authorized providers across practices and health organizations to provide ongoing continuity of care.

An EHR can be shared with clinicians and organizations involved in a patient's care, such as labs, specialists, imaging facilities, pharmacies, emergency facilities, and school and workplace clinics. When the facility records are seamlessly integrated with other members of the health care community, it helps to improve coordination of care, improve the quality of patient care, and increase efficiencies and cost savings for the facility.

Additionally, an EHR is necessary to meet Meaningful Use requirements. Meaningful Use is a Medicare and Medicaid program that supports the use of an EHR to improve patient care. To achieve Meaningful Use and avoid penalties on Medicare and Medicaid reimbursements, eligible providers must follow a set of criteria that serve as a roadmap for effectively using an EHR. CMS has renamed the Medicare Meaningful Use program as Merit-Based Incentive Payment System (MIPS) and the Medicaid program as Promoting Interoperability.

Benefits of a long-term care EHR software can include:

- Residents' personal and medical records are more secure than paper records.
- Clutter, liability, and storage concerns with paper systems are eliminated, especially with long-term storage of resident records required by states, most averaging 7 to 10 years after discharge.

- Digital files are easier to search, sort, store, and access when you need them.
- It provides critical data that inform clinical decisions and help coordinate care between all providers in the health care ecosystem.
- It documents residents' health information over an extended period, allowing health care providers to identify trends and make better-informed treatment decisions.
- Compared to paper records, a digital patient-record (EHR) system can add a variety of information management tools to help provide better care by more efficiently organizing, interpreting, and reacting to data. All data entered are time-stamped and cannot be manipulated after being saved without creating a trail. This adds to the integrity of the records.
- The more interactive an EHR system is, the more it will prompt the user for additional information. This not only helps collect more data but also enhances their completeness.
- It can improve family communications and resident relations with modules that share activity levels, resident heath trends, and family concerns and contact.
- EHRs can alert providers to potential drug interactions and other safety concerns in real time to avoid any potential harmful incidents.
- EHR systems focus on the total health of the patient. EHR software is built to share information with caregivers in same facility, outside health care providers, and specialty services, as they contain information from everyone involved in the patient's care, improving care coordination.
- The information moves with the patient—to the specialist, the hospital, the nursing home, the next state, or even across the country. EHR systems are designed to be accessed by all people involved in the patient's care—including the patient.

While there are many advantages to having an EMR or EHR system, there are some disadvantages as well.

- They are typically much more expensive to implement initially, as providers must invest in the proper hardware, training, and support on top of the software. But as EHR technologies have become more commonplace over the past decade, the initial cost of systems has come down dramatically.
- The maintenance cost of an EHR can also be costly. Hardware must be replaced, and software must be upgraded on a regular basis. In addition, providers must have ongoing training and support for the end-users of an EHR.
- Unless properly built, there's also the chance the system will malfunction, destroying all data.

Ultimately though, the world is being radically transformed by digital technology in our daily lives and the way we communicate. With the advent of EHRs, communication and information can be readily available and accessible when and wherever it is needed, resulting in more efficient, cost-effective, safe, and higher quality care. With the advent of Medicare reform and the growth of accountable care organizations, there will be an increasing need for providers across the continuum to share medical records, and account for services to avoid duplication. When used properly, EHRs enable memory care and assisted living communities to create a truly comprehensive picture of their residents' well-being, and even the well-being of the entire community.

STAFF TRAINING

Training personal care aides never seems to receive the attention it deserves. Many companies talk about training, but few perform much of it. Some states, such as Colorado, require eight hours of dementia care training before a personal care aide can work with memory care residents, then eight hours of dementia care training annually thereafter. Virtually all states require an orientation to safety, emergency plan and building evacuation (or shelter in place), resident rights, and infection control within three days of employment. Although this can become expensive, it represents an investment in employee satisfaction and, ultimately, longevity. It is up to the management to teach employees about the expectations of their jobs and to eliminate guesswork.

Many textbooks, training manuals, and videos are on the market. Each community should develop its own training program consistent with its management and care philosophy, a program that can be easily communicated in several short orientation sessions. The program should include the following topics:

- Philosophy of independent living in an assisted living community
  - Choice
  - Dignity and respect
  - Right to privacy
  - Fostering independence
  - Promoting individuality
  - Resident freedom
  - Responsibility of sharing information
  - Expectations of quality and service outcomes
  - The role of the personal care aide and how it looks when it is done well
  - Overview of the job's specific requirements
  - A place to call home: the residential environment
  - Involvement of the resident and family
  - Relationship to the wider community
  - Confidentiality
- Residents' bill of rights
  - Residents' rights and responsibilities
  - Grievance procedures
  - Ombudsperson
  - HIPAA rules for protecting privacy
- Communicable diseases (including AIDS/HIV and hepatitis B); infection control and universal precautions
  - Defining a communicable disease
  - Examples of communicable diseases
  - Guidelines for infection control
  - Universal precautions
  - Sanitation
  - Basic personal hygiene
- Communication skills
  - Changes due to aging that affect communication
  - Communicating appropriately with residents
  - Communicating with families
  - Communicating without words; nonverbal tools
  - Barriers to communication
  - Talking about death and losses
  - Listening skills
  - Handling residents' complaints
- The aging process
  - Normal versus pathological changes in aging
  - Common diseases and issues
  - Common myths and stereotypes
  - Coping with loss and the grieving process
  - Dealing with sensory loss

- Death and dying; dying as a stage in life; the needs of the dying resident; hospice care
- Dementia and cognitive impairment
  - Overview of Alzheimer's disease and related dementias
  - Effective communication techniques, verbal and nonverbal
  - Safety and environmental issues
  - Coping with difficult behaviors
  - Stress and taking care of yourself as a caregiver
  - Role of the caregiver
  - Resident transfer and body mechanics
  - Depression and elderly people
  - Nutrition, weight loss, and hydration for people with dementia
  - Avoiding the need for restraints
- Managing medications
  - Common geriatric medications
  - Medication reminders
  - Abuses of medications
  - Liability
  - Documentation
  - Medications and people with cognitive impairment

Topics such as these can provide employees with an understanding of their position and of the needs of the residents they serve. The more vividly expectations are communicated, the more likely it is that they will be met. There are numerous online resources for subscription to training designed to meet state qualifications. Relias.com features online training and tracking software to provide personalized learning plans for companies with multiple employees. Mycaregivercoach.com is a YouTube channel with pragmatic, free, downloadable training videos for individuals or groups.

MANAGEMENT OF MEDICATIONS

In most assisted living communities, an essential element of personal care services involves the management of self-administered medication. A quarter of all prescription and nonprescription drugs in this country are consumed by only 12 percent of the population—people over the age of 65. Approximately two-thirds of the residents in a typical assisted living community require some help with their medications. As residents age, the complexity of their care and medication regimens typically increase. In turn, the exposure to and responsibility for medication errors increase for the owner and manager of the community, regardless of who administers the medications. The more involved the assisted living community is with its residents, the greater its potential liability.

State regulations vary widely concerning the distribution, administration, and delivery of medications to residents of assisted living communities. Any true regulation of medical services, and especially the flow of medications, remains nebulous. One study found that 73 percent of the staff members who reported passing medications in an assisted living setting were not licensed nurses (RNs or LPNs) and that 28 percent of the staff giving injections were not licensed nurses.[4] The researchers also tested those who passed or administered medications to residents on correct procedures and recognition of signs and symptoms of adverse reactions. Only 14 percent of the operators and staff scored 75 percent or higher, and 39 percent of the staff scored less than 50 percent.

Approximately 25 percent of all medications are inappropriately selected and dosed in elderly patients. Of the patients who receive inappropriate drug therapy, an estimated 28 percent require hospitalization.[5] In fact, more than one in six older Americans are taking prescription drugs that are not suited for elderly people and may lead to physical or mental deterioration and even death.[6]

Usually in assisted living communities, staff are permitted to manage the administration of medications but may not dispense or administer them directly. Most states define medication management to include the tasks of reminding or cuing residents to take their medications at the appropriate time, opening containers, reading labels, and observing, checking, and reassuring residents. Medications can be administered through crushing and mixing with food, injection, topical lotion, nasal spray, eye drops, gastrointestinal tube, intravenous line, or other methods. Those that cannot be self-administered are administered by licensed staff, and that service is generally contracted for by the resident. Some states, such as New Jersey, certify nurses' aides to administer medications on completion of a 40-hour course. Some communities insist that the pharmacy deal directly with each resident and deliver medications directly; others accept medications centrally and distribute them from medication carts.

Errors in the administration and documentation of medications arise when there is a difference between the dose dispensed and the dose prescribed. Such errors often involve omission or the use of the wrong drug, dose, or schedule; in some cases they involve deliberate misuse of a drug by the resident or another person. Clearly, the more medications a resident takes, the greater the likelihood of errors.

A number of options are available to minimize the risks of medication errors and misuse of drugs. Instead of using traditional pill bottles, pharmacists can dispense prescription medications in ways that portion out individual doses into clearly labeled compartments with a soft foil backing, printed with the day and time of dosage. These are often referred to as bingo cards or foil packs. Strip packs can also be set up that package pills into a roll like old-time penny candy. The prepackaged individual dose is simply torn off the roll, opened, and taken. The contents of each pack, along with the dose amount, patient, physician and patient names, frequency, and other information are printed on the packaging. The disadvantage with this system is that, unlike foil packs, which allow the caregiver to easily see whether the medication was taken by inspecting the empty compartments, the strip packets are discarded after use.

Medication boxes are another tool for managing medications. A medication box is a plastic pillbox with individual compartments for every day of the week. The medications are usually taken from their individual containers at the beginning of each week and distributed into the compartments according to the frequency and time of dose. The disadvantage to the boxes is that there is no way for the pharmacist to guarantee that the medications are correctly distributed and taken. Until recently, the family or home health agency had to accept the responsibility for setting up a resident's medications, for this service is beyond the license capability of assisted living staff in most states. With several different people handling medications, there is a wide margin for error. Pharmacists eager to capture business within the assisted living market are now more willing to dispense unit doses into medication boxes, unit-dose packets, or customized blister packs that can hold several different medications.

Exhibit 18.1   Standard of Care Issues

- Failure to adequately address patient risks in care plan.
- Failure to develop individual care plan (ICP) within seven days of occupancy with signature of resident or responsible party and administrator or designee. Failure to revise ICP semiannually or if there is a change in condition. Facility must provide services and activities to attain or maintain the highest practicable physical, mental, and psychosocial well-being of each resident in accordance with a written plan of care—Quality of Life.
- Failure to review and revise care plan subsequent to event (see change in condition).
- Failure to update care plan for change in condition. Change in Condition? = Assessment -> Care Plan -> Interventions -> Verify implementation
- Failure to notify family and physician.
- Failure to implement interventions to prevent further events (strategy change, refer to PT, OT, dietary, psych nurse, physician).
- Failure to communicate risks to all staff.
- Nursing notes document a problem or risk without notification, solution, and reassessment or follow-up.
- Failure to supervise or anticipate preventable events.
- Failure to have adequate staffing necessary to provide safe and appropriate care matching the level of care required.
- Failure to follow physician's orders for medication and treatments.
- Failure to provide a safe environment. Appropriate safeguards should have been put into place with interventions to address these risks, including hourly checks, remove visual barriers, clear pathways, frequently used personal items within reach, move room closer to nurses station, provide bed/chair alarms.
- Failure to recognize risk and anticipate injury and intervene in a timely manner.
- Failure to have adequate and or trained staffing to serve the care needs of the residents. For example: failure to ensure patient was properly supervised by competent nursing personnel who had the training and ability to recognize the significant risks of falling, particularly as functional assessment documented that patient required extensive assistance with bed mobility, locomotion on unit, locomotion off unit, and assistance with transfers, dressing, toilet use, personal hygiene.
- Acts and omissions amounting to negligence; recklessness and a willful and wanton disregard for the health and well-being of resident.
- Notes of observation of resident not being conducted at least monthly, or if a condition or incident occurred requiring more frequent documentation, not being done.
- Falsifying records: checking off that medication was administered or that care was provided when resident was absent from the building.
- Failure to maintain building and equipment in a safe and working order.

Other complications arising from medications include interactions with certain foods that can result in gastric disorders, undesirable weight loss, poor appetite, chronic infection, or insufficient caloric or protein intake, with insufficient vitamins and minerals necessary to ensure nutritional balance. Temporary imbalances such as dehydration may significantly affect an individual's response to a standard dose of medication. Outdated medications that a resident is reluctant to discard may be ineffective or even dangerous. A resident may refuse or be unable to take certain medications.[7]

Many commercial pharmacies that specialize in long-term care may offer to provide a consultant pharmacist, a fax machine, and a fax line at no cost to the community. A consultant pharmacist manages the entire medication program for residents. The services provided can include answering questions about

medications, checking that residents are taking their medications as prescribed, and checking for incompatibilities between different medications, other contraindications (such as reactions with food or drink), and adverse side effects. Consultant pharmacy services, especially review of drug regimens, can significantly improve the accuracy and suitability of medication management in the assisted living community. In addition, consultant pharmacists are often aware before physicians of new drugs that might be more effective, easier to administer, or less costly for residents.

Provisions of the Omnibus Budget Reconciliation Act of 1987 require that state Medicaid programs have prospective and retrospective drug-use review programs in place. These programs require pharmacists to screen prescriptions for therapeutic duplication, drug-disease contraindications, incorrect dosage or duration of treatment, drug allergies, and clinical abuse or misuse. An integral part of the law is a requirement that pharmacists offer to counsel all Medicaid patients about their prescription medications. Since the law was enacted, many states have amended their pharmacy practice acts to require that pharmacists offer these same services to all patients, not just those covered by Medicaid.

As the assisted living industry continues to expand rapidly and competition forces providers to retain their residents longer, it is inevitable that medication-related incidents will occur. In the assisted living environment, individual independence is often emphasized over safety. Implementing a comprehensive system of managing and monitoring medications can help reduce the operation's liabilities, as well as help the community retain clients by preventing unnecessary hospitalization due to adverse drug reactions.

Several excellent training programs are available. The state of New Jersey has developed a medication training program and procedures manual for personal care aides that is a first-rate resource for familiarizing laypeople with common medications and their effects on elderly people. Most institutional pharmacies also have reference libraries with videos and guides to common geriatric medications that can be checked out for the training purposes.

As families become increasingly familiar with the assisted living industry, communities have encountered increasing scrutiny toward the quality of care provided. As the communities struggle to maintain occupancy, they are less likely to discharge medically complex residents whose care needs often exceed the community's expertise to care for them. This can result in accidents or care issues, which can lead to poor outcomes for the residents. These poor outcomes are often met with legal action designed to recover dam-

ages from substandard care and demand more and better operational safeguards from providers. Lost or settled legal actions will translate to much higher liability insurance premiums for the communities. Often communities repeat common mistakes that could easily have been avoided. Exhibit 18.1 is a list of typical standard of care issues that plaintiff lawyers often focus upon to establish culpability.

NOTES

1. ConsumerAffairs, Assisted Living Statistics, updated March 17, 2023, https://www.consumeraffairs.com/assisted-living/statistics.html.
2. See B. Pearce and T. Grape, "Checks and Balances," *Assisted Living Today* 4, no. 2 (Winter 1997): 30.
3. P. Garrett and J. Seidman, Health IT Buzz, January 4, 2011, https://www.healthit.gov/buzz-blog/electronic-health-and-medical-records/emr-vs-ehr-difference.
4. C. Hawes, V. Mor, J. Wildfire, et al. *Analysis of the Effect of Regulation on the Quality of Care in Board and Care Homes* (Washington, DC: US Department of Health and Human Services, Office of the Assistant Secretary for Planning and Evaluation, 1995).
5. S. F. Clackum, "The Quest: Preventing Adverse Drug Events," *Provider* 22, no. 8 (August 1996): 58–59; US General Accounting Office, *Prescription Drugs and Medicaid: Automated Review Systems Can Help Promote Safety, Save Money*, GAO/AIM-96-72 (Washington, DC: GAO, 1996). Available online at: https://www.gao.gov/assets/aimd-96-72.pdf.
6. US General Accounting Office, *Prescription Drugs and the Elderly: Many Still Receive Potentially Harmful Drugs Despite Recent Improvements*, GAO/HEHS-95-152 (Washington, DC: GAO, 1995). Available online at https://www.gao.gov/products/t-hehs-96-114.
7. J. W. Cooper, *Drug-Related Problems in Geriatric Nursing Home Patients* (Binghamton, NY: Haworth Press, 1991).

19

Caring for People with Memory Impairment

Dementia care has evolved from treatment in a nursing home to programs in environments created especially for people with this disease. Demographics will continue to fuel growth in this critical component of care. Health care providers will adapt their programs to this population, add dementia care components to existing facilities, and develop additional freestanding homes to accommodate this burgeoning demand. Providing dementia care is much more complex than offering traditional senior living. Operators who develop expertise in this component of care will prosper, while others may become overwhelmed.

Aging is a natural and universal process of change. Our bodies show this change in various ways: hair turns gray, skin texture and elasticity alter, muscle tone decreases, and bodily functions slow and weaken. Advancing age may also bring about subtle changes in memory.

Until recently, there was a widespread belief that "senility" was a natural part of old age, as the word itself bears witness. The term *senility* is not a medical diagnosis but has been used to cover a variety of symptoms and behaviors, including forgetfulness, confusion, lack of responsiveness, and depression. In fact, many of these symptoms can be brought on by reversible causes such as malnutrition, anxiety, alcohol abuse, or adverse reaction to medications.[1]

We now know that loss of mental capacity with age is not inevitable. Not all older people develop memory impairment; however, short-term memory does tend to decline with age. The main complaint of most older people with respect to the aging process is changes in cognitive ability.

DEMENTIA

Dementia is a neurological disorder that affects the ability to think, reason, remember, speak, and move. While Alzheimer's disease is the most common cause of dementia, many other conditions also cause these symptoms. Some of these disorders are progressive and incurable; others can be treated and reversed. Because more than 50 diseases can cause dementia or similar symptoms, a thorough medical evaluation is needed.[2]

The three most common forms of dementia are Alzheimer's disease, vascular dementia, and Lewy body dementia. Sometimes a person can have more than one of these problems.

Alzheimer's disease, first described by the German neurologist Alois Alzheimer in 1906, is a debilitating and ultimately fatal illness. It involves a loss of nerve cells in areas of the brain that are vital to memory and other mental functions. The first sign of Alzheimer's disease is usually forgetfulness. As the disease progresses, it affects language, reasoning, and understanding. Eventually, people with Alzheimer's disease lose the ability to care for themselves.

The risk of developing Alzheimer's disease increases with age. Ten percent of individuals over the age of 65 have the disease. After age 65, the percentage doubles with every decade of life.[3] Nearly half of individuals over 85 have Alzheimer's disease.

Until recently, Alzheimer's disease was difficult to diagnose and could be positively confirmed only by examining the brain after death to identify the abnormalities which characterize the disease: protein deposits, referred to as plaques, and neurofibrillary tangles. According to the Alzheimer's Association, there is no single diagnostic test that can determine if a person has Alzheimer's disease. A number of dementia screening tests have been marketed directly to consumers. None of these tests has been scientifically proven to be accurate. Furthermore, the tests can have false-positive results, meaning that individuals can have results saying they have dementia when in fact they do not. This is extremely unlikely to happen if the individual visits a physician to seek care and potential diagnosis. For these and other reasons, the Alzheimer's Association believes that home screening tests cannot and should not be used as a substitute for a thorough examination by a skilled doctor. The whole process of assessment and diagnosis should be carried out within the context of an ongoing relationship with a responsible and qualified health care professional.[4] Physicians will evaluate medical history, perform a physical exam and diagnostic tests, perform a neurological exam, administer cognitive status tests, perform brain imaging, and conduct cerebrospinal fluid tests and blood tests. The currently available tests may predict the presence of amyloid changes in the brain or the presence of neurodegenerative disease or neuronal damage. Blood tests cannot be used as a stand-alone test to diagnose Alzheimer's disease or any other dementia; they will be used as part of a diagnostic workup with other exams.

Vascular dementia occurs when arteries in the brain become narrowed or blocked. The onset of symptoms is usually abrupt, following a stroke. But some forms of vascular dementia progress slowly, making them difficult to distinguish from Alzheimer's disease. Some people have Alzheimer's disease and vascular dementia at the same time. Vascular dementia often causes problems with thinking, language, walking, bladder control, and vision. Preventing additional strokes by treating underlying conditions, such as high blood pressure, may halt the progression of vascular dementia.

In Lewy body dementia, abnormal round structures—Lewy bodies—develop within cells of the midbrain, beneath the cerebral hemispheres. Like Alzheimer's disease, Lewy body dementia causes confusion and impaired memory and judgment. It often produces two distinctive physical signs typical of Parkinson's disease: a shuffling gait and flexed posture. Lewy body dementia can also cause hallucinations.

Lewy bodies contain a protein associated with Parkinson's disease and often are found in the brains of people who have Parkinson's disease or Alzheimer's disease. This suggests that the three ailments are related or that Lewy body dementia and Alzheimer's disease or Parkinson's disease sometimes coexist. Some people with Lewy body dementia experience a modest improvement in symptoms when treated with Alzheimer's or Parkinson's medications.

Several less common brain disorders also can result in dementia:

- **Frontotemporal dementia.** Because it affects the lobes of the brain that are responsible for judgment and social behavior, frontotemporal dementia can result in socially inappropriate behavior. Symptoms of this form of dementia usually appear between the ages of 40 and 65. The disease appears to run in families.
- **Huntington's disease.** Symptoms of this hereditary disorder typically begin between the ages of 30 and 50, starting with mild changes in personality. As the disease progresses, the person develops involuntary jerky movements, muscle weakness, and clumsiness. Dementia commonly develops in the later stages of the disease.
- **Parkinson's disease.** People with Parkinson's disease may experience stiffness of limbs, tremors, speech impairment, and a shuffling gait. Some people develop dementia in late stages of the disease.
- **Creutzfeldt-Jakob disease.** This extremely rare and fatal brain disorder belongs to a group of human and animal diseases known as the transmissible spongiform encephalopathies. A variety of Creutzfeldt-Jakob disease has emerged, particularly in Great Britain, that is believed to be linked to

human consumption of beef from cattle with mad cow disease (bovine spongiform encephalopathy).

Many other conditions, some reversible, can cause dementia or dementia-like symptoms:

- **Reactions to medications.** Some medications have side effects that resemble the symptoms of dementia. A single medicine may trigger such a reaction in an older person or in someone whose liver fails to eliminate the drug properly. Interactions among two or more drugs may lead to reversible symptoms of dementia.

- **Metabolic abnormalities.** Decreased thyroid function (hypothyroidism) can result in apathy, depression, or dementia. Hypoglycemia, or low blood sugar, can cause confusion or changes in personality.

- **Nutritional deficiencies.** Chronic alcoholism can result in deficiencies of certain B vitamins, which may lead to symptoms of dementia. Pernicious anemia, an impaired ability to absorb vitamin B_{12}, can also cause changes in personality. Dehydration also can cause confusion that may resemble dementia.

- **Emotional problems.** The confusion, apathy, and forgetfulness associated with depression are sometimes mistaken for dementia, particularly in older individuals.

- **Infections.** Meningitis and encephalitis, which are infections of the brain or the membrane that covers it, can cause confusion, memory loss, or sudden dementia. Untreated syphilis can damage the brain and cause dementia. People in the advanced stages of AIDS also may develop a form of dementia.[5]

Because researchers have mapped where alterations occur in the brains of people with Alzheimer's disease and have begun to associate locations of changes with clinical symptoms, schematic associations between brain area and functional capacity are possible. Such associations can be useful for diagnosis, family counseling, and treatment. Alzheimer's disease tends to begin in the temporal lobe, which controls new learning and short-term memory, then spread to other regions of the brain. The motor cortex and sensory areas are less affected.

Dementia usually begins with memory deficit or difficulty performing routine tasks. Early in the dis-

ease, individuals can adjust their lifestyle by making notes to supplement memory loss and establishing routines for taking medications and for locating keys, glasses, dentures, and other important items. Many behaviors, such as paranoia, agitation, pacing, and wandering, are common to people with dementia, but each person exhibits different symptoms to different degrees.

Early diagnosis can be devastating to those who have the capacity to understand what it means. Families are often concerned that the diagnosis itself may trigger panic or depression and hasten the degenerative process, but for many the opposite may be true. A person who is kept in the dark about the source of the problems may become frustrated, agitated, and possibly depressed when he feels he should be able to remember things and cannot. He needs to know that his problems are due to a disease, not simply to growing old. The ability to identify a particular disease can help equip those involved to understand the disease process, respond to the changes they are seeing, and make appropriate plans for care.

With the progression of dementia, a person may become increasingly dependent on the caregiver for even the most basic tasks. The caregiver should reconsider the range of acceptable activities for the person as the impairment progresses. The management of financial affairs and previously safe activities such as driving and preparing meals, taking medications, or going for unaccompanied walks may become hazardous. In later stages of the disease, matters such as daily hygiene and dressing may be beyond the person's capabilities and will become the caregiver's responsibility.[6]

The first symptom noticed is usually loss of short-term memory, as a person becomes forgetful, loses things, and has trouble remembering recent events. Some individuals who are newly diagnosed with dementia experience depression. Symptoms often include withdrawal, crying, agitation, anxiety, changes in eating habits or sleeping patterns, feelings of worthlessness, and disruptive behavior. Depression, which can significantly lower a person's cogitative capabilities and resistance to disease, is the single biggest factor influencing quality of life. Depression is treatable with medications and therapy, and socialization can help. Some people with dementia tend to focus on their own limitations. In social situations such as day care or senior living homes, their focus can be directed outward toward their environment.

People with dementia often experience word-finding problems, especially when they become fatigued or are emotional. Many people will ask the same question repeatedly. This indicates that the person is trying to remember something that is important to him or her. Changes in the brains of people with early-stage dementia cause impairments in memory, reasoning, and judgment, rendering it difficult for them to make decisions. Many feel overwhelmed when asked to make choices, and this inability in turn causes them to feel ashamed.

For many adults, driving represents independence, freedom, competence, and control, and giving it up can be a deeply emotional issue. Concerns about driving are likely to surface during early stages of dementia, when individuals are still socially engaged and able to manage other daily activities. Disorientation and changes in memory, visual perception, and reaction time make driving dangerous for the individual and everyone else on the road. In most states, the Department of Motor Vehicles offers a competency test.

As the disease progresses, individuals may undergo severe changes in personality and experience confusion. When an individual can no longer care for herself, 24-hour supervision becomes necessary, with eventual transfer to a special care facility.

Alzheimer's disease steadily takes away a person's identity. The feeling of loss is overwhelming in the beginning and confusing as the disease progresses. The individual is not only robbed of his sense of self, but he also loses his connection to his loved ones. He doesn't know who he is, who his loved ones are, whom he can relate to and who he can trust. It's a frightening world he lives in. Changing the way you think about providing care is the first step in building the foundation of the person-centered care approach. No longer is it just about getting the bathing done. Now it's about the quality of the time you spend with each resident and learning what strategies work on each individual. Share residents' sensitivities and the solutions or approach that you find are effective with all the caregiving staff. Involve everybody who provides care for the residents. Person-centered care requires knowing the person, noticing subtle changes, and adapting your approach.

Dementia strikes families particularly hard. The complex needs of a person with dementia and the emotional distress of watching that person decline can exact a huge toll. It is normal for caregivers to feel helpless, angry, fearful, upset, and bewildered. They should remember, however, that their reactions can either calm the person with dementia or create bigger problems. It is critical for the caregiver to act with warmth and tenderness.[7] The Alzheimer's Association can provide families with educational materials and advice.[8]

HOUSING AND CARE OPTIONS FOR PEOPLE WITH MEMORY IMPAIRMENT

An estimated 6.2 million Americans age 65 and older are living with Alzheimer's disease dementia today. This number could grow to 13.8 million by 2060. Unpaid dementia caregiving was valued at $256.7 billion in 2020. Its costs, however, extend to family caregivers' increased risk for emotional distress and negative mental and physical health outcomes—costs that have been aggravated by COVID-19. Average per-person Medicare payments for services to beneficiaries age 65 and older with Alzheimer's disease or other dementias are more than three times as great as payments for beneficiaries without these conditions, and Medicaid payments are more than 23 times as great. Total payments in 2021 for health care, long-term care, and hospice services for people age 65 and older with dementia were estimated to be $355 billion.[9]

Until the late 1980s, virtually all dementia care was provided either by caregivers in the home or in skilled nursing facilities. With the advent of assisted living, families with sufficient funds were attracted to this alternative. Today, care for seniors with memory impairment is offered in a variety of settings.

Caregiving at Home

More than 40 percent of family caregivers provide some type of nursing care for a loved one, such as giving medications, changing bandages, managing medical equipment, and monitoring vital signs.[10] Many family members who are caring for a loved one eventually find the associated strains and stress overwhelming. Elderly spouses who are experiencing caregiving-related stress and who have a history of chronic illness themselves have a 63 percent higher mortality rate than their noncaregiving peers.[11] This is especially true of individuals who started out providing intermittent assistance with simple tasks such as shopping, errands, or bill paying and end up providing physically demanding personal care such as bathing and dressing. In many cases, caregiving responsibilities obliterate what was once a normal routine. Burnout may be gradual and insidious in its onset but devastating in its consequences. The caregiver may wake up one morning, look in the mirror, and not even recognize the person she sees.

Burnout can cause helplessness, depression, and a constant sense of fatigue. Caregiving may force a withdrawal from social contacts and friends who are the primary support structure, or even cause the caregiver to lose interest in work, where he may receive professional validation. Some caregivers may experience a change in eating habits or increase their use of stimulants and alcohol. While most people can endure and recover from these symptoms, in others they may accumulate and worsen over time. Eventually, they may have a dramatic impact on the health of the caregiver and his ability to provide effective care and even turn the caregiver into a patient himself.

Part of the art of being a successful caregiver is the ability to set expectations, recognize one's limitations, and learn to care for oneself as well as for others. Varying the responsibilities of the caregiver is a way to stay fresh. Rotating tasks among family members or taking advantage of day care programs can give the primary caregiver some time off. Most senior living facilities offer respite programs providing short-term residency with professional supervision while caregivers take a well-deserved rest or vacation. Respite can also serve to introduce the person with dementia to the concept of assisted living so that she can overcome fears of living in such a community one day. Once the person sees that others have made the choice to live there and that their lives and family relationships have improved as a result, she might consider the option more willingly.

At-home care using home companions or home health aides is the single largest system for the delivery of health care services in this country. Families hire caregivers or outside contractors such as home companions or home health aides to perform a variety of services. Families must carefully screen such personnel before hiring. Unfortunately, they may be exposing themselves to financial risks that are not covered by homeowner's or general liability insurance. Knowl-

edge of the pitfalls of home care can help families to prepare for these liabilities and equips the senior living professional to advise families of their risks.

Elderly people been taken advantage of, robbed, and verbally and even physically abused by those paid to look after them. Long-term care ombudsperson programs in the United States investigate thousands of complaints of abuse, gross neglect, and exploitation on behalf of nursing home and board-and-care residents each year. Physical abuse was the most common complaint.[12] Recognizing mistreatment is often difficult. The older adult may be unable or unwilling to provide information because of a cognitive impairment or fear of retaliation. Older adults are often fearful of being placed in a nursing home, and some may prefer to be abused in their own homes rather than move to such a facility. Most states now require employers to check criminal offender record information before employing a caregiver. It is also important to verify whether the person is certified and trained to provide the services needed.

While most home health agencies usually carry comprehensive general liability insurance and professional liability insurance (each with separate limits of $1 million per occurrence) and workers' compensation insurance, most independent home companions do not. This means that if the home companion is injured on the job while providing care, the employing family may be personally liable for the injury. Several states mandate insurance coverage. If the injury results in a disabling condition, the employer may be liable for long-term loss of income. Additionally, if no workers' compensation insurance is in place, the injured caregiver's remedy could entail a lawsuit against the employer, claiming negligence, and typical homeowner's policies will not cover injury to an employee.

Domestic employees must be paid at least the federal minimum wage. Live-in employees must be paid for every hour worked; all employees must be paid overtime for any hours exceeding 40 hours per week. If the person lives on site, the Department of Labor assumes 8 hours sleeping or 16 hours working per day, or 112 working hours per week. Because all work in excess of 40 hours per week is required to be paid at time and a half, this situation would result in 72 weekly hours of overtime. This translates to several thousand dollars per month for 24-hour coverage, not including payroll taxes. This amount is comparable to the cost of assisted living. For a live-in aide, the fair value of room and board can be deducted from straight pay. Failure to observe employment regulations relating to the payment of overtime can subject the employer to multiple damages for the unpaid amounts. Also, the employer is legally required to verify the candidate's eligibility for employment under immigration laws using form I-9.

The Internal Revenue Service requires that a domestic employer who pays a caregiver more than $2,400 cash wages in a calendar year pay payroll taxes. These payroll tax obligations may include Social Security and Medicare taxes (7.65% of gross wages), federal unemployment tax (FUTA), state unemployment and disability insurance taxes levied on the employer, and advance payment of earned income credit for eligible employees. The employer is required to collect the employee's Social Security and Medicare taxes. If the employer fails to collect, he or she is still responsible for remitting these taxes for the employee.

Congress revised the "nanny tax" legislation in 1994, offering employers alternative means to remit the federal payroll taxes for wages paid. This legislation requires employers to disclose the wages paid to household staff on the employer's personal income tax return. Failure to disclose this information compromises the integrity of the tax return. There is no statute of limitations on the failure to report and remit federal payroll taxes. Families are most likely to be caught when a former employee files for unemployment, disability, or Social Security benefits and it becomes apparent that the person was receiving unreported compensation. Employers are generally required to pay back taxes, penalties, interest charges, and professional fees for an accountant or attorney.

Senior Housing Options

Providers of senior housing generally offer three choices for dementia care: as a component of traditional assisted living in a secured unit, in a stand-alone dementia care facility, or in a skilled nursing facility.

SPECIAL-CARE UNIT WITHIN TRADITIONAL ASSISTED LIVING. Approximately 42 percent of residents living in assisted living experience Alzheimer's disease or related dementia.[13] Traditional assisted living facilities have recognized the value of incorporating a separate dementia care component

into their existing communities. Such a unit enables the facilities to relocate a resident who becomes unsafe or unable to live with residents who do not have dementia. These special-care units typically consist of 25 to 40 apartments clustered in a separate part of the property, with their own common areas and grounds. Usually the unit has its own manager or director and activity staff. The special-care unit typically has staff-to-resident ratio of 1:6 to 1:8 during the day and up to a 1:15 ratio at night. If needed, additional staff members can be drawn from the assisted living component of the building, and staffing or management is often shared, especially at night.

Most units have a private room with a bathroom or a double room or suite with a shared bathroom. Meal service is provided from the main kitchen and delivered to a pantry or warming kitchen in the special-care unit. Most facilities have a secure, fenced outside area with a walking path or garden area for residents to enjoy during good weather. Dementia residents are normally prohibited from using common areas outside the dementia care unit, which may cause some residents with early-stage disease to feel discriminated against.

Residents are often admitted to special-care units when they are in the early stages of dementia. As the level of disability increases, so does the level of care and the corresponding monthly cost. A resident who enters the unit paying a base monthly rate may find the cost increasing by as much as 60 percent as the level of care needed increases over time.

STAND-ALONE DEMENTIA CARE. Some operators have developed a stand-alone model for the delivery of dementia care. These small, highly specialized units seek to imitate the home environment that residents have been accustomed to so that the connection to familiar things helps them maintain their independence as long as possible. These homes typically have fewer than 20 residents, some as few as 8.

There are many advantages to this setting. The homelike environment encourages building relationships. Meals are social occasions, and relaxing on the covered porches offers a familiar and peaceful time for socialization. The staff-to-resident ratio is much lower than that of special care units in traditional assisted living, which results in employee longevity and facilitates easier recruitment. Long-term employees become familiar with the needs and preferences of each resident, ensuring the best care possible. Smaller populations enable the staff to customize the care plan, the activity program, and even the food service to each individual. Over time, symbiotic relationships develop between the residents and the staff. Residents can often be seen helping in the kitchen, setting tables, folding laundry, or even helping other residents. Many of the tasks that would be impossible for residents in large assisted living environments are encouraged in these smaller settings.

Smaller homes usually have an all-inclusive flat rate structure, which means that rates do not increase with the level of care. Because the staff ratio is high, the cost to provide the care does not generally increase as the resident's disability increases. This is an attractive feature for families on a fixed income and for residents needing more care.

Residents usually have a private apartment and shared bathing arrangements, which are preferable for this population because of the inherent risk of falls. People with dementia often have problems with mobility and should be assisted in toileting and bathing. Residents suffering from dementia are highly susceptible to falls because they are often driven by impulse and do not exercise the same caution as a cognitively alert person. Facilities have therefore offered families a shared-risk agreement for falls to avoid institutionalization, while some courts have found that these operators may not be able to negotiate away liability for resident accidents.

Meal service in the stand-alone setting is usually offered from a central kitchen and cooked by a caregiver from a menu created by a dietitian. In smaller settings, employees are often multitask workers. While their primary function may be providing care to the residents and assisting with activities of daily living, they can also be found preparing meals, administering medications, participating in activities, and doing residents' personal laundry and light housekeeping.

When assisting with activities of daily living (ADLs), the staff should try to help the residents help themselves. "People with Alzheimer's disease can retain certain living skills that they would normally lose if caregivers let them perform those skills regularly," note researchers in the Occupational Therapy Department at the University of Pittsburgh. Their study found that encouraging people with Alzheimer's disease to perform certain ADLs for themselves allows them to retain skills they might otherwise lose. "Typically, individuals with Alzheimer's disease have not been able to gain access to a great deal of rehabilitative care because it was felt that the disease is a progressively degenerative disease, and they would not benefit from the care," explains Joan Rodgers, the leader of the study. "What our study demonstrated is that when people with Alzheimer's disease are provided with the appropriate support they can improve their ability to participate in ADLs."[14] The appropriate support described by these researchers involves behavioral intervention, a research term for cuing.

Rogers explains, "If nursing staff or an in-home caregiver does things for people that they can do for themselves, you run into a condition called 'excess disability' which is an inability to do things that's caused by the caregiver, not necessarily the disease." Caregivers need to resist the temptation to simply perform these tasks themselves for the sake of efficiency. If the staff can provide cuing to start and finish some challenging tasks, such as dressing, while encouraging residents to attempt to complete some portion of the task themselves, it can help build confidence and maintain independence longer.

This type of intervention puts demands on people with dementia and can create frustration that leads to disruptive behavior. Staff members who ask a resident to do something must first determine whether the person can do it successfully, to prevent a negative response. Operators must attempt to create a failure-free environment. Residential settings foster independence as an outcome and make coping with the disease more manageable for residents.

DEMENTIA CARE IN A SKILLED NURSING FACILITY. In skilled nursing facilities, dementia care is provided predominantly to residents with behavior challenges that cannot be managed at home or in assisted living or those whose financial resources have become exhausted. Some nursing homes attempt to place residents with dementia in special sections or on separate floors and have activities designed specifically for them. But as these facilities reorient themselves toward providing more acute care and rehabilitation services, separation is not always possible.

Most skilled nursing facilities focus on providing high levels of care rather than specialized dementia care. State regulations require skilled nursing facilities, unlike assisted living communities, to offer specific recreational therapy for the residents, supervised by licensed activity professionals. Therefore, programming for residents in nursing homes can be more sophisticated than in some assisted living facilities.

Some continuing care retirement communities with a nursing component have special care units designed to accommodate residents who develop dementia and can no longer live safely in their apartments. These units are generally shared with residents from the community who need higher levels of care as a result of other conditions.

SPECIALIZED PROGRAMS FOR DEMENTIA CARE ENVIRONMENTS

Operators who specialize in dementia care can create an integrated approach, recognizing that body and mind—physical and emotional health—are interrelated. Treatment for dementia employs nutrition, environment, activities, communication, and programs to maximize the use of the cognitive capabilities that remain intact while compensating for those that decline.[15] Specialized programs, such as nutritional support and evaluation, treatment for critical issues such as depression, failure-free activity programming, and aromatherapy, can be created to cater to the specific needs of this population.

Nutritional Support

Anorexia is an overall decline in appetite leading to decreased food intake and inadequate consumption of calories. It is the major cause of weight loss and poor nutritional status in elderly people.[16] Malnutrition and dehydration are associated with susceptibility to infections, cognitive impairment, poor skin and bone integrity, pressure sores, and hip fractures. These serious consequences, along with comorbidities from chronic illness, often lead to mortality.[17] A protocol to screen and assess elderly residents for nutritional risk is essential to forestall the serious health effects of malnutrition.

Researchers followed the weight loss trends of 1,000 nursing home residents across the United States. They found many elderly residents to be undernourished. During a six-month period, 30 percent of the residents who continued to lose weight died. The study also found that 16 to 18 percent of elderly

people living in communities consume fewer than 1,000 calories per day.[18]

In 1997, the Collaborative Studies of Long Term Care initiated a series of multiple-state projects that studied almost 5,000 residents in more than 350 retirement and assisted living communities. Their findings, published in a special issue of the *Gerontologist*, showed that low food intake was common in 54 percent of the participants and low fluid intake was prevalent among 51 percent of those studied in long-term care, particularly those with cognitive impairment.[19] They also found that residents who are closely monitored by staff during meals are significantly less likely to have low food and fluid intake. Similarly, residents who eat in a central dining area are much less likely to have low intake than those eating in their bedrooms. Often in large facilities mealtimes are set, and residents have limited time to consume their food. Staff members may mistakenly assume that a slow eater is not hungry and remove the uneaten food before the resident can finish.

Many signs of weight loss are visible. Pronounced indentations at the temporal lobes (commonly referred to as temporal wasting), loss of muscle mass, loose and elastic skin, and decreased functional ability are all early indicators. Causes of anorexia are numerous and can include swallowing difficulties, poor dentition, mouth pain, psychological disorders, depression, impaired mobility, and loss of appetite. Residents who lose 5 percent of their weight in one month, or 10 percent over 6 months, or those who eat less than 75 percent of their food at mealtimes should be considered for a complete nutritional evaluation by a registered dietitian.

Operators should routinely evaluate body weight at the time of admission and monthly thereafter. Use of the body mass index (BMI) can help establish a baseline.[20] Residents who are determined to be at high risk for weight loss can be identified in their charts and with silicon bracelets. A registered dietitian should develop individualized food plans for them. Angela G. Sullivan, a consultant dietitian who specializes in dementia care nutrition, claims, "The specific nutritional recommendations we make are *in addition* to a liberalized menu, offering favorite foods, and routine mealtime practices.... The strategies and protocols for the resident at risk address prevention of continued weight loss and dehydration." The goal is to optimize food and fluid intake at each opportunity.[21] "Simply adding supplements is not enough to prevent weight loss," Sullivan warns. Recommendations might include adjusting food texture for residents who have difficulty swallowing. Cutting up food rather than pureeing it, and adding sauces and gravy or fruit smoothies can offer additional hydration while making caloric intake easier to manage. "Allowing residents additional time to complete their meal, offering assistance with feeding, using words of encouragement in addition to nutritional supplements and calorie-dense snacks are protocols that can really make a difference."

Once individuals at risk for weight loss have been identified, individual nutritional protocols can be established, with recommendations documented in a format accessible to the staff in the meal-preparation areas. All employees should be trained in the implementation of the protocols for these residents. Each at-risk resident should be weighed weekly and monitored for intake. After 60 days, 90 percent of the at-risk residents should respond to the nutritional intervention, either maintaining their weight or gaining weight. After implementing this program in one community, employees and families found the residents to have more energy, less depression, and higher participation in community socialization.

Clearly, identifying and treating elderly people at risk for weight loss can be beneficial, even preventing nutritionally triggered catastrophic health failures. By recognizing at-risk residents early, operators can improve the overall quality of life of their residents and help reduce the level of care needed in their communities.

Managing Depression, Delirium, and Dementia

In a study by Baldini-Gruber and colleagues, researchers found that symptoms of depression were more than twice as common among assisted living residents with mild or moderate dementia than among those without dementia. Depressed residents often do not have positive outcomes and are at greater risk of discharge to nursing homes or death. Chronic depression can lead to declining appetite, weight loss, lethargy, and a host of premature health complications. The study documents the high prevalence of depressive symptoms among those with dementia, as

well as problems with diagnosis. About 54 percent of the depressed and 33 percent of the nondepressed participants were taking antidepressant medication.[22] Many of the participants were depressed but had received no formal mental health treatment. Depression was more common among participants with severe dementia, behavioral symptoms, and pain. The study also found that more than half of the depressed participants were not identified as such by the staff.

These results indicate a strong need to properly assess residents for depression, seeking interventions for those whose depression has not been diagnosed and corrective actions for those being treated unnecessarily or inappropriately. Identifying these at-risk residents and advising attending physicians and family members may help operators avert unnecessary mental health–triggered discharges and improve the quality of life for each individual.

The Cornell Scale for Depression in Dementia (CSDD) is a tool for diagnosing depression in elderly populations with dementia.[23] This simple 19-question tool offers physicians a nationally recognized diagnostic means of evaluating and prescribing for their patients, rather than relying on sporadic and subjective observations from caregivers and family members. See also chapter 17 for details on this and other assessments.

Using the CSDD, operators can create a team of nurse's aides, licensed practical nurses (LPNs), and registered nurses (RNs) familiar with the residents. The team should review their impressions of each resident to identify characteristics of depression in each of the 19 symptom areas. This information can then be tallied and charted to evaluate potential risk. The dose, frequency, and indication information for medication is also collected to help evaluate the adequacy of any treatments currently in place. The resident's physician or a consultant psychologist or neuropsychologist reviews this information and evaluates the treatment options, including a multidisciplinary review if appropriate.

The Baldini-Gruber study found that depression was the quality-of-life domain with the lowest perceived treatment success.[24] Perhaps the main reason is that a high percentage of dementia care residents have depression that is not diagnosed or appropriately treated. The survey results facilitate development of a treatment protocol for each resident now properly diagnosed, and the staff can be trained to recognize and deal effectively with the symptoms of depression. Further, involvement from mental health professionals can contribute significantly to residents' wellness. These interventions are simple and can significantly enhance residents' overall quality of life and well-being.

Delirium is defined as a disturbance in consciousness or change in cognition with a relatively sudden onset (hours or days). Delirium is often confused with dementia and depression. Table 19.1 differentiates these conditions, which are both common in elderly people. Delirium should be treated as a medical emergency because it has a 65 percent mortality rate. It is associated with poor outcomes, such as prolonged hospitalization, functional decline, and increased use of chemical and physical restraints, and it increases the risk of admission to a nursing home. Individuals at high risk for delirium should be assessed daily using a standardized tool to facilitate prompt identification and management. Risk factors for delirium include age, prior cognitive impairment, presence of infection, severe illness or multiple comorbidities, dehydration, use of psychotropic medication, alcoholism, impaired vision, and fractures. The Confusion Assessment Method (CAM) includes two parts: part 1 is an instrument that screens for overall cognitive impairment, and part 2 includes only the four features that most accurately distinguish delirium or reversible confusion from other types of cognitive impairment.[25]

Failure-Free Enrichment Programs

Therapeutic, multifaceted, interdisciplinary approaches to activities and social and leisure programming for dementia patients must be goal-oriented. The goal is to provide specialized stimulation to create structure and support in meeting each resident's physical, psychosocial, cognitive, and spiritual needs. All components of the program should be designed according to each resident's abilities in order to provide failure-free stimulation. Programming should focus on the resident's wellness and needs, rather than the losses that the disease causes.

Residents should be assessed on admission and periodically thereafter, combining a personal history with leisure interests and an activity interest inventory. These interests are then considered along with cognitive status to develop a leisure interest and social stimulation plan for each resident. Programs are specifically designed to promote communication, which helps to maintain social skills while improving self-esteem and dignity. Because many residents face serious difficulty in initiating and maintaining interest in daily activities, the staff need to provide structure and stimulation.

Aromatherapy

Fragrance consists of volatile molecules that float in the air. Millions of olfactory receptor cells line the human nose, and aroma causes these nerves to fire and send messages to the limbic area of the brain. From there, the messages travel to other parts of the

Table 19.1   Differentiating Dementia, Depression, and Delirium in Elderly People

Characteristic	Dementia	Depression	Delirium
Onset	Chronic, gradual	Often abrupt	Acute, subacute
Evolution	Months to years	Weeks to months	Hours to days
Awareness	Clear	Clear	Reduced
Alertness	Generally normal	Normal	Fluctuates
Attention	Generally normal	Minimal impairment	Impaired, fluctuates
Orientation	May be impaired	Some disorientation	Impaired, fluctuates
Memory	Recent, remote impaired	Selective impairment	Recent, immediate impaired
Mood	Labile	Consistent	Fluctuating
Progression	Ongoing	Resolves with treatment	Resolves with treatment
Answers	Response incorrect	"Don't know"	May be incoherent
Mini mental state examination	Stable, downward trend	Fluctuates	Severe fluctuations

Source: Adapted from M. Forman, K. Fletcher, L. Mion, and L. Trygstad, "Assessing Cognitive Function," in *Geriatric Nursing Protocols for Best Practice*, 2nd ed., ed. M. Mezey, T. Fulmer, I. Abraham, and D. Zwicker (New York: Springer, 2003), 102–3.

brain, activating thought and memory. The pituitary gland is also stimulated to release chemicals that travel via the blood to glands and organs that react. This means that a scent has the potential to activate a number of physical and emotional responses.

Aromatherapy is the use of essential oils to benefit physical, spiritual, and psychological well-being. Essential oils are stored in minute quantities in special cells, ducts, or glandular hairs in the roots, leaves, bark, stems, and flowers of a plant. They are complex molecules that may trigger a number of responses in the human body. They have been used for centuries to promote health and relaxation and to guard against bacteria, molds, fungi, and other microorganisms. Essential oils can be diffused in the air, applied to the skin, and even used as dietary supplements.

Ample research has demonstrated the human response to essential oils.[26] Some oils, such as peppermint, rosemary, jasmine, lemongrass, and grapefruit, stimulate and have an uplifting effect. Others, such as lavender, rose, geranium, sandalwood, and ylang-ylang, have a relaxing or sedating effect. All of these may have applications in the care of residents with dementia, to stimulate appetites and energy levels, to relieve anxiety, and to promote sleep.

Other oils can be used to boost self-esteem and create a grounding effect for tearful residents. A blend of spruce, rosewood, and frankincense has been used to restore confidence and well-being. Another blend, using cloves, rosemary, lemon, and cinnamon oils, was tested at Weber State University in Ogden, Utah, and was found to have a 99.96 percent effective rate against airborne bacteria.[27] Diffusing these oils can be effective during the cold and flu season. Many hospitals in Europe routinely diffuse essential oils to purify the air.

In summary, providing high-quality dementia care in a cost-effective way in smaller settings is challenging but achievable. Success in this area requires specialized knowledge and a commitment among the management and staff to providing a comfortable, safe, and supportive environment for residents, as well as appropriate medical supervision and monitoring. As the number of seniors with dementia increases in the years ahead, this form of specialized care will be in high demand.

NOTES

1. R. N. Butler, *Why Survive? Being Old in America* (New York: Harper & Row, 1975).

2. P. Davies, "Alzheimer's Disease and Related Disorders: An Overview," in *Understanding Alzheimer's Disease: What It Is; How to Cope with It; Future Directions*, ed. M. K. Aronson (New York: Scribner's, 1988), 3–14.

3. National Institutes of Health, National Institute on Aging, *Progress Report on Alzheimer's Disease* (Bethesda, MD, 1995).

4. Alzheimer's Association, "Medical Tests for Diagnosing Alzheimer's," https://www.alz.org/alzheimers-dementia/diagnosis/medical_tests.

5. Alzheimer's Association, "Types of Dementia," https://www.alz.org/alzheimers-dementia/what-is-dementia/types-of-dementia.

6. A. Raia, *Common Problems in Early Alzheimer's Disease* (Cambridge, MA: Alzheimer's Disease and Related Disorders Association, 1995), 1–5.

7. H. A. Crystal, "The Diagnosis of Alzheimer's Disease and Other Dementing Disorders," in Aronson, *Understanding Alzheimer's Disease*, 15–33.

8. The Alzheimer's Association can be reached at 800-272-3900, https://www.alz.org. The Alzheimer's Disease Education and Referral Center, part of the National Institute on Aging, provides excellent resource materials; call 800-438-4380 or visit https://www.nia.nih.gov/health/about-adear-center.

9. National Library of Medicine, "2021 Alzheimer's Disease Facts and Figures," https://pubmed.ncbi.nlm.nih.gov/33756057/.

10. National Family Caregivers Association, *Random Sample Survey of Family Caregivers* (Kensington, MD, 2000); C. Levine, *Rough Crossings: Family Caregivers' Odysseys through the Health Care System* (New York: United Hospital Fund, 1998).

11. R. Schulz and S. R. Beach, "Caregiving as a Risk Factor for Mortality: The Caregiver Health Effects Study," *Journal of the American Medical Association* 282, no. 23 (December 15, 1999): 2215–19.

12. *National Ombudsman Reporting System Data Tables* (Washington, DC: US Administration on Aging, 2003).

13. C. Samuels, "Assisted Living Statistics: Population & Facilities in 2022," A Place for Mom, last updated April 21, 2022, https://www.aplaceformom.com/caregiver-resources/articles/assisted-living-statistics.

14. J. C. Rogers and M. B. Holm, "Activities of Daily Living Intervention," *Alzheimer's Care Quarterly* 2, no. 4 (2001): 66–69.

15. J. Zeisel and P. Raia, "Nonpharmacological Treatment for Alzheimer's Disease: A Mind-Brain Approach," *American Journal of Alzheimer's Disease* 15, no. 6 (2000): 331–40.

16. D. R. Thomas and J. E. Morley, "Regulation of Appetite in Older Adults," *Clinical Strategies in LTC: A Supplement to Annals of Long-Term Care* (July 2002): 4.

17. D. R. Thomas, "Progress Notes: Nutrition and Chronic Wounds," *Supplement to Annals of Long-Term Care* (November 2004): 1–12.

18. P. S. Reed et al., "Characteristics Associated with Low Food Intake in Long-Term Care Residents with Dementia," *Gerontologist* 45 (October 2005): 74–80.

19. Reed et al., "Characteristics Associated with Low Food Intake."

20. BMI is calculated using a mathematical formula that takes into account both height and weight: a person's weight in kilograms is divided by height in meters squared ($BMI = kg/m^2$). A BMI of 18.5 or lower is considered underweight; 18.5–24.9 is normal; 25–29.9 is overweight; and greater than 30 is considered obese. K. L. Mahan and S. Escott-Stump, *Food Nutrition and Diet Therapy*, 9th ed. (Philadelphia: Saunders, 1996), appendix 18, 950–51.

21. "Liberalization of the Diet Prescription Improves Quality of Life for Older Adults in Long-Term Care," *Journal of the American Dietetic Association* 105, no. 12 (December 2005): 1955–65.

22. A. Baldini-Gruber et al., "Characteristics Associated with Depression in Long-Term Care Residents with Dementia," *Gerontologist* 45 (October 2005): 50–55.

23. G. S. Alexopoulos, R. C. Abrams, R. C. Young, and C. A. Shamoian, "Cornell Scale for Depression in Dementia," *Biological Psychiatry* 23 (1988): 271–84.

24. Baldini-Gruber et al., "Characteristics Associated with Depression."

25. CAM instrument and algorithm adapted from S. Inouye et al., "Clarifying Confusion: the Confusion Assessment Method," *Annals of Internal Medicine* 113, no. 12 (1990): 941–48.

26. *Essentials Oils Desk Reference*, 3rd ed. (Orem, UT: Essential Science Publishing, 2004), 6–13.

27. *Essentials Oils Desk Reference*, 6–13.

20

Architectural Design Considerations

This chapter details design features and suggestions from an operator's perspective. The author has been directly involved in the development, from scratch, of over 50 new independent, assisted living, and memory care communities. Post-opening site visits were conducted with community staff to determine specific strengths and weaknesses in the design. Those responses combined with the author's 40 years of operating experience across 37 states were incorporated into this chapter to assemble the best practices in design and construction of new senior living communities from an operator's perspective.

KEY PLANNING AND DESIGN PRINCIPLES

A predictor of the success of assisted senior living communities has been the degree to which they have been able to embody a residential environment while still providing supportive services. By involving experienced operators in the design of a new project, architects will create a more user-friendly environment. Design teams who incorporate operational input during planning stages will provide a more efficient floor plan that will operate at a lower cost once the facility is occupied.

Design the Building to Be a Luxury Residential Setting

The layout of spaces is an important ingredient in designing a building to be a residential setting.

When one walks into a residential setting, one typically sees residential spaces off the entry foyer, not a reception station with glass looking into an office space. The selection of artwork and appointments for finishes should be as residential as possible. Common examples include the elimination of fluorescent lighting, the absence of institutional reception desks, and the design of public toilet rooms resembling powder rooms. Most important, a residential environment can be achieved with a commitment at the outset not to include anything that would not be found in one's own home.

Design the Facility for a Frail Elderly Population

Consider the walking distances from the farthest apartment to the common areas. Maximizing indoor spaces that relate to the outdoor spaces will make the outdoors seem more accessible. Layouts that allow residents to preview activities taking place in a room without having to enter that room are popular. A host of considerations in the configuration of apartments are appropriate for a frail elderly population, most notably in the layout and design of bathrooms. (See resident rooms design specifications below.)

Customize the Project to the Local Market

The local sponsors of a project should be able to provide some ideas on interior and exterior design that reflect the history, traditions, and preferences of the community. The architecture should incorporate spaces that are unique to the area. The selection of local artwork and accessories will reinforce the feeling of familiarity and local sensitivity. Most public libraries have period photographs of the township during the residents' younger days. These photos can often be professionally printed and attractively framed to hang in the facility's library or lounge.

Remember What Consumers Are Buying

While it is important to design a building that offers a long-term competitive advantage, remember that fundamentally what consumers are buying is a solution to a problem or challenges they may face in the future, and provide access to those services on-site. Senior living providers who develop care continuums that link to these physician and hospital payers and referral sources through IT connections and on-site medical clinics will be drawing patients from both ends of the continuum. By adding more medically oriented assisted living and on-site clinics to a resort campus, the campus is providing residents a rental aging-in-place alternative that enables them to potentially utilize their Medicare benefits.

BUILDING LAYOUT
Exteriors

- The porte-cochère at the entry must have adequate clearance to accommodate a rescue van, fire trucks, and ambulance with a normal maximum height of 12 feet (recommend to build to 14 feet clearance).

- Walking paths should be paved, concrete, or compacted stone dust. They should be a minimum of 6 feet wide to accommodate golf carts and maintenance carts and be able to pass someone walking without leaving the path.

- Minimize the planted areas that require weeding. Because mowing is easier than weeding, lawn area is easier to maintain. These areas may require an irrigation system.

- Consider including benches and raised-bed garden areas as many residents love to garden. The addition of a perennial herb garden can provide fresh materials for use in aromatherapy with the residents. The addition of a cutting garden can offer opportunities for residents to harvest fresh flowers to decorate the building interior areas all summer.

- Social distancing in patio areas can create even more space and functionality. Converting a patio area into extra dining is a great way to take advantage of outdoor space and natural air circulation. Adding outdoor kitchens, including a grill, a cooler and mobile bar, a warming cart, and a buffet can offer a unique dining experience and reduce the number of trips to the kitchen for staff.

- Water ponding can occur at the foundation of a building due to the manner in which it was graded. The roof line and gutters should be designed to channel water into proper drainage. This is a particular concern in areas where ice can accumulate on eaves and build up at exit doors. Pressure-treated plywood for the bottom run of underlayment can help avoid rot from splash up while providing a protective barrier against insect infestation.

- Emphasize adequate parking, recognizing the unique problems presented by the site limitations. According to a parking study conducted by the American Seniors Housing Association (ASHA), the total traffic volume for senior housing is 1.72 trips per unit, compared to 9.57 trips per unit for single-family detached housing and 4.20 trips per unit for a high-rise apartment. Visitors represent 29 percent of total traffic, service vehicles 15 percent, and employees 56 percent. Based upon their traffic data, assisted living residences require 0.22 parking spaces per unit. Also consider additional parking for any outpatient therapy and holistic medicine components that may be offered.

- Hallways between buildings with natural lighting, nature sounds, and music can be used to communicate your brand and showcase artwork while offering a sheltered connection.

Interiors

- There should be one main entrance to the building where all traffic is funneled past a grand lobby and concierge reception. Avoid repetition in the layout, which can be disorienting. Provide landmarks in the building circulation to serve as cues for location or orientation. Some facilities have even developed themes for resident areas in the building and have used interior design features to accentuate these neighborhoods, such as pictures of fish or flowers or hearts. Painting or wallpapering feature walls at each corridor or elevator lobby can help residents easily identify their neighborhood in the building.

■ Locate elevators near an exterior door to promote more efficient move-in or move-out of residents' belongings. Avoid a design that requires moving in or out through the main lobby. This also applies to the removal of trash from the resident floors. At least one elevator car must be large enough (at least 6 feet) to accommodate a gurney and two EMTs for emergency transport and located so that any sick or deceased residents do not need to be transported through the main lobby. Minimize travel distances to elevators and include seating in all elevator lobbies on each floor. For the most efficient movement of residents at mealtimes, locate elevators adjacent to the main dining room. Residents often transport food and beverages with their walker. Upon entering or leaving the elevator car, the walker wheels will bounce when going over the tracks, causing their beverages and food to spill. To avoid damage, avoid carpet on elevator floors and design a ceramic tile walk off outside the elevator door where possible in each elevator lobby.

■ High-end sound systems throughout the building can be used to communicate warmth, add to festive occasions, and even manage behaviorally challenged residents using delta tones. Delta tones are a brain-calming binaural audio component embedded within music.

■ For uncarpeted areas with high traffic or spill potential, such as physical therapy, exercise, activities, or crafts rooms, consider using high quality luxury vinyl tile (LVT).

■ Position the kitchen and dining areas on the same side of the core area so that food carts will not need to be transported through the foyer. Food carts typically pick up grease from the kitchen floor, and their wheels will soil common area carpeting.

■ Handrails that can be built to look like chair rails can give an upscale appearance in the hallways while at the same time providing a needed safety feature. These can be purchased with an antimicrobial agent imbedded.

COMMON AREAS
Reception and Concierge

■ This area needs designated spaces for any package deliveries and/or pickups, guests' coats, and other storage; avoid cluttering this area. Closets are helpful for visitors, residents, wheelchair storage, and UPS packages. Security monitors and remote door openers can be helpful equipment.

■ Incorporate a separate circuit for the Ecall system computer to avoid interference from the other equipment that can produce false alarms. Consider Ecall systems with pendants.

■ At the entry, consider recessing the ceiling and installing acoustical tile to dampen noise in this busy area. The concierge should focus their attention on residents and family. Have limited seating at the entrance; avoid decorating with sofas and overstuffed chairs, as residents tend to congregate here and may fall asleep. This would leave an undesirable impression for guests and marketing prospects. Consider the placement of a circular table for a large floral display. Front lobbies that feature a water feature or fountain as well as streamed music that can be controlled by the receptionist make a nice first impression to visitors and guests. Also consider a sanitation station with an infrared thermometer, temperature log, and hands-free sanitizer.

■ Lighting technology provides opportunities to control the intensity, distribution, and spectrum of light in health care. Tunable white LED luminaires, rather than fluorescent systems, can save energy up to 68 percent based upon the LED's reduced power and automatic dimming features.[1] Studies have also shown a direct correlation between color technology and mood and behaviors in the elderly. Research has shown marked improvements in depression, mood stabilization, and even healing with the effects of correlated color temperature on older adults.[2] (See also WELL v2, below.)

Executive Director Office

This office should be large enough for a desk and separate seating area with coffee table for family and staff meetings, approximately 175 to 200 square feet. It may also have a separate small conference room with a four-top round table that can be shared with the business office or human resources, used as work space for assembling mailings and handouts, and so on.

Work Room

Located adjacent to the business office, the work room should include practical countertops for assembling projects, with locking cabinets for storing paper, marketing collateral, and office supplies. This room can be equipped with a fax line, and internet ports in order to utilize the main copy machine as a central printer. This is also a good place to install the electronic time clock so that it can be supervised by the office manager. It is a good idea to install a four-socket GFI outlet near the desk.

Business Office

This office can be similar in size to the executive director's office but should feature a separate lockable file room to secure business office files. This office also needs a fax line and internet in case you use banking auto deposit or electronic time machines. There should be a separate key for this office.

Set up a phone system equipped for 12 lines, wired for 16, and with a capacity of 24 (modem/fax lines included). At least 4 lines should be equipped with power-fail bypass trunks (for the fire alarm system). The single-line phones are largely placed in the public areas and therefore should offer simple access to internal and external calling. Voice message capability is desirable. Incorporate a separate circuit for the emergency call system computer to avoid interference from other equipment which can produce false alarms. The emergency call system should incorporate a check-in feature. This system should also be capable of annunciation to a handheld unit.

Marketing Office

This office should also be similar in size to the executive director's office and feature a small seating area large enough for four people to sit around a round table. Some larger facilities also have a marketing coordinator (who could also be receptionist) with her own desk who handles inquiries and manages the computer database. Also set up a vacant fully decorated apartment with comfortable seating for a private post-tour-close room. A wall-mounted TV is useful for showing videos of resident events, activities, webinars, virtual tours, menus, and food displays.

Post Office/Mailboxes

This can either be a separate area or on a wall in the country kitchen. Eighty percent of all resident mail is junk, and since you do not want the residents taking this trash up to their room where it will just need to be dealt with by housekeeping later, provide a recycle bin where it can be easily discarded. Be sure to number the boxes such that the handicap room boxes are located along the bottom row of the panel where they can be accessed while seated. Pigeonholes for internal mail are very helpful for communicating special events and activity programs.

General Store

This is a very small store for the sale of convenience items and crafts to the residents and visitors; 75 to 100 square feet is sufficient. This should be lockable and feature glass display cabinets.

Private Dining

Family parties sometimes involve 20 people or more and often cannot be accommodated in the private dining room. These functions can be handled in a main dining room if it can be divided. This room can also double as a conference room. A retractable screen can be very useful for small training, marketing events, training presentations and webinars.

Provide a hutch for storage and a buffet server top with an four-socket outlet behind for a coffee warmer and IT equipment. This area is useful for small functions and meetings. This could be done as an extension of the main dining room rather than a separate room. The hutch should be large enough to accommodate a chafing dish and platters (see specifications for the bistro, below).

Main Dining Rooms

- The dining room design should minimize barriers to traffic flow in and out of the kitchen and allow easy access to all tables for wait staff. Incorporate 20 to 25 square feet per diner into the dining room space allocation for efficient traffic and access to the tables by residents with supportive devices. Incorporating a beverage station in a servers' alcove outside the kitchen will facilitate more rapid service and less congestion with food prep and plating.
- To promote privacy and social distancing, consider the addition of decorative room dividers. These can be mobile full-height panels that separate tables or even tabletop acrylic clear dividers that provide protection for residents sharing a table.
- Specify wood laminate tables so that placemats can be used for breakfast and lunch if desired;

they should also feature a different color laminate edge for visual cuing. This can save considerably on linen costs. Cloth placemats can be laundered in the community machines and look very nice. Dining room tables should be square with a square edge so that they can be ganged (laid end to end). This way they can be used to seat larger groups or be covered, skirted, and used as banquet tables. Many residents will prefer a table for two (30×36 inches) especially when they first move in and have not established dining companions. The other tables should either seat four (42×42, 36×36, or 30×42 inches) or be convertible from square to round to accommodate additional diners. Round tables should be large enough for six diners (54 inches in diameter). In addition, it is useful to have several 29-inch high tables that can be raised to 31 inches to accommodate wheelchairs. Also order several banquet tables and half- or quarter-rounds to be used for parties and events. Specify metal bases for all tables to avoid damage from wheelchairs.

- Silvertex fabrics, which are treated with silver ion technology to provide a germaphobic defense, can help safeguard against odor and bacteria. Chair fabric should be treated for moisture resistance. Faux-wood metal is a very durable material for tables and chairs that can easily be cleaned with strong disinfectants without damaging the finish. Seamless thermo-laminate countertops assembled from one piece are preferred to prevent bacteria from collecting in cracks.

- Dining room chairs should all have cross-braced construction. They can feature casters on the legs to enable residents to seat themselves and scoot their chair toward the table, while still remaining relatively stable. Most chairs should have arms, but include some armless chairs for larger residents. They should feature open sides rather than closed arms that create pockets where food particles can collect.

- The dining room needs to be large enough to accommodate at least 75 percent of the residents plus 10 percent allowance for guests, unless you want to do two seatings. There should be a minimum of two feet of aisle space between the backs of two chairs plus 18 inches of table space for each chair. There should be a parking area for wheelchairs and walkers.

- Consider installing a see-through gas fireplace or bubble aquarium in the middle of the dining room to break it up and add ambiance. The dining room should be organized into separate seating areas. Consider a separate space for a yogurt bar at breakfast and lunch, as these are very popular and inexpensive to deliver.

- Consider adding a busing station with silver/glassware storage in the dining room. There should be outlets to accommodate coffee warmers and soup kettles if desired. It should be plumbed for a water line for the coffee maker with a shutoff valve for easy servicing.

- There should be cabinet room dividers which can store additional china, silver, linen, and glassware so residents' requests can be immediately handled and the dining room reset quickly. This also helps break up the room for more intimate dining experiences.

- Do not run carpeting to the kitchen access doors as staff will pick up grease from the kitchen floor and walk it off onto the carpet, causing it to look constantly dirty. Instead install a tile or vinyl walk-off outside each swinging door. Always put interior locks on these doors to prevent access to the kitchen after hours.

- Consider adding a PA system to these areas so that the residents can easily be communicated with during meals.

Bistro-Style Restaurant or Country Kitchen

A separate restaurant apart from the main building with an enclosed walkway can really give the appearance of going out to dinner (if there is sufficient land). Creating adaptable spaces with flexible design features will enable the community to respond with greater flexibility. Adaptable spaces allow resident socialization while being able to easily separate or convert spaces in a crisis. Intentionally designing amenity spaces that can be converted to additional dining spaces can help adapt to unforeseen situations. This area is great as a waiting area and gathering area for residents and staff. Be sure to keep walking distances from the farthest apartment to the restaurants under 250 feet.

It would be desirable to have a counter so that cooking demonstrations and Iron Chef–style competitions could be held.

Common area open kitchens are highly versatile. Grab-and-go items (salads and sandwiches) can be offered here. It can be also used for baking and cooking by residents and staff. Consider a large kitchen table that seats eight with a hanging fixture for good reading light. With a bistro design, a long bar across the front with seating can double as the main service station for parties. The countertops need to be large enough to accommodate a standard eight-quart chafing dish (24½ × 13½ × 9½ inches) for snacks and small parties. The front dimension of the bistro area should be long enough to accommodate one 60-inch half-round and one 8-foot by 24-inch rectangular banquet table (about 15 feet total). These are very useful for a quick set up for marketing events or holiday function parties. If the country kitchen is large enough, it can be set up each morning for continental breakfast, then the restaurant can be used for lunch and dinner. Extra covered meals, sandwich platters, and desserts can be stored in the refrigerator for residents who may have missed a meal.

Consider adding a reach-in refrigerator in the country kitchen for sodas, milk, juice, and other perishables that can be purchased by the residents. Also consider an ice cream freezer to hold supplies for ice cream socials.

Kitchen (Commercial)

A well-designed kitchen will require a minimum of 1,800 square feet for an efficient operation. This space needs to be professionally designed by a kitchen designer. Below are some operational recommendations.

- Incorporate two doors—in and out of the kitchen— for the best flow of service personnel. This kitchen should ideally be positioned so that it can service both both independent living and assisted living or memory care dining rooms. Walk-off mats at kitchen exits can save wear and tear on dining room carpets. Wait staff will pick up anything spilled on the kitchen floor with their shoes and walk it into the dining room.
- Windows in the kitchen are helpful for ventilation and promote a more enjoyable work environment. Dry storage areas should be lockable and an area needs to be reserved for clean dishes, party supplies, banquet tables and skirting, and linen storage. Fiber-reinforced plastic or Plexiglas wall protection behind the dishwashing area and stainless

steel behind the cooking line can increase wall life and promote better sanitation.

- The minimum kitchen cooking line equipment suggested for a dish-up-to-order operation should include the following: tilt-skillet, double convection oven, convection steamer or slow cooker, six-burner range, charbroiler grill, and a deep-fryer (optional). A steam-jacketed kettle is also a nice feature. Consider a salamander for finish work or to char up-charged items such as filet mignons and tiger prawns.
- Large kitchens will require separate walk-in refrigeration and freezer capacity. The walk-in refrigerator must have a ramp or level entrance and space to accommodate both three-tier standard wall-hung shelving as well as at least two rolling rack carts. It will also require a reach-in cooler on the cooking line and a stand-up server reach-in for condiments, salads, desserts and specialty drinks and wine.
- The kitchen serving line should feature a six-well steam table, a sandwich unit, a cooks' reach-in refrigerator, and an overhead warmer. It should have a separate storage area for warming plates (do not hard-wire the plate warmer so it can be used for banquets) and shelving on the server side. This counter also needs a four-socket outlet for the blender, belt toaster, Robot Coupe, and other powered devices.
- Nonslip tile in the kitchen should have dark grout to promote a consistent appearance over time.
- There should be a large prep table either behind or adjacent to the cooking line and on the opposite side of the kitchen from the dishwashing area. The prep area needs to be convenient to the walk-in and dry goods storage areas. Consider a towel warmer for scented hot towels, which communicates a first-class service style.
- As an option, consider wiring the kitchen for sound so staff could drop in their iPods to have their own music instead of the elevator music the residents listen to. Consider the addition of an outdoor cart/wheelchair washing station for pressure-washing equipment and sanitizing residents' durable medical equipment (DME). This can feature an outdoor outlet (for electric pressure-washer), faucet, and floor drains. This can easily be added to the loading dock.

Beauty/Barber Shop

Normally two chairs and drop sinks for hair washing are minimum, with a separate chair for a hair dryer. A mirrored wall above the sinks allows residents to view the progress of their hair styling. Be sure to add waterproof backing below sinks to protect the wall. Several side chairs are nice for residents to congregate in this area and a single-cup K-Cup coffee maker is useful. It is vital to install upgraded ventilation in this room, and it should feature a glass front window that can be decorated like a commercial salon. There should be a separate beauty shop for independent living and assisted living areas if possible.

Activities Room

Be sure to provide adequate seating and storage in this area. This room requires upgraded lighting. Cabinetry should be lockable for storage of supplies. A countertop with a sink is helpful. Washable, non-slip tile or luxury vinyl tile flooring is best for this room. The closets in the activity room should have floor-to-ceiling shelving with some open space for the storage of seasonal decorations.

Lighted glass display cases are useful for displaying residents' handiwork or personal collections and provide evidence of an active lifestyle for marketing to showcase. Through-wall cases facing the hallway are very effective and can help bring light into corridors, which is a great marketing feature.

Library

This room should feature floor-to-ceiling bookshelves in a dark wood color such as cherry and be furnished with comfortable chairs. Upgraded ceiling lighting should be provided to allow adequate lighting for reading. There should be a square table with flip-up wings to convert it from four-person to six-person in case a card game breaks out.

Also install two workstations where permanent iPads or other tablets can be mounted with iBooks and Kindle installed. These units can be adjusted to feature extremely large print for the visually impaired. Studies have found that e-readers can improve reading speed from an average of 120 words per minutes to 140 simply due to the availability of larger fonts and sharper contrast of the words against the page.

Wi-Fi access will be needed here. Consider adding a pool table area in the library as a dual use for the room, which is a nice selling feature. You can also join in partnership with the Library of Congress or establish an account with Audible (audible.com) to have audiobooks available.

Living Room TV and Card Room

A separate area with sofas and recliners should be provided for residents to sit and socialize and watch TV. Often one spouse likes to watch TV while the other plays cards or assembles puzzles, so a few four-top tables (which can flip up and convert for six persons) are a great idea adjacent to the TV area. The TV should be wall-mounted with an internet connection available as well as Apple TV or similar. Install four-socket outlets with GFI protection. This room can also include gaming consoles for the residents to play.

Piano Bar/Cocktail Lounge

Facilities that feature a bar/lounge area with a happy hour each night staffed by the dining room manager prior to dinner will attract a more active clientele. This can have a walk-up bar with stools and a couple of cocktail tables with stuffed chairs. This feature really shows well and is appealing to prospects who are used to a country club and do not wish to be placed in a "home."

This area should have lockable storage for alcoholic beverages and a mini-fridge for mixes. A player piano would be nice here and even a glass-enclosed gas fireplace. Preferably this room should have a view. It could be located adjacent to and pushed out into the pool area so it can serve a dual purpose. Generally, residents prefer to sit in chairs rather than on stools at the bar as they are more stable and easier to use for people with limited mobility. Avoid table lamps and low tables as they can be a tripping hazard for those with poor eyesight.

Theater/Conference Room

It's not necessary to have separate rooms for these two functions, so a combination of functions is recommended. The theater should accommodate about 30 percent of the assisted living population as that's about the most you will get on any one night. The room should be wired for internet and surround sound with a docking station for guest speakers who use a laptop. Morning stand-up meetings with department heads can happen here, so provide a space in front for them to stand.

Dimmable lighting should be provided through wall sconces and also directional ceiling lights for the front speaker. A standing popcorn machine cart can add to the character of this room. If possible, locate this room adjacent to the kitchen and main dining room. It could also be converted to be used as a community room that can be separated with air walls or French doors, which will provide flexibility to accommodate large functions. Wire this room for public address and a ceiling-hung LED projector with hidden remote control jack at the front stage. This room can also be designed to accommodate a golf simulator.

Internet Cafe/Resident Business Center

This is a must and should feature one computer for every 25 independent living residents. There should also be at least two printers, one of which could be a black/white copier.

A single serving coffee maker should also be available here with a fruit bowl or snacks and an adjacent bathroom. It would also be ideal to have two iPads or tablets permanently mounted here as well, one of which is wirelessly connected to a music source for this room alone. This room should feature eclectic design found in internet cafes in Europe. Be sure to include four-socket GFI outlets and a charging station all electronic devices. This area can also be utilized by a travel agency for booking trips.

Great Room

The great room (not the same as the great lobby) can be used for parties, outside entertainers, guest speakers, training, art exhibits, fundraisers, intergenerational programs, marketing networking events, and conferences. This room should have excellent lighting, perhaps a small collapsible stage at one end, plenty of stacking chairs on a rolling caddy, and a half dozen banquet tables suitable for covering and skirting for formal events. This room needs to be large enough to gang-up at least six banquet tables. Wire this room for internet and public address. Some designs add an air wall of movable panels on a track to allow even more flexibility in this room. When not in use, the air wall panels fold neatly into a closet at one end. It's possible to make this in combination with the theater.

Public Washrooms

Public washrooms close to the dining room are essential—wall-hung, raised toilets are preferred. These washrooms can be unisex and should be strategically located outside the main dining areas and near the rehab area and beauty shop. It's a good idea to equip these washrooms with an emergency call feature on a pull cord that *reaches to the floor*. Install a wall-mounted mirror that is *tilted down* for wheelchair-bound residents. Color-coding of doors with similar functions helps to identify service areas from public areas. Install all hands-free fixtures for infection control. All public bathrooms must be wheelchair accessible.

■■■■ INDEPENDENT LIVING
Golf Simulator (in Theater)

Installing a golf simulator both creates value and communicates an active lifestyle. Golf simulators have a small footprint and their compact size allows for a beautiful custom install in any location. The simulator scape can also be groomed for multiuse, including a floor-to-ceiling movie theater with surround sound, or it can be used to project educational programs and community marketing presentations, like a virtual tour of future construction and campus development concepts and design.

Boutique

This area can be used as retail space to offer upscale clothing or even consignment. Basics should include a bathroom and back area storage, dressing room, high flood lighting, a platform front window, adjustable wall racks, sales counter with four-socket GFI outlets and charging station. Minimum of 375 square feet. This space could be leased out to an outside vendor.

Medical/Therapy Offices—Leased Spaces and Retail

This area could be created for home health, hospice, pharmacy, durable medical equipment, all unfinished with a 12-foot ceiling height. This space could be leased out to an outside vendor. The tenant can build this out within the owner's design restrictions. The use of telehealth will continue to grow in popularity well after the current pandemic, as payors like Medicare offer reimbursement to physicians and other health professionals to bill under these platforms. The community will require high-speed internet and private space for this function to prevent disclosure of protected health information.

Swimming and Aquatic Therapy Pool

Aquatic exercise is a low-impact activity that takes the pressure off bones, joints, and muscles. Water offers natural resistance that can help strengthen muscles. Aquatic exercise can have health benefits such as improved heart health, reduced stress, improved endurance, and strength. Aquatic therapy pools can be any size but need to have sufficient water depth (four to five feet) so that a person standing in chest-deep water will become buoyant. In conjunction with the community therapy services, deep water therapy can be offered. Deep water therapy normally depends on a flotation device attached to the user. This therapy is offered in depths in excess of six feet. An in-ground pool (covered with a sunshade sail) with a continuously sloping or tiered floor offering multiple water depth options is ideal. The pool can be equipped with a ramp or walk-in access, which can also accommodate wheelchairs for maximum flexibility. The pool could also feature a swim-up cocktail or nutritional smoothie bar.

The pool should have a water treatment system that offers redundancy. This can be accomplished with a chemical sanitizer, such as chlorine or bromine, and also with ozone gas, which is a powerful sanitizer and oxidizer of contaminants.

Social distancing in patio areas can create even more space and functionality. Converting a patio area into extra dining is a great way to take advantage of outdoor space and natural air circulation. Adding outdoor kitchens, including a grill, cooler and mobile bar, warming cart and buffet can offer a unique dining experience and reduce the number of trips to the kitchen for staff.

Day Spa

There will be some residents who will require water bath therapy, and it would be handy to have one area in the building suited for this therapy. The room should be large enough for a dressing area and bench with cubbies and hooks for clothing. A heat lamp in the ceiling would be helpful, and a small linen closet for clean and dirty towels. A heated rack for towels and a heated floor would be memorable for prospects touring. A toilet is a must and a bidet would be impressive and useful for residents with bowel inconti-

nence to sanitize them prior to their bath. Adjacent to this room, a 50-square foot room for massage therapy would be nice, wired for access to the internet to find sources of spa music, such as Pandora or Spotify.

ASSISTED LIVING
Exercise Room Convertible to Therapy Room (CORF)

A fully appointed rehab center will enable the facility to serve both inpatient and outpatient clients while utilizing their Medicare eligibility. Equipment requirements (provided by therapy company leasing this space):

- Step bike
- Mirrors on one wall with handrail for gait and balance exercises
- Two matte tables ($4' \times 5'$)
- Electrical stimulation (ESTIM) and ultrasound
- Hydrolator: Hot and cold packs
- Weights and rack, dual sides, hand and ankle weights
- Parallel bars for gait training
- Stair unit with three-step platform (or in multi-story building can use emergency stairwell)

The following services can be offered in this room:

- Physical therapy services are those services necessary for the diagnosis and treatment of impairments, functional limitations, disabilities, or changes in physical function and health status.
- Occupational therapy services are those services necessary for the diagnosis and treatment of impairments, functional disabilities, or changes in physical function and health status. Occupational therapy is medically prescribed treatment concerned with improving or restoring functions which have been impaired by illness or injury, or, where function has been permanently lost or reduced by illness or injury, to improve the individual's ability to perform those tasks required for independent functioning.
- Speech-language pathology services are those services necessary for the diagnosis and treatment of speech and language disorders that result in communication disabilities and for the diagnosis and treatment of swallowing disorders (dysphagia),

regardless of the presence of a communication disability.

- A pulmonary rehabilitation (PR) program is typically a physician-supervised, multidisciplinary program individually tailored and designed to optimize physical and social performance and autonomy of care for patients with chronic respiratory impairment. The main goal is to empower the individual's ability to exercise independently. Exercise is combined with other training and support mechanisms to encourage long-term adherence to the treatment plan.

- Cardiac rehabilitation (CR) services mean a physician-supervised program that furnishes physician-prescribed exercise, cardiac risk factor modification, including education, counseling, and behavioral intervention, psychosocial assessment, outcomes assessment, and other items/services.

The rehab area, if it is to be eligible to be licensed as a comprehensive outpatient rehabilitation facility (CORF), must have a handicap accessible toilet and hand sink, emergency lighting, and at least one door that will accommodate a wheelchair or stretcher. Separate the rehab area into a PT section and an OT section with a sink and stove/range top connections along with a small desk for charting. A wall-mounted TV/DVD combo would be helpful here for people using the room for fitness or to play instructional videos to train residents regarding the use of durable medical equipment (DME) equipment and stretching exercises. It is a simple matter to install the plumbing and electrical during construction which can later convert the exercise room to a therapy center (or vice versa) if needed under Medicare reform.

WELLNESS CENTER

This area will be staffed on a weekly basis where nurses and/or the medical director will be available for the residents to participate with health care visits. This area will serve as a resource center and be a private venue to answer any health-related questions.

This room should feature a small reception desk and a small seating area for a relaxed conversation. It should be located next to the exam room, which should have the physician's office on the opposite side.

This area could also be used as a hub for telehealth monitoring. Telehealth technologies can identify critical changes in key health indicators and dispatch health professionals to assess trouble as the very first signs arise. As with any health condition, the sooner the response, the better the outcomes. Telehealth will enable staff to accommodate residents' needs in their existing apartment as they age in place and alert caregivers whenever resident vitals signify a change in condition. This way residents can be accepted directly back from the hospital and receive all the services they will normally encounter in a rehab or LTC facility. This program can be charged separately to the residents and generate ancillary revenue. Telehealth can have a dramatic impact on resident turnover to higher levels of care by catching issues early and providing intervention before they become catastrophic.

EXAM ROOM AND OFFICE

This room should feature a hand sink and countertop with wall-hung cabinets, an exam table, and swivel chairs for the doctor with a side chair for a guest. A lockable mini-fridge should also be mounted in this room. A wall-hung blood pressure cuff and exam light would be useful. The exam room should be located in the middle between the wellness center and the physician's office and should have access doors to allow movement between all three rooms without exiting into the hallway. This room will also be used for rehab therapists, podiatrists, telemedicine, and other visiting professionals.

TV LOUNGE/WAITING AREA

A small TV lounge/waiting area would be useful on the health and fitness floor to provide a place to queue residents and outpatients. This should have a health care "theme" and be decorated like you might find in an upscale doctor's office. Wall murals of nature scenes are very popular and inexpensive. A brochure rack to organize and display collateral material of senior-related health topics here would help prevent this material from being scattered all around the furniture and looking like clutter.

ALL FLOORS
Housekeeping and Trash

A small closet would be useful to store housekeeping supplies and the housekeeping cart when not in use. Having one of these on each floor avoids the need for housekeepers to chase after supplies and PPE, lowering their productivity. These rooms must be lockable. It is preferred to have a trash chute on each floor for residents to dispose of refuse and recyclables. In independent living areas, they have a tendency to put their bagged trash outside their door, which leaks and stains the carpet.

Laundry Rooms

One laundry room on each floor enables residents and/or families to do their own personal laundry if they choose or allow their aides to do it at night. Incorporating a recessed drop-down ironing board (with outlet) is a nice addition and shows well during a tour. It is recommend that wiring be suitable for a stacking washer and dryer in each unit as these are a highly desirable marketing feature.

Public laundry rooms can be troublesome for the following reasons:

- They must be equipped with a heavy fire door with strong self-closer that many residents can't open.
- It's embarrassing for residents to launder clothing in a public area if they are incontinent.
- It's difficult for many frail residents to physically carry their laundry basket safely to these public areas and back to their unit.

Do not use vinyl coated tile (VCT) floor tile in any laundry room as the washers will have a tendency to "walk" during the spin cycle if unbalanced and damage the walls. Nonslip plank flooring works best in these areas.

BACK OF THE HOUSE
Staff Lounge

Employees need lockers in the lounge (enough for two-thirds of the employees per shift). The staff lounge should have a refrigerator, a sink with a small counter, a microwave, and room for one vending machine. A unisex bathroom will work, but separate bathrooms with changing areas are preferable. This is where staff can shed street clothes and change into PPE in the event of another pandemic. Consider a phone charging station for phones, walkie-talkies, and facility tablets. The staff lounge should be decorated with company mission statements and feature motivational artwork and a wall large enough to display OSHA and other required postings. (Wall letters can be purchased at https://www.craftcuts.com/wall-letters .html). This room should also be equipped with Wi-Fi and wiring for a time clock. The space should incorporate an area for a communication board.

Maintenance Office

Maintenance needs an area to store tools, supplies, parts, light bulbs, filters, and the like. Some metal shelving can accommodate this need. They also need a workbench with a vice for repairing equipment safely without straining their back. An air compressor with a hose reel is recommended. A small metal desk and file cabinet with upgraded lighting are helpful.

This area should be furthest from resident areas so as not to disturb them with tool noise. This room must be lockable. It would be handy for the maintenance director to have an internet connection at his desk so he can watch instructional videos or order parts from the work area rather than running to the internet café in his dirty clothes to use that computer. Consider several four-socket outlets for the recharging of battery-operated tools and walkie-talkies.

Central Laundry

Dirty laundry must be separated from clean to avoid cross-contamination. This can be accomplished with carts or separate rooms. Ideally, dirty laundry should come in through one set of doors and clean laundry exit through another in a semicircular setup—a separate sorting room or section for dirty on one side, and the drying and folding area for clean on the other. A wall-hung flushable sink can be installed in the dirty area for rinsing extremely soiled clothing prior to washing.

Floor covering is essential to prevent-cross contamination; rubberized tile floors are the easiest to clean and disinfect. Untreated concrete floors are the worst. In independent living, this could be simply two heavy-duty washers and dryers for doing house and kitchen linen. There should be some stainless-steel shelving on the clean side. The dining room linen will likely be sent out for cleaning and pressing.

Mechanical/Emergency Generator

In most applications where frail elderly will be living, it is essential to provide a mechanism for backup protection of the essential building components relating to the health and safety of the residents. This can be accomplished with the addition of an emergency generator. The generator can be either diesel or natural gas operated depending upon service availability, site, and environmental restrictions. Some communities prewire a split phase or three-wire single phase separate panel with the appropriate circuits which can then be connected to a portable generator that can be rented and delivered to the site in the event of a prolonged outage. There should be one outlet in each room tied to this to operate oxygen concentrators, CPAPs, and patient monitoring devices.

The following circuits should be rough-wired to the emergency power panel for the future use of emergency generators:

Emergency call system
Fire alarm
Kitchen equipment (coolers, freezer, etc.)
Emergency lights
Elevators (at least one)
Phone systems
Main office (computers), two circuits only
Delay egress system (Alden locks, if any)
Circulator pumps (heater)
Boilers
Electric fire pumps—water pressure
Heaters above ceiling (if any)
Jockey pump (if any—water pressure).

Storage

A separate lockable area in the back of the house would be nice for the storage of food and beverage equipment such as banquet tables, linen, table skirts, chafing dishes, display platforms and molds, roasters, paper goods, china/silver/glassware inventory, party items, and mandatory emergency dry food and water required in various state regulations.

Building Components

There needs to be good access to the HVAC units. There also is a need for lockable programmable thermostats in all common areas. Keying and lock systems must operate smoothly and not require jockeying from the opener. Have the general contractor create a notebook with all cut sheets and equipment manuals. They should also provide two copies of the "as-built" drawings. It is helpful to create a video of maintenance/operational procedures on all physical plant systems and kitchen equipment using the manufacturer's representative or the mechanical engineer at the time of building turn over.

Brick, wood siding, sloped roofs, covered porches, shutters, fireplaces, staircases, lamp posts, and circle driveways are homelike materials and details. Choose materials and design standards from single-family home construction to maintain that impression for the building.

INFECTION CONTROL: PUBLIC AREAS

The development of multiple, smaller ecosystems throughout the community can provide flexibility when facing uncertain health conditions. Each ecosystem can include enhanced amenities to support them, such as smaller satellite dining and lounge areas, a room for virtual visits, telehealth, and private fitness. These spaces would also include tenets of biophilic design by adding access to outdoor areas and natural light. This strategy helps build adaptability while allowing socialization with the ease of conversion to private areas during a health crisis.

- Consider hands-free screening at the front desk for visitors. Also separate the visiting room for family communication with negative pressure ventilation. Separate public restrooms for visitors only with fixtures to include hands-free sinks, toilets, and soap and towel dispensers. Install hands-free power-operated doors into resident areas. Arrange a separate entrance and storage area for deliveries. This entry should feature touchless access control and security systems. Consider increasing freezer/cooler space so that inventory can be stocked up during shortages and employee take-home meals can be stored.
- Health screening technology using thermal temperature scanners can be employed in the main vestibule and at the staff entrance. This technology can collect personal information and conduct automated screening on all entrants to the community.
- The staff lounge should include separate bathrooms and one shower allowing staff to decontaminate prior to starting their shift if needed. During a health crisis, this would also be an excellent location to distribute PPE. Consider adding a secure area with limited access for the storage of PPE and sanitary supplies. Infection control

measures generate significantly more trash, so easy access to trash removal in the resident areas will be needed.

- As online medical records and medication administration will compete with resident communications for bandwidth, upgraded Wi-Fi will be required throughout the building.

- In the resident units, consider adding 1 percent isolation rooms. These should be equipped with an entry vestibule (or anteroom) with a damper switch for energy recovery or exhaust ventilation only with negative pressure. Consider a modular construction so that an isolation room can be created if needed or converted if not.

- Outdoor areas will be increasingly important and should feature areas where large group activities and entertainment can be brought in while residents can maintain social distancing.

- High-touch surfaces can be painted with Linetec with Microban technology. These products can be specified for high-touch exterior or interior surfaces, such as handrails, doors, windows, curtain walls, entranceways, and countertops. This system meets the requirements of AAMA 2605. Also, copper is a highly antimicrobial surface that kills germs on contact. Needlepoint bipolar ionization (NPBI) technology has been shown to inactivate 99.4 percent of the viruses that cause COVID-19 in just 30 minutes in lab tests. This technology can be added to existing HVAC systems, with no filters that would provide extra strain on your system.

ALL RESIDENT ROOMS—DESIGN SUGGESTIONS

- Bathrooms should be fully accessible by those in wheelchairs and walkers, and should contain design features that support self-bathing and self-toileting, Toilets in the resident units should be tank type, 17-inch height preferable. The common area toilets should be 19 inches in height. This way, resident toilets can be exchanged for a 19-inch or equipped with a toilet riser for easier access on and off the toilet.

- All showers should be roll-in with a sloping tile floor to the central drain. All shower stalls should feature a pull-down seat, and extra blocking behind the walls to secure grab bars. Install additional blocking behind the shower at the time of construction to allow for additional supports, if

needed. Some prefabricated shower units come equipped with wooden blocking built into the fiberglass. The mixing valve should be firmly attached to blocking on installation, as residents often depend on this fixture to support their weight; it should have an antiscald device. Consider installing the mixing valve close to the outside edge of the shower. This allows the personal care aide easy access without getting wet. It is much faster to shower someone if a shower chair can be rolled into the shower rather than requiring a transfer over a lip. All showers should use a handheld wand that can be turned on and off at the wand and can be on a slider.

- Hinged doors work well for closets in the apartments and require less maintenance than bifold or pocket doors. There needs to be a logical mix of apartment sizes (i.e., studio versus one bedroom versus two bedrooms). Studios may be easier to market in price-sensitive areas and produce the most revenue per square foot. The smaller the unit, the more revenue per square foot as a general rule.

- Mount electrical outlets 24 inches above the floor. Mount a thermostat with large numbers at 48 inches.

- Consider audiovisual fire alarms in all apartments, not just in accessible apartments.

- Bedrooms need a headboard wall that will accommodate a full-size bed and a nightstand. One-bedroom apartments should be able to accommodate twin beds. This needs to be measured.

- Adequate closet and storage space is important. Two-bedroom units need two closets in each bedroom (walk-in closets would be best). Add overhead light in closets for better visibility of colors. Install L-shaped handles (not knobs) on all doors for persons with limited dexterity. Consider adding a small linen closet in the larger one-bedroom, den, and two-bedroom apartments. Consider a custom closet organizer upgrade.

- Stove and oven combination should have auto shutoff for safety. iGuardStoves have a motion-sensor device that automatically shuts off the stove after five minutes of no one being in the kitchen. This device can be conveniently disabled and even remotely disabled. Provide a separate circuit for this appliance so that it can be disconnected if needed. Allow adequate space and ventilation for a microwave oven. Microwave ovens should never be mounted at eye level; mount at chest height or lower to prevent scalding. Incorporate at least one drawer for utensils.

- The refrigerator should be capable of storing a half-gallon of ice cream in the freezer.
- The ILF apartments will require a full kitchen (30-inch slide-in range, 28-inch-wide refrigerator and dishwasher).
- Add wall-mounted task lighting at the kitchen sink area to eliminate shadows.
- Use single-lever faucets at the kitchen sink and in the bathroom for a residential appearance and non-grip operation. Motion-detection faucets are confusing for the elderly and require maintenance.
- Bathrooms should be situated for easy access from the sleeping area and be convenient to living area. Toilets that are visible from the bed offer visual cuing. Equipping bathrooms with motion-activated lighting can significantly reduce the occurrence of falls (which can lead to discharges) and are worth the small additional investment.
- Some larger unit designs often feature a walk-in closet between the master bedroom and the master bath. While this is a nice feature, the shortest distance between the bed and bathroom will reduce the number of falls. Residents should not need to walk through the closet to get to the bathroom in the middle of the night, which poses an additional tripping hazard.
- Locate emergency call stations in the bedroom and bathroom.
- Bathrooms should be fully accessible by those using a wheelchair or walker, should contain design features that support self-bathing and self-toileting, and should be sized to allow for assistance by staff or family members.
- Surround the wall-mounted bathroom sink with a countertop. Many residents have health and beauty supplies (shaver, hairbrush, dentures, etc.) that do not lend themselves to storage in the medicine cabinet.
- Medicine cabinets are a must for storing prescriptions in independent living. Be sure to include two in semiprivate units.
- Consider a robe hook on the back of the bathroom door (screwed, not glued).

- Grab bars by toilets that can double as towel racks are preferred; be sure to add blocking behind the sheetrock for support.

MEMORY CARE

Snoezelen—Quiet Room

Snoezelen rooms are designed for later-stage residents, but others may also enjoy the soothing environment of this sensory room. Each room is equipped with the following: One stationary rocking chair, a small comfortable couch (love seat), a table, and a credenza, a variety of lights, bubble tubes and other visual movement pieces, a music player and relaxation CDs and "new age" repetitive music.

Another nice feature to have is a Snoezelen cart. This is a portable activity station with lighted bubble towers, projector, mirrored panels, and fiber optics. These stations provide sensory stimulation for late-stage and end-of-life residents.

The goal is to help the resident "experience" the light and sounds. Residents do not need to be actively involved in the experience; all they need to do is use their senses as they watch the soothing lights and water bubbles, and listen to the music. Because the room is darkened, the resident should not be distracted by other noises or activities. They should be encouraged just to enjoy this relaxing experience.

Nurses Station

The space should be lockable and afford views of the common areas and ideally down the hallways. It must be equipped with high-speed internet to allow the use of electronic medical records (EMR) and a laptop computer. There must also be a storage area for the med cart, a lockable mini-fridge to store refrigerated medications, a cabinet for bandages and first aid supplies, a counter for charting, and some file storage area. A second separate mini-fridge in the room is preferred as foods needed for administering medications are not allowed to be stored with medications.

Warming Kitchen—Memory Care Dining Area

This can be designed as a standard household kitchen with a full-size refrigerator (with ice maker), stove top, oven, sink (two wells), and cabinets to store dry food and snack items. A high-temperature dishwasher will be required by most sanitation regulations. These cost about twice as much as the household type but can complete a cycle in about two minutes instead of two hours, as well as sterilize the tableware. There needs to be a convenient place to plug in hot carts that delivers food from the main kitchen to any satellite memory care kitchens. Other plug outlets are useful for the soup kettle and for residents who are on pureed diets and require their food pureed. A bi-level high/low breakfast bar with stools is handy to serve some residents, and with a flip-up countertop access to the back it can discourage residents from getting into the stove and refrigerator. The dining area should feature both four-top tables and at least one two-top table (deuce) for residents who are agitated and not appropriate to sit with other residents. Ideally a dining room for memory care should not serve more than 16 residents. The stove needs to have a separate shutoff breaker so that the residents cannot turn it on if temporarily unsupervised. Use of induction cooktops would be preferred as they operate with a different technology than either gas or electric stovetops. These features make them safer and easier to use—rather than depending on flames or hot coils, induction cooking elements heat pots and pans with magnetic fields.

Laundry

The laundry room for personal laundry is most efficiently handled by nurses' aides on the units. This way residents' clothing never leaves the unit, and the aides can easily run laundry during their shift, especially at night. Install one washer and one dryer for every 10 residents. A flushable floor-mounted service sink is a must for precleaning linens and clothing prior to putting them into a washing machine. This room must be lockable to secure laundry chemicals from the residents.

Living and Activity Room—Each Pod

This area should feature a large (50-inch or larger) smart TV with an internet connection and a hunt-board server below for activity storage. Cabling should be run behind the wall and a double outlet provided below or one behind the TV and another below. This area must have Wi-Fi internet access.

There should be a mix of sofas and recliners with two square tables for projects. Sofas should be skirted in front so that the resident's heels can fit underneath, which aids them in standing up. Sofa cushions need to be double-stuffed and removable. Recliners may be provided to discourage some residents from wandering and providing them a secure and comfortable place to sit. There needs to be a small closet with shelves on each unit to store activity supplies and comforters.

Memory Care Units

■ A plate rack in each room located just above eye level allows residents to display personal items for cuing as well as keeping them out of reach of other residents who may browse from room to room.

■ The addition of a drinking fountain with a cup dispenser can cue residents to keep hydrated. The fountain should be pressure activated with a bar device or a turn handle.

■ Toilet tank covers need to be secured to prevent removal. This is needed for the safety of the resident and to prevent breakage. Arm rails on toilets are beneficial to assist with the visualization of the toilet and safe seating. Toilet lids and seats should be a contrasting color to direct residents to its location.

■ Other articles that resemble a commode, such as waste cans and plant pots, should be removed, as visual perception is diminished with Alzheimer's disease.

■ Lighting of the environment needs to be nonglare, consistent, and have the ability to simulate daylight. Dimmer switches are very helpful. Chandeliers and other decorative lighting need to be in addition to quality lighting, not the main source of light.

■ A delayed egress system is an essential piece of the system for providing safety and security to the residents in the unit. It helps to control resident access to outside areas, yet complies with building and fire codes. The system needs to be UL-approved and conform to NFPA-101. The system should feature a keypad control, but doors will open when the fire alarm system is engaged or (after 15 seconds) when 15 pounds of pressure are applied to the door.

■ Adequate individual rooms are needed for activities, visiting, dining, preparing or distributing meals and snacks, and laundry.

■ It is essential that the laundry room be located on the unit so that caregivers can do laundry while supervising the residents. Laundry facilities off the unit will require additional staffing resources to complete this task. Dementia residents are often recruited to help fold clean linen.

- Avoid the use of coffee tables and end tables. They are too low and frequently are not seen by the resident. Glider rocking chairs are safe and work well with this population. They provide comfort and motion; footstools should be avoided.

- All wall decorations need to be touchable, and any framed pictures need to have Plexiglas rather than glass for safety. The colors need to contrast with the wall colors and be warm in nature. It is also a good idea to have contrasting colors where the walls meet the floor. This can easily be accomplished with cove base molding.

- Because residents do not spend much time in their rooms, accessible public bathrooms need to be provided in common areas. The visual cue is important to them to minimize accidents and cleanup. Tilt-down mirrors and touch-less fixtures are needed.

- Lamps on bedside tables can create shadows and present a hazard even when attached to the table. Consider wall-mounted sconces with open bottoms to prevent bug collection.

- For outdoor areas, see-through fencing at least six feet high is best. Also consider outdoor benches and raised-bed garden areas as many residents love to garden.

WELL BUILDING STANDARD VERSION 2

The WELL Building Standard version 2 (WELL v2) is a vehicle for buildings and organizations to deliver more thoughtful and intentional spaces that enhance human health and well-being. WELL v2 includes a set of strategies, backed by the latest scientific research, that aim to advance human health through design interventions and operational protocols and policies and foster a culture of health and wellness.[3]

The WELL Building Standards highlight 10 major concepts. Each concept consists of features with distinct health intents. Features are either preconditions or optimizations. Preconditions define the fundamental components of a WELL Certified space and serve as the foundation of a healthy building. WELL v2 offers a universal set of preconditions for all projects. All preconditions are mandatory for certification. Optimizations are optional pathways for projects to meet certification requirements in WELL. Project teams may select which optimizations to pursue and which parts to focus on within each optimization.

Air: The WELL Air concept aims to achieve high levels of indoor air quality across a building's lifetime through diverse strategies that include source elimination or reduction, active and passive building design, operation strategies, and human behavior interventions.

Water: The WELL Water concept covers aspects of the quality, distribution, and control of liquid water in a building. It includes features that address the availability and contaminant thresholds of drinking water, as well as features targeting the management of water to avoid damage to building materials and environmental conditions.

Nourishment: The WELL Nourishment concept requires the availability of fruits and vegetables and nutritional transparency. It encourages the creation of food environments where the healthiest choice is the easiest choice.

Light: The lighting environments where humans spend their time impact their visual, circadian, and mental health. Currently, lighting conditions in most spaces are designed to meet the visual needs of individuals but do not take into account circadian and mental health. This presents an opportunity for projects to provide lighting conditions required by humans for improved health and well-being.

Movement: The WELL Movement concept aims to promote movement, foster physical activity and active living, and discourage sedentary behavior by creating and enhancing opportunities through the spaces where we spend our lives.

Thermal Comfort: The WELL Thermal Comfort concept takes a holistic approach to thermal comfort and provides a combination of research-based interventions to help design buildings that address individual thermal discomfort and support human health, well-being, and productivity.

Sound: The WELL Sound concept aims to bolster occupant health and well-being through the identification and mitigation of acoustical comfort parameters that shape occupant experiences in the built environment.

Materials: The WELL Materials concept advances two strategies for selecting building materials and products. One is to increase literacy on materials by promoting ingredient disclosure whereas the second is to promote the assessment and optimization of product composition in order to minimize impacts to human and environmental health.

Mind: The WELL Mind concept promotes implementation of design, policy, and programmatic strategies that support cognitive and emotional health through a variety of prevention and treatment efforts. In combination, these interventions have the potential to positively impact the short- and long-term mental health and well-being of individuals of diverse backgrounds throughout a community.

Community: The WELL Community concept promotes the implementation of design, policy and operations strategies that focus on addressing health disparities and promoting social diversity and inclusion. Providing access to health services, inclusive and health-promoting policies, and design that enables all individuals to access, participate and thrive within a space can build a foundation for truly equitable, diverse, and healthy communities.

■■■■ BIOPHILIA: DESIGNING BIOPHILIC ENVIRONMENTS

Older adults who move into senior living communities may find that their connection to the outdoors changes depending on their acuity level, their mobility, or their age. While some of this access to see and experience the outdoors depends on the level of care they need, architecture and design can help play a part in ensuring that the benefits of the outdoors are accessible in different ways and for different population.

Clearly the best way to experience the outdoors is to design pathways for access to it. But the climate outside may not always be conducive to experiencing it personally. Also, for those who aren't able to move or achieve that traditional access, the challenge is to bring the outdoors in.

In the industry, this is known as biophilia. Biophilic design promotes elements that allow the outdoor natural world to be brought inside, or provide views to the outside and access to sunlight from within. Here are a few ways to achieve this in senior living.

Enhance the visual experience. One way to help achieve the benefit of the outdoor experience is visually. This concept lends itself to designs with as much glass as possible to visually let in the light and the view outside.

The typical older-adult residence may have a traditional residential window centered in a room. If the glass can instead extend from floor to ceiling, it allows for a better sightline to vegetation and sun for both a person standing and someone in a wheelchair. Careful selection of window coverings can maximize visibility out while also helping control glare and harsh direct sunlight.

Enhancing the visual experience with intentional views out the window is important not only for the resident but also for the caregivers and staff.

In higher acuity situations such as skilled nursing or memory support environments, the staff are frequently engaged within the unit. Place windows so that when a caregiver enters their focus is out the window, giving the staff a glimpse of the outdoors and a pleasant visual pause from the day's tasks as they visit each resident's room.

Consider the window design. Thoughtful window design is part of improving this process. A common residential-style window is often three feet wide by six feet tall. But these windows usually have multiple frame elements, which can obstruct the view.

Design utilizing a window that is unimpeded in the middle where a person would center themselves on the opening can offer a more transparent view to the exterior, which can make all the difference to a person who has limited access to the outdoors.

It's important that the views from those windows lead to something beautiful and eye-catching outside. Resorts do this well, often positioning trees or brightly colored flowers outside a window to draw the eye from the indoors out. Dense, tall vegetation, eye-catching trees, mountain views, and even natural textures like wood or rock can draw the eye and give the person inside more satisfaction when they look out.

Create a tangible experience. Creating the feeling of being in nature can provide healing qualities. Taking the visual experience a step further, such as turning a window into French doors that open to a Juliet balcony, can get people even closer to an outdoor experience. This way, even the wheelchair bound would have the opportunity to lean out, feel the breeze, and potentially even touch real plant material.

Inserting a person in an environment with the opportunity to feel the heat of the sun, the breeze in the air, or the plants or rocks in the natural environment can have a powerful effect on the brain and outlook. In fact, we are often naturally drawn to textures like wood, stone, or vegetation. Inserting these touchable textures inside the building—in the floor, along the wall, in furnishings, or in a touchable art fixture—can help create that organic outdoor feel indoors.

NOTES

1. US Department of Energy, "Tuning the Light in Senior Care," August 2016, https://www.energy.gov/sites/prod/files/2016/09/f33/2016_gateway-acc.pdf.

2. Effects of illuminance and correlated color temperature oof indoor light on emotion perception. National Institute of Health, https://www.ncbi.nlm.nih.gov/pmc/articles/PMC8275593/.

3. For more information and a description of each of the standards, visit https://www.wellcertified.com.

Appendixes

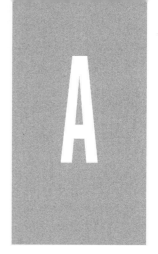

Sample SWOT Analysis and Strategic Plan

Company:	Sample Assisted Living and Memory Care	Updated	01/01/2023	
	STRENGTHS / OPPORTUNITIES		WEAKNESSES / THREATS	

	STRENGTHS / OPPORTUNITIES	WEAKNESSES / THREATS
Status Quo	**Strengths:**	**Weaknesses:**
	→ Located on river with mountain views	→ Penetration into the affluent markets
	→ Experienced clinical team with outstanding reputation	→ Lack of physical therapy program and restorative exercise equipment
	→ Unique experiences / activities program permeates the community	→ Lack of sufficient outdoor areas for events and gatherings
	→ Full dining service with gourmet and farm to table options using CSAs	→ Staff shortages in marketplace
	→ Attractive and desirable product, only MC in the marketplace	→ Strong competitors
Targets	**Opportunities:**	**Threats:**
	→ Differentiate programmatically from competitors	→ Size of geographic marketplace
	→ Increase Google reviews capitalizing on positive family feedback	→ Highly Competitive employment market
	→ Build family referral program	→ New competitors opening bringing rate compression and employee wage expansion
	→ Build lead volume across town toward city center	→ Management of high acuity in memory care
	→ Create a sense of innovation in the industry to make competition irrelevant	→ Building FFE aging

Major Objectives	How We Are Going to Do It	Frequency / Due Date	Responsible
1. *Build professional referrals*	→ Professional open house and tour events	Monthly	**MD**
	→ Track outreach communication in CRM	Weekly	**MD**
	→ Weekly outreach to professional offices to relationship build and foster awareness of our advocacy efforts	Complete & ongoing	**MD / OD**

Major Objectives	How We Are Going to Do It	Frequency / Due Date	Responsible
	→ Improve lead generation through grassroots efforts: roll out one new educational program monthly	Revisit	**Agency / MD**
	→ Outreach Fax Blast weekly	Weekly	**MD / ED**
	→ Outreach to promote continuing education opportunities for referral sources	Monthly	**MD / ED**
	→ Continue building relationships with local physicians and the hospital, hospice, home health	Montthly	**MD / ED / WD**
	→ Track community outreach efforts by prioritizing potential to refer (1, 2, 3) and by relationship (green, yellow, red)	Complete & ongoing	**MD**
2. *Build family satisfaction and referrals*	→ Conduct Monthly family night with educational series presentations	Complete & ongoing	**ED / VPO**
	→ Formalize onboarding process for new residents	Revisit	**ED / VPO**
	→ Continue monthly wellness update to families from wellness director using care plan and collaborative care dashboard	Complete & ongoing	**ED / WD**
	→ Promote family feedback loop through the QR codes on the doorframes	Restart	**ED / WD**
	→ Dementia support group for family and care provider's holistic support	Ongoing	**ED / WD / EC**
	→ Biweekly newsletter to families: birthdays, upcoming events, showcase special events and activities, "What's new," Constant Contact	Complete & Ongoing	**MD / ED / VPO**
	→ Invite families to senior seminar series and preexisting collaboration events	Monthly	**MD / ED / VPO**
	→ Conduct family opinion survey online with SurveyMonkey	July	**ED / VPO**
3. *Differentiate from competitors*	→ New messaging on website and collateral, new branding to attract upscale prospects for a distance	Completed	**ED / VPO**
	→ Offer experience-based programs to engage residents, families, and staff	Need more	**ED / VPO**
	→ Bring community artisans, chefs, and musicians into the community to broaden experiences and perception of change	Restart	**ED / VPO**
	→ Communicate value added of collaborative care dashboard	Quarterly	**ED / VPO**
	→ Promote clinical staff RN, executive director, and wellness director with emergency management expertise	Ongoing	**ED / VPO**
	→ Promote short-term stay through respite, transitional care, step-down, and hospice care	Complete & Ongoing	**ED / VPO**
	→ Follow up to verify competition of each (140) items on prep survey to ensure complete compliance with state regulations	Ongoing	**ED / VPO**
	→ Specialized training of memory care staff and dementia care certifications	Ongoing	**ED / WD**
	→ Create desirable logo items for staff achievement gifts	Complete & Ongoing	**CEO**
4. *Operator branding*	→ Event-driven marketing program: senior seminar series, senior productions, chef workshops, community advocacy from residents	Restart	**Agency / MD**
	→ Create content library for use on website, social media, advertising, commercials of experts and interior / exterior footage	Complete & Ongoing	**Agency / MD**
	→ Wellness program space with physical fitness and therapy offerings	August	**Agency / MD**

Major Objectives	How We Are Going to Do It	Frequency / Due Date	Responsible
	→ Create radio and TV familiarity in the marketplace with interviews, features, and commercials	Completed	**Agency / MD**
	→ Create geofencing advertising targets surrounding key referral sources and develop cell phone and iPad compatible ads	Completed	**Agency / MD**
	→ ED and MD luncheon meetings monthly to build brand identity and foster professional referrals	Restart	**MD / ED**
	→ Continue process by which caregivers and staff get to know the residents & families	Ongoing	**ED**
	→ Community advocacy (Alz org, blood drive, community fundraisers, Meals on Wheels), Eblasts	Incomplete	**VPO**
	→ Website upgrades to state-of-the-art, which engages and educates visitors—link to eBook as a contact information harvesting tool	Completed	**VPO**
5 *Build inquiry volume and tours*	→ Create networking group to drive lead volume and share referrals	First Quarter	**MD**
	→ Provide value-added informational PDFs as fulfillment piece for each follow-up contact	Completed	**VPO**
	→ Identify the top 50 referral sources and customize meaningful offerings to each	Started	**VPO**
	→ Sponsorship of hospital newsletter and discharge collateral	Second Quarter	**CEO**
	→ Email and print media blasts to newspapers and Constant Contact list	Complete & Ongoing	**Agency / MD**
	→ Create video brochure and 360 tour for top prospects and referral sources	Hold	**Agency**
	→ Advertising plan to include monthly infomercial on key age-related topics	Second Quarter	**ED / MD**
	→ Create media blasts for community events (outside and inside the facility)	Ongoing	**Agency**
6. *Build employee satisfaction*	→ Create employee benefit brochure	First Quarter	**Agency**
	→ Recruitment and retention of high-quality employees	Ongoing	**VPO / ED**
	→ Implement operational absolutes with department heads	Follow up on POC	**VPO / ED**
	→ Competitor benefits matrix analysis and wage survey	First Quarter	**ED / VPO**
	→ Create benefit portal and communicate value and access ease to all employees	Complete & Ongoing	**MD / ED**
	→ Offer partial pay for PTO	Hold	**CFO / BOM / ED**
	→ Procure new radios and pendants for better staff communication	Completed	**ED / VPO**
	→ Conduct associate engagement survey using SurveyMonkey online	Third Quarter	**VPO / ED**
	→ Monthly associate feature—doing something for their community	Revisit	**ED / MD**
	→ Create employee exit interview to evaluate terminated employees' perceptions	Complete & ongoing	**ED / VPO**
	→ Create formalized employee engagement program	Revisit	**ED / VPO**
	→ Upgrade quality of caregiver staff, recruit from competitors	Ongoing	**ED / DON / BOM**

Major Objectives	How We Are Going to Do It	Frequency / Due Date	Responsible
	→ Develop monthly training calendar with video, handouts, and certificates each month for 12 months, create links for online access	Second Quarter	**ED / DON**
	→ Biweekly meetings: Staff achievements, tips and tricks, policy changes / reminders	Complete & Ongoing	**ED / DON / VPO**
	→ Establish preceptor status training aide position and specialist accreditation classes	Revisit	**DON / VPO**
	→ Upgrade employee break room and add motivational slogans there and in back-of-the-house areas	Thirty Days	**ED / VPO**
7. *Physical plant*	→ Create and implement preventive maintenance plan	Thirty Days	**ED / VPO**
	→ Consider adding Alexa to foster communication with remote families and assist staff with music and information	Hold	**ED / VPO**
	→ Model furniture and set up two respite apartments	Hold	**CEO / VPO**
	→ Create interior design upgrades for resident units and common areas	Hold	**VPO**
	→ Clean and reorganize maintenance storage	Hold	**CEO / VPO**
	→ Create outdoor event space	Hold	**CEO / VPO**
	→ Build storage area inside activity center	Hold	**ED / VPO**
	→ Purchase and install storage shed	Hold	**VPO**
8. *Leadership development*	→ Implement training and process FYI (For Your Improvement) to develop management skills inventory	Review	**ED / VPO**
	→ Survey prep checklist to verify that all regulations are in full compliance and all checked boxes in prep survey have been verified	Ongoing	**ED / VPO**
9. *NOI management*	→ Aggressively manage vacant unit pricing—utilize staged release technique to create urgency on pricing	Ongoing	**ED / VPO**
	→ Reprice every unit in the building based upon desirability—identify unique feature of each	Ongoing	**ED / MD**
	→ Implement overtime reduction policies, approvals, and tracking	Revisit	**ED / VPO**
	→ All new hires must have separate and individual approval, if not in the budget	Ongoing	**ED / VPO**
	→ Redeploy assets to slow turnover—e.g., hospital visits, video get-well cards, AAOA, county nurse, hospice controls, Quarterly assessments and interventions for all residents	Restart	**ED / VPO**
	→ Revise spend-downs to reflect actual occupancy vs budget and adjust to appropriate staffing levels	March	**ED / VPO**
	→ Create recruitment and retention plan to match expected staffing demands with occupancy growth	Ongoing	**ED / VPO**
	→ Variance reports should be required on all expenditures that exceed budget by $500	Completed & Ongoing	**ED / VPO**

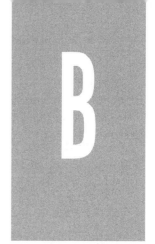

Senior Living Metrics Glossary

■■■■■■ OPERATING METRICS

REVPOR = Total revenue all resident sources per occupied bed. This is a good indicator of growth in rent per unit plus level of care fees. Increase demonstrates growth in actual rents or LOC, decrease indicates discounting or loss of heavy care resident.

Operating margin = The operating margin reflects the portion of total revenues retained as operating income, and it relates solely to the operations. This ratio is also referred to as the operating profit margin. The operating margin can also be calculated by subtracting the expense ratio from 1. Operating ratios will vary with the type of community. According to a CBRE study, independent living should target 48%, assisted living and memory care 39%, and skilled nursing 17% for Class A CORE communities. OM = NOI (net operating income) / gross revenue.[1]

Expense ratio = The operating expense ratio is a useful tool to determine overall operational efficiency. An expression of the proportion of operating expenses to gross revenue operating expenses, it should include management fees but should be net of depreciation, real estate taxes, capital improvements and debt service. Expense ratio = operating expenses / gross revenue. Expense ratios will vary with the type of community. According to a CBRE study, independent living should target 52%, assisted living and memory care 61%, and skilled nursing 82% for Class A CORE communities. Nonprofit communities will have expense ratios close to 100%.

Net occupancy = Month-end financial occupancy. This means the unit produced revenue at the end of the month whether physically occupied or not.

Total patient days = Total days during the month times the number of financially responsible residents paying during those days whether physically present or not.

Revenue PPD = Total revenue (all sources from residents) / Total patient days.

Expenses PPD = Total operating expenses revenue (includes management fees but should be net of depreciation, real estate taxes, capital improvements and debt service) / Total patient days. For assisted living, an industry target for this is $100; for memory care, $120 assuming stabilized occupancy.

NOI PPD = Revenue PPD − Expenses PPD.

Total labor = Total labor includes all paid regular wages, overtime, and PTO. Does not include payroll taxes, workers' compensation, medical and dental insurance, physicals and TB tests, payroll prep fees, 401K, or background checks and hiring costs.

Labor PPD = Total labor / total resident patient days for the same period (typically monthly). For assisted living, an industry target for this is $60; for memory care, $70 assuming stabilized occupancy.

Wellness labor = Total wellness labor (including nursing aides, nurses, and supervisors). Does not include payroll taxes and benefits.

Wellness labor PPD = Total wellness labor in dollars including wages, salaries, overtime, paid time off, bonuses, and any retro pay (including nursing aides, nurses, and supervisors) / Total resident patient days for the same period (typically monthly) For assisted living, an industry target for this is $30; for memory care, $40 assuming stabilized occupancy. The same job categories are also used to calculate nursing hours per patient day. To calculate this, take total hours per month and divide by total patient days per month.

Overtime = Total overtime dollars paid during the month, which could include 2 and sometimes 3 pay periods / Total labor. For a well-run operation, target no more than 6%.

Food cost PPD = Total cost of raw food for the month / Total number of residents physically present. Cost per meal is often confused with the daily food cost. Depending upon utilization, a continental breakfast costing approximately $2.00 per person to produce, combined with a lunch of $3.00 and a dinner of $5.00 can yield a combined daily food cost of $10.00, but when averaged on a per-meal basis it comes to $3.33 per meal. Industry averages per patient day for a low-end product is $3.50 to 5.00; a moderate program will range from $5.00 to $7.00; and a high-end program can run up to $8.00 to $12.00.

■ MARKETING METRICS

Inquiries per month = Total qualified leads per month from all sources. Does not include inquiries not qualified medically or financially.

Tours per month = Total physical or virtual tours of a qualified prospect or family. This does not include professional, vendor, contractor, regulatory, investor, or non-prospect event tours.

Total move-ins = Total residents who took financial responsibility anytime during the month. This number includes respite and second occupants paying additional fees. It does not include guest and visitor stays. A single resident paying for both sides of a semiprivate unit counts as 1. This can include residents who moved in and then moved out the same month. You can estimate future move-in volume by taking the historical average number of inquiries and multiplying it by the historical move-in per inquiry ratio.

Total move-outs = Total persons who cease to be financially responsible during the month. This can exclude deaths from a prior month who have not turned over their unit.

Net occupancy gain (loss) = Total move-ins − Total move-outs.

Marketing spend = Total nonlabor dollars spent on marketing during the period. Includes all marketing costs, advertising, print media, sponsorships, social media, online advertising, branding, paid referral fees, outreach costs, collateral, marketing signage, promotion items, travel, and meals. Does not include sales commissions.

Cost per lead = Total marketing spend / Total qualified inquiries during the same period.

Cost per move-in = Total nonlabor marketing spend / Total move-ins during the same period.

Tour per inquiry = Total qualified tours / Total qualified inquiries for the same period. Target = 50%. This metric is a measure of the effectiveness of the marketing program to attract qualified leads that are interested in touring the community.

Total move-in per tour = Total persons who became financially responsible / Number of qualified tours given during the same period. Target = 30%. The metric is a measure of both the quality of the lead toured and the ability of the salesperson to close that lead.

Move-in per inquiry = Total number of persons who became financially responsible / Total number of qualified inquiries during the same period. Target = 15%. This metric is a measure of all components of the marketing and sales program. The ability to attract qualified leads and to convert them into paying residents. This metric can be used in planning to predict the total lead volume necessary to generate the desired move-ins. This ratio can also be impacted by market conditions beyond the control of management, such as price wars and pandemics.

Total sales contacts = Total number of face-to-face, phone calls (where someone was spoken to or left voice mail), emails, letters sent, follow-up cards. Average sales contacts per person per day = 25–50. Industry averages: Number of contacts per sale = 3–5; number of days from first contact to sale = 60; number of days from sale to move-in = 30; percent of sales generated within 30 days of inquiry = 50%.

FTF outreach visits = In-person contact with referral source or source representative such as nurse, office manager and leave collateral information. This can include Zoom calls or virtual tours where social distancing is required as long as personal contact is made.

Referral Sources

Priority 1 = Capacity to refer to facility immediately and ongoing. Frequency = Weekly. Targets are hospitals, psychiatric physicians, rehabs, cardiologists, orthopedics, geriatricians, neurologists, oncologists, APFM, caring.com, geriatric care managers, senior living private agencies, area agency on aging, discharge planners, geriatric specialty physicians, pharmacists, skilled nursing centers, social workers

Priority 2 = Capacity to refer to facility every 60–90 days. Frequency = Monthly. Targets are family general practitioners, adult day care centers, hospice agencies, home health agencies, Alzheimer's Association, chiropractors, elder-law attorneys, financial advisors.

Priority 3 = Capacity to refer to facility annually. Frequency = Every other month. Targets are chamber of commerce, churches, alumni associations, council on aging, family counselors, funeral directors, grief support centers, women's clubs, Jewish federation, moving companies catering to seniors, Red Hat Society groups, senior centers, Veterans Affairs.

Relationship definitions = Goal is to move relationships to green status.

Green = Reliable and consistent lead source with committed relationship.

Yellow = Potential to become a consistent lead/referral source but not reliable currently.

Red = Potential to become a referral source but currently unresponsive.

Outreach call outs = All contact with professional or paid referral sources that was not in person. This can include phone calls, emails, text messages, fax bombs, office visits where only information is left or refreshed without personal contact.

EVENT METRICS

Event attendees = Total number of in-person or virtual persons attending a marketing event, educational series, seminar, or sponsored outing. This does not include staff, residents, resident families. It is intended to track prospect and referral traffic attracted to the event.

New leads generated = New qualified leads who attended or were referred by an attendee to an event and became a workable lead.

Contacts collected = Number of business cards, raffle entries, names and addresses collected from sign-in log at an event or seminar.

Referral source attendees = Number of existing or potential professionals who have the ability and capacity to refer qualified prospects to the community that are workable.

▬▬▬ PROPERTY METRICS

Building condition = Visual evaluation of physical plant in terms of marketability, functionality, and deferred maintenance.

Grounds condition = Visual evaluation of building exterior and grounds/landscaping, signage, parking structures in terms of marketability, functionality, and deferred maintenance.

Rent-ready units = Units that are currently showable and move-in ready immediately. This should be maintained at approximately 90% to have on hand sufficient variety of each unit type to show prospects and families. Average cost of apartment turn should be less than $1,000. If over this amount, prior occupant may have left damages beyond normal wear and tear and should be charged from security deposit. Units should be turned within 36 hours of vacancy. Vacant units should never be used to store maintenance, kitchen, or marketing supplies, and never durable medical equipment, hospital beds, wheelchairs, and former resident furniture.

Capital expenditures = Fixed asset capitalization, also known as capital improvement, as a process of assessing the current and projected physical state of a property, establishing the cost of maintaining or modernizing it, and planning for needed improvements. All expenditures for new assets and permanent improvements can be capitalized if they increase the value of the property, clearly have a benefit that extends three or more years, and generally have a minimum purchase of $200 per invoice with a unit cost of at least $50 and do not fall within the classification of repair and maintenance. Expenditures made for the purpose of keeping the property in ordinary, efficient operating condition, which do not add value or appreciably extend the useful life of the asset, are repair and maintenance expenses. The facts and circumstances surrounding the expenditure often determine whether it is capital in nature or an ordinary expense. Expenditures that can be capitalized should be. Expenditures such as these are generally not planned for in the operations budget but are dealt with separately in a fixed-asset capitalization budget. The priority system should be defined to establish a comparative relationship between capital needs to facilitate informed decisions during the budgeting process. For example, those expenditures that are required for health and safety reasons normally would be assigned top priority. Second priority could be assigned to projects that facilitate a more efficient operation, thereby reducing the cost of operations. Third priority could be assigned to projects designed to meet company standards. Fourth priority could be reserved for major renovations, and fifth could be assigned to elective projects that may simply promote community enhancement or "wish list" items. Payback periods should be calculated on all items, including installation, that are intended to save operating money. The payback period is the time it takes for the cumulative operating savings to exceed initial total costs (calculate by dividing the initial cost by the annual operating savings).

▬▬▬ REPUTATION AND REGULATORY METRICS

License in good standing = License is current, without restrictions of any kind, such as an admission hold, building safety hazard, certificate of occupancy, life safety, or financial mandates.

Regulatory = Review last clinical and life/safety surveys for deficiency-free status or plan of correction accepted by the state. There should be a detailed plan of correction accepted by the state for any violations. There should not be any immediate jeopardy (IJ) violations, which put resident health or safety at risk and normally mandate a temporary admissions hold or "stop placement."

Legal cases/litigation = Total of the following during the last 12 months: medical record requests from a family's attorney, lawsuits filed, cases settled, cases lost. This is often a reflection of poor operations, unfit or inadequate staffing, family dissatisfaction, poor communication with families. Publicity from these lawsuits and online reviews can severely impact marketability and referrals.

Ombudsman activity = The typical duties of an ombudsman are to investigate complaints and attempt to resolve them, usually through recommendations (binding or not) or mediation. Ombudsmen sometimes also aim to identify systemic issues leading to poor service or breaches of people's rights. Typically, they are called in to investigate family complaints and produce a report with findings to either substantiate the complaint or unsubstantiate it.

HUMAN RESOURCE METRICS

Staff turnover = Total staff terminated / total employees + new hires. Staff turnover rates in senior living typically run 90% or more. Employee longevity translates directly to quality of care. The longer an employee is in his or her job, the more familiar he/she becomes with each resident and can manage their needs over time as they become increasingly complex. The formula for staff retention is: Proper orientation + frequent and respectful communication + ongoing training + fair treatment + career development + fair pay and benefits = Staff retention.

DOL audits = The Wage and Hour Division conducts audits to enforce federal labor law (namely the FLSA). During a Wage and Hour Division audit, the DOL investigator will review payroll, employment records, and overall employee rights in the workplace. These are normally triggered by a complaint from an employee or multiple employees.

EEOC cases = An employee can file a formal job discrimination complaint with the EEOC whenever they believe they are "Being treated unfairly on the job because of your race, color, religion, sex (including pregnancy, gender identity, and sexual orientation), national origin, disability, age (age 40 or older) or genetic information; or being harassed at work for any of these reasons; or being treated unfairly or harassed because you complained about job discrimination, or assisted with a job discrimination investigation or lawsuit." This complaint is called a "Charge of Discrimination." "All of the laws we enforce, except for the Equal Pay Act, require you to file a Charge of Discrimination with the EEOC before you can file a job discrimination lawsuit against your employer." Presence of these in the community is normally a sign of incompetent or prejudicial leadership at the facility.

Workers' compensation mod rate = The experience mod rate, or EMR, is an important component of your company's workers' compensation program. The basic tenant of the EMR is that it uses an employer's past experience—your losses—to project future losses. It is a calculation using actuarial rates to compare a company's experience to state averages for similar companies. Once calculated, the rate is utilized to modify a company's workers' compensation premium. If you have an average EMR of 1.0, no modification is made to the premium. If your EMR is over 1.0—let's say 1.10—your premium would be assessed a 10% debit. Conversely, if your EMR was under 1.0—let's say 0.90—your premium would be assessed a 10% credit. Typically a high mod rate relates to high incident frequency of work-related injuries. Sometimes in bad work environments employees will push this to receive income protection.

NOTE

1. BRE Valuation & Advisory Services and BRE Research, April 2019, https://www.cbre.com/insights#sort=%40publish date%20descending&numberOfResults=9.

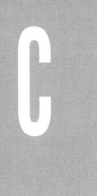

Operations Audit

This operations audit is designed to assist executive directors and their staff in attaining excellence in all aspects of managing a senior living facility. It should be used as a self-evaluation tool to help managers and department supervisors understand the performance expectations and provide high-quality services for residents. Rate each line item from 0 to 10, with 10 being best and 0 being poorest. In some instances, an item may have multiple parts. For example:

- Staff meetings and department head meetings are held regularly.
- Minutes of all meetings are kept on file.

If both statements are true, a score of 10 would be appropriate. If the second statement is not true, then perhaps a score of 5 would be appropriate.

Each section of the survey is scored separately and rated as follows:

92%–100%	Excellent
83%–91%	Good
74%–82%	Fair
65%–73%	Poor
0%–64%	Disaster

Use the final page of the survey to total the results and arrive at a rating in the same way.

Where improvement is needed, the department head is responsible for preparing and implementing a plan of correction. This plan should be proactive and address the performance standards alone, not the behavior or personality of the employees. People work best when expectations are clearly defined, standards are communicated, and consistency is the norm. The more managers can take the guesswork out of what they expect of the staff, the better the job the staff can do.

▬▬▬▬ EXECUTIVE DIRECTOR

Category	Standard	Score
1. **Goals and objectives**	All departmental prior-period goals and objectives have been met.	_____
2. **Budget**	All departments consistently meet their budgetary guidelines.	_____
3. **Revenue**	The community maintains occupancy levels as budgeted. All rollover units are repriced at the maximum marketable value.	_____
4. **Regulations**	The community fully complies with all governmental laws and regulations regarding the operation of the facility.	_____
5. **Management**	The executive director monitors departmental systems, goals, and objectives designed to report on and analyze the performance of all service components and individuals under direct supervision.	_____
6. **Delivery of services**	The executive director monitors all aspects of delivering services to the residents and makes changes to ensure resident satisfaction and achieve optimal profitability.	_____
7. **Business plan**	The facility has a SWOT strategic plan that is being followed and updated quarterly for the current fiscal year. (See Appendix A.)	_____
8. **Hourly wage plan**	The facility has an hourly wage plan that is being followed for the current fiscal year. Benefit matrix is updated annually with competitor data.	_____
9. **Policies and procedures**	The facility has a full set of departmental policy and procedure manuals. The manuals are kept current, are used for training new management staff members, and are referred to before contacting the corporate office.	_____
10. **Analysis**	Relevant metrics are promptly, consistently, and effectively analyzed, with recommendations and conclusions offered. Reports are clear, concise, and thoroughly researched. (See Appendix B.)	_____
11. **Competition**	Consumer purchasing behaviors, pricing sensitivities, and differentiation of facility services from competitors' services are reviewed and evaluated semiannually.	_____
12. **Communication**	A formal system of communication is in place to ensure that routine and emergency information is efficiently distributed to the staff, the residents, and the corporate office.	_____
13. **Meetings**	Weekly department-head meetings, monthly all-staff meetings, and all resident meetings are held consistently and with an appropriate agenda. Minutes are taken, and copies are distributed and kept on file.	_____
14. **Resident survey**	The management scored acceptably on the resident opinion survey. There is a written plan of corrective action to address any negative responses	_____
15. **Consistency of communication**	All staff members are fully informed and rehearsed on appropriate responses to the questions that prospects, residents, and their families frequently ask about the facility and its services.	_____
16. **Community relations**	Community relations functions for the facility (with particular attention to the medical, legal, financial, and religious communities who influence the senior market) are carried out in a focused and systematic manner.	_____
17. **Motivation and discipline**	All management staff members are challenged and motivated using a systematized approach with regularly scheduled follow-up. Staff members are disciplined, if necessary, in a proactive and positive manner, using a written success plan and review.	_____
18. **Sales management**	Sales department performance is monitored daily. The executive director meets weekly with the marketing and sales staff to review and strategize on the closure of all hot leads.	_____
19. **Marketing**	All staff members are fully informed and rehearsed quarterly on their role in marketing the community. Monthly training in all staff meetings emphasizes the importance of marketing.	_____

Category	Standard	Score
20. **Employees' files**	All employees' files are current and complete. All new employees are interviewed in person before hiring. Vacant positions are filled on a timely basis.	_____
21. **Job description and orientation**	Each employee has a current job description and employee handbook. Each employee has been thoroughly oriented to the job expectations and resident relations. Supporting documentation for the orientation is in each employee's file and is current. Executive director responsibility checklist is used consistently. (See Appendix D.)	_____
22. **Performance appraisal process**	All employees understand the appraisal process and have an annual appraisal before receiving any merit increase.	_____
23. **Merit increase process**	All employees understand the merit increase process. Announcements of increases are made in a timely manner.	_____
24. **Employee opinion survey**	A high level of employee participation is achieved. Survey results are communicated to all employees, and plans for improvement are developed and implemented.	_____

Departmental score _____ Percent _____ Rating _____

▮▮▮▮ PROPERTY ACCOUNTING

Category	Standard	Score
1. **Rents**	All rents are current and agree with the lease. Ancillary and level of care (LOC) charges are tabulated for the prior month and included in the posted charges.	_____
2. **Billing**	Monthly billings are correctly prepared and released before the twenty-sixth of the month. Copies of bills and supporting documentation are properly filed.	_____
3. **Deposits**	Revenue collected is properly recorded.	_____
4. **Collections**	After the rent-due date specified in the lease, all uncollected balances are resolved and late charges are billed.	_____
5. **Approve invoices**	All invoices are validated with packing slip and statement and properly approved.	_____
6. **Payments**	All invoices are paid on a timely basis.	_____
7. **File invoices**	Checks and canceled invoices are filed properly and on a timely basis.	_____
8. **Labor Report**	A monthly recap of payroll by position compared to budget is prepared and forwarded to the corporate office on a timely basis.	_____
9. **Food cost**	The food cost report is accurately prepared and submitted on a timely basis.	_____
10. **Regulations**	The accounting staff understand all changes in local, state, and federal laws as they relate to wage and labor issues.	_____
11. **Benefits**	Monthly employee contributions are accurately calculated and withheld from paychecks.	_____
12. **Reconciliation**	All bank accounts are reconciled on a timely basis.	_____
13. **Transactions**	All transactions are properly documented, posted, and filed	_____
14. **Prepaid and accrual**	All prepaids and accruals are calculated, supported, and posted.	_____
15. **Month-end schedules**	All supporting month-end schedules are prepared and updated by the tenth of the month.	_____
16. **Monthly statements**	Profit and loss, rent roll, balance sheet and A/R statements are finalized by the tenth of the month.	_____
17. **Cash projections**	By the ninth of the month, cash projections are calculated for the remainder of the month and a check issued for the excess or a cash call requested from the owner.	_____
18. **Capital expenditures**	All capital expenditures are processed each month according to the capital expenditure procedure for the site.	_____

Departmental score _____ Percent _____ Rating _____

▰▰▰▰ HUMAN RESOURCES

Category	Standard	Score
1. **Interview process**	All applicants are provided an equal opportunity. All new employees are interviewed thoroughly, and documentation of reference checks is kept on file.	_____
2. **Hiring procedures**	The executive director interviews all final candidates and approves all hires.	_____
3. **I-9 verification**	No employee works more than three days without presenting proper I-9 identification. I-9 information is complete, current in compliance with federal law, and filed separately from the personnel file. Expiration dates on documents are tracked.	_____
4. **Deadline for orientation**	No employee works more than seven days without receiving a proper orientation.	_____
5. **Status change and W-4**	All employees on payroll have completed and authorized status change and W-4 forms.	_____
6. **Handbook**	Each employee's file contains the handbook's last page, signed by the employee and confirming the receipt of a handbook.	_____
7. **Employee files**	Employee files are audited annually. Each file has a completed and signed application. All personnel and payroll information is current and kept in a secure area. A separate file is maintained for employee benefits and other information that is not appropriate for a personnel file.	_____
8. **Benefits enrollment**	Benefits are clearly explained to all eligible employees, and employees are enrolled in a timely manner. The benefit plan is perceived as an added value and part of the total compensation.	_____
9. **Policy for resolving disputes**	All employees and management staff members understand the policy for resolving disputes.	_____
10. **Disciplinary procedures**	Disciplinary procedures are applied fairly and consistently. All managers, supervisors, and department heads are constructive when taking disciplinary action. Success plans for corrective action are used to improve performance. All disciplinary decisions are properly documented. There is a proper follow-up to disciplinary discussions.	_____
11. **Organizational chart**	The facility and corporate organizational charts are explained to new staff members in the orientation. Direct-line and dotted-line responsibilities are communicated where appropriate.	_____
12. **Labor notices**	All federal, state, and local labor notices are posted and updated as necessary.	_____
13. **Time clock**	All employees understand the time clock procedures. Employees who consistently punch in too early or punch out too late without authorization are disciplined.	_____
14. **Overtime**	All employees understand the overtime policy. Any overtime is approved in advance and in writing by the employee's supervisor.	_____
15. **Payroll**	The executive director reviews and initials all payroll printouts before they are submitted for processing	_____
16. **Company property**	Uniforms, keys, tools, manuals, etc., are all distributed with a property receipt form in the personnel file. Company property is returned on termination of employment.	_____
17. **Risk management**	All human resources staff understand and follow risk management procedures. They know the liability insurance carrier and follow reporting procedures. Shared risk agreements for elopement, falls, and skin breakdown are in place for appropriate assisted living and dementia care residents.	_____
18. **Unemployment compensation**	All terminations, whether voluntary or involuntary, are reported to the corporate office. Reports are reviewed for accuracy and filed appropriately.	_____
19. **Incident reports**	All employees are aware that injuries and incidents are to be reported to their supervisor immediately. In-house accident report, state report, and OSHA logs are completed as appropriate. OSHA reports are completed annually.	_____
20. **Workers' compensation**	All employees are aware of their rights under the Workers' Compensation Act. All supervisors are familiar with workers' compensation procedures and reporting.	_____

Category	Standard	Score
21. **Human resources reports**	Human resources monthly summary reports are completed and submitted to the management. Federal EEO-1 reports (for private employers who are subject to Title VII of the Civil Rights Act of 1964 who have 100 or more employees) are completed annually.	_____
22. **Employee opinion survey**	A high level of survey participation is achieved. Survey results are communicated to all employees. Plans for improvement are developed and implemented. Grievance procedures are maintained and consistently administered.	_____
23. **Performance appraisal process**	All employees understand the appraisal process and have an annual appraisal before receiving any merit increase.	_____
24. **Merit increase process**	All employees understand the merit increase process. Increases are announced in a timely manner.	_____
25. **Hourly wage plans**	The wage plan process is updated at least annually and completed in a timely manner for all hourly positions.	_____

Departmental score _____ **Percent** _____ **Rating** _____

▰▰▰ CONCIERGE

Category	Standard	Score
1. **Reception**	The concierge gives a warm, friendly, professional greeting to all who enter the community. The concierge staff have been trained on and routinely follow procedures outlined in the concierge manual.	_____
2. **Security**	All concierge staff members are trained in emergency response. All are knowledgeable in the use of security systems. All visitors are sanitized, screened for current illness and contact tracing and offered PPE where needed.	_____
3. **Incident reports**	Incident reports are maintained and copies distributed to appropriate management staff. The log book is maintained in a complete, professional, and informative manner.	_____
4. **"I'm OK" procedure**	The resident "I'm OK" list is carefully completed every day, and follow-ups are made in a timely manner.	_____
5. **Emergency contacts**	An up-to-date emergency contact list is maintained, containing emergency phone numbers of all management staff and vendors.	_____
6. **Work orders**	Work orders and transportation requests are completed and properly distributed to the appropriate department head.	_____
7. **Night staff**	Night concierge staff are used to the maximum potential. Projects are scheduled and completed to ensure maximum productivity on this shift.	_____
8. **Notification**	A log is kept of all packages delivered to the front desk, and residents are notified of their arrival.	_____
9. **Guest rooms**	All guest room check-ins and check-outs are properly handled.	_____
10. **Marketing**	All concierge staff members are fully informed and rehearsed in their role in marketing the community.	_____
11. **Resources**	A directory of local area resources is maintained and updated, including transportation, emergency services, entertainment, hotels and restaurants, and recreational and exercise facilities to serve the needs of residents and their guests off-site.	_____

Departmental score _____ **Percent** _____ **Rating** _____

RESIDENT RELATIONS

Category	Standard	Score
1. **Goals and objectives**	All departmental prior-period goals and objectives are met.	_____
2. **Budget**	The department consistently meets its budgetary guidelines.	_____
3. **Programming manual**	The programming manual is current and is used as a reference and training tool.	_____
4. **Job description and orientation**	Each staff member has a current job description and employee handbook. Each has been thoroughly oriented and evaluated with an appropriate technical skills supplement.	_____
5. **Training**	Within the department, staff members are cross-trained.	_____
6. **New residents' orientation**	Each new resident receives a formal orientation. A support group is formed to address move-in concerns and relocation trauma. Each resident receives a copy of the resident handbook and reviews its contents. The move-in coordinator meets with each resident and family on the day of move-in to greet and assist where needed. Within twenty-four hours of move-in, the functions of apartment equipment are reviewed with the resident, and the resident is given a building tour. The resident's adjustment to living in the community is monitored, and assistance is provided as needed.	_____
7. **Communication with residents**	The facility has an organized and consistent way of communicating with residents. Resident meetings are held monthly. Minutes of council meetings and resident meetings are kept on file and current.	_____
8. **Handling concerns**	All residents' concerns are handled in an efficient and timely manner. Concerns are communicated to management staff in writing.	_____
9. **Resident survey**	The department scored well on the resident opinion survey. There is a written plan of corrective action for any negative responses.	_____
10. **Events**	Staff work closely with the marketing department on marketing events and functions to promote the community.	_____
11. **Marketing**	All staff members are fully informed and rehearsed in their role in marketing the community.	_____
12. **Emergency call system**	The emergency call system is checked quarterly. Calls are answered promptly, and all activations of the call system are properly documented in the log book.	_____
13. **Library**	The library and all reading areas have a current and accurate inventory of books. Only hardcover books are on display in public areas. All magazines and newspaper subscriptions are kept current, organized, and orderly.	_____
14. **Volunteers**	Volunteers are solicited to aid with community projects. An annual social event is held to recognize volunteers, and gifts are given at this event. Residents are educated about opportunities to volunteer in the outside community.	_____
15. **Counseling move-outs**	The staff work with families to handle residents who have special needs and problems. When applicable, they recommend a move to a greater level of care. Move-out assistance and a move-out package are provided to families.	_____

Departmental score _____ **Percent** _____ **Rating** _____

TRANSPORTATION

Category	Standard	Score
1. **Budget**	The department consistently meets its budgetary guidelines.	_____
2. **Maintenance**	Vehicles are in safe working order. They are regularly maintained, cleaned, and waxed. A daily checklist is used to document deficiencies. Vehicle fire extinguisher inspection tag is current.	_____
3. **Transportation**	All driving request forms are correctly completed. The resident is contacted personally on the day the request is made, and all requests are met.	_____

Category	Standard	Score
4. **Service**	The driver maintains a record of punctuality, and no unscheduled drop-offs and pick-ups are made.	_____
5. **Schedule**	A monthly transportation schedule is issued to the residents and strictly adhered to. Transportation requests outside scheduled times are referred to Uber, Lyft, or non-emergency medical transportation resources.	_____
6. **Records**	Transportation employees' driving records are verified in written form with the state in accordance with OSHA rules, with a copy to the insurance company. The drivers are considered safe drivers by the residents.	_____
7. **Assistance**	Residents receive assistance in getting into and out of all vehicles, and separately with their parcels when required.	_____
8. **Deliveries**	Resident-requested deliveries are taken to their rooms, and delivery is arranged at convenient times that do not conflict with the driving schedules.	_____
9. **Safety**	The driver makes sure that residents use seatbelts in all vehicles at all times and is aware of individual residents' needs, such as assistance in walking. The driver reports noticeable changes in residents' functioning to the director of resident relations.	_____
10. **Accidents**	The driver knows how to handle an accident or emergency situation. Reporting procedures are followed at all times.	_____

Departmental score _____   **Percent** _____   **Rating** _____

■ ACTIVITIES/ENRICHMENT

Category	Standard	Score
1. **Budget**	The department consistently meets its budgetary guidelines.	_____
2. **Resident survey**	The activity department scored well on the resident opinion survey. There is a written plan of corrective action for any negative responses.	_____
3. **Files**	An activities resource file is kept and updated.	_____
4. **Participation**	Programs maximize resident participation. Residents are motivated and encouraged to attend events and programs whenever possible. Activities are designed to be failure-free.	_____
5. **Newsletters**	A newsletter and/or calendar of events are issued each month. They are of good quality and legible for older adults, and can be used as marketing tools. Monthly reminders of special events are sent to all family members.	_____
6. **Bulletin boards**	The facility is decorated for special events and holidays. Decorations are tasteful and adult-oriented. Bulletin boards are changed monthly; they reflect a theme and are attractive and current.	_____
7. **Supplies**	The department has all necessary equipment and supplies, properly maintained, stored, labeled, and inventoried.	_____
8. **Activity setup**	There is a variety of common spaces for the scope of activities, such as a card room, exercise room, bar or lounge, and library. These are properly set up with assistance from housekeeping and food and beverage at least thirty minutes before an event.	_____
9. **Leisure interests**	All residents have had leisure interest interviews. The interview information is used to program activities. Residents are individually invited to activities in which they have expressed interest.	_____
10. **Planning**	All major activities or events are planned and budgeted at least sixty days in advance, using a function sheet distributed to the management staff. Monthly programming includes a variety of therapeutic environments.	_____
11. **Continuing education**	Programs for the continuing education of the residents are well received, and marketing prospects are involved in the program.	_____

Category	Standard	Score
12. **Transportation**	Transportation for all resident functions is arranged in advance. Where possible, costs are billed appropriately to resident accounts.	_____
13. **Measurement**	Residents are regularly surveyed for input and opinions on programs and classes. Participant numbers are measured, statistics are kept, and activities are planned to encourage optimal involvement.	_____
14. **Marketing**	All activity staff members are fully informed and rehearsed in their role in marketing the community. They work closely with the marketing department on events and functions to promote the community. They are aware of publicity possibilities.	_____

Departmental score _____ Percent _____ Rating _____

▓▓▓▓ FOOD AND BEVERAGE

Category	Standard	Score
1. **Goals and objectives**	All departmental prior-period goals and objectives are met.	_____
2. **Budget**	The department consistently meets its budgetary guidelines.	_____
3. **Food and beverage manual**	A copy of the food and beverage manual is kept in the chef's office. All managers have a working knowledge of all concepts, procedures, and directives.	_____
4. **Health department**	Health department inspection records are kept on file in the chef's office. Department scores are above 90 percent on all inspections. All kitchen staff members have current food-handler permits.	_____
5. **Job description**	Each food and beverage employee has a current job description that outlines all aspects of the daily responsibilities and accepted standards of performance.	_____
6. **Schedules**	All staff schedules are prepared, calculated in FTEs, and posted at least one week in advance. Schedules are approved by the executive director and strictly comply with labor budget. Any overtime is approved in writing by the executive director.	_____
7. **Inventory of food**	The chef and the property accountant take physical inventory of the storeroom and freezer on the last day of the month (or the next working day when applicable). Perpetual inventory from the daily food-cost report (book value) and physical count are within 5 percent of each other.	_____
8. **Maintenance of equipment**	All kitchen equipment is maintained in working order. Work orders are completed for any equipment in need of maintenance.	_____
9. **Uniforms**	Cooks and utility workers wear uniforms that are clean and complete.	_____
10. **Sanitation**	All cooks, prep people, and utility workers are completely trained using the company sanitation program and video. Employees are retrained, tested, and monitored on a quarterly basis as directed by the corporate office.	
	All cooks, prep staff, and utility workers complete daily sanitation side-work task sheets to assist in maintaining the health and sanitation of food products and the kitchen environment. These are distributed by the manager and kept on file in the food service office.	
	All equipment, such as walk-in and reach-in coolers and freezers, cooking equipment, and food-processing equipment (mixers, slicers, etc.), has a daily or weekly sanitation plan that specifies how and where food is to be stored, cooked, and held. All sanitation procedures are detailed in task sheets.	
	All cooks, prep staff, and utility workers are trained by managers in the correct health and sanitation procedures for all equipment and procedures before task sheets are distributed.	_____
11. **Warewashing**	The dishwasher is cleaned and maintained regularly. All cookware is cleaned thoroughly and not allowed to soak overnight. All china and glassware is checked for chips and cracks and taken out of service as needed. Dishwasher chemical levels and water temperature are checked at frequent intervals during the day. The machine is drained and cleaned after each meal.	_____

Category	Standard	Score
12. **Resident survey**	The kitchen scored well on the resident opinion survey. There is a written plan of corrective action for any negative responses.	_____
13. **Menu planning**	Menus are planned thirty days in advance and sent to the corporate office for review. Each meal includes one health-smart entrée and dessert.	
	The chef reasonably accommodates residents with special dietary needs.	
	The menu includes one special food and beverage event and at least two theme meals per month.	_____
14. **Purchasing plan**	Weekly purchasing plans precede all orders. All high-cost items, such as fish and meat, are put out to bid and ordered at the most competitive price. A purchasing plan with all pertinent information is kept visible in the food service office to be used when receiving products.	_____
15. **Production plan**	Production plans are coordinated with the purchasing plan and menu, and explicit instructions are given to all food service employees involved with daily production in the kitchen. Production plans are issued on a weekly basis so that staff members can work on production several days in advance of need. All production and purchasing plans are kept on file. Clear, simple, standard recipes accompany the production plan where applicable.	_____
16. **Reports**	Receiving, payroll, food-cost analysis, requisitions, and other reports are completed on a daily basis.	_____
17. **Implementation**	All food is served at the correct temperature: hot food on hot plates covered with plate covers, and cold food on cold plates.	
	Plates are designed to have color, texture, and variety. Each plate is garnished.	
	Room service meals are always timely and appetizing. All trays, dishes, and glassware are retrieved at the end of each shift. Dietary preferences are maintained for all active residents.	_____
18. **Banquets**	The cost of all banquets is estimated in advance of commitment to ensure that the profit margin is met.	_____
19. **Storage**	All food storage, both dry and refrigerated, is organized to ensure that like items are stored together; cross-contamination does not occur; products are appropriately covered, rotated, dated, and priced; and no food product is stored on the floor.	_____
20. **Resident relations**	Staff members routinely visit with residents in the dining room, solicit input from residents, and make every effort to implement suggestions within budgetary limitations.	_____
21. **Marketing**	All kitchen staff members are fully informed and rehearsed in their role in marketing the community.	_____

Departmental score _____ Percent _____ Rating _____

▃▃▃▃ DINING ROOM

Category	Standard	Score
1. **Goals and objectives**	All departmental prior-period goals and objectives are met.	_____
2. **Budget**	All supervisors fully understand how to follow the budget in hiring, staffing, and purchasing operating supplies and revenue. Monthly labor costs are consistently in line with the budget.	_____
3. **Food and beverage manual**	All managers have a working knowledge of all concepts, procedures, and directives in the food and beverage manual.	_____
4. **Job description and orientation**	Each dining room staff member has a current job description and employee handbook. Each has been thoroughly oriented to the job expectations and resident relations.	_____

Category	Standard	Score
5. **Sanitation**	All dining room staff members are completely trained in proper sanitation practices. Employees are retrained, tested, and monitored on a quarterly basis.	_____
6. **Uniforms**	All servers on the floor area wear uniforms that are clean and complete. Grooming standards are enforced as part of the uniform. Name tags are always worn.	_____
7. **Work schedules**	All staff schedules are prepared and posted at least one week in advance. Schedules are approved by the executive director and comply with the labor budget. All overtime is first approved by the department head in writing.	_____
8. **Function sheets**	Each day, the chef and the dining room manager review the function sheets for that day and the following day. Equipment lists and special side-work assignments accompany the function sheets.	_____
9. **Side work and dining room maintenance**	Each server receives a task sheet, specifying task completion times, during the scheduled shift. All employees are checked out by their managers or shift supervisors before the end of the shift. The manager and the employee sign off for the work completed each day.	_____
10. **Linen control**	All linen is counted and sorted nightly. An inventory is prepared for any laundry sent to an outside laundry service. All deliveries are counted to verify the delivery receipt.	_____
11. **Breakage control**	All broken or chipped items are accounted for daily. Chipped china is retained for reimbursement from the china company.	_____
12. **Inventory**	Quarterly inventories of china, glass, silverware, and linen are sent to the corporate office. Operational losses do not exceed 25 percent annually.	_____
13. **Walk-through**	The manager walks through the dining room before opening and after closing each meal period to check for and correct any deficiencies.	_____
14. **Premeal meetings**	Daily meetings are held to discuss the menu with the manager, chef, and servers. Servers are aware of menu choices and specials.	_____
15. **Reservations**	Dinner reservations are reconfirmed with each resident by a return phone call from the shift supervisor. The reservation policy is enforced to ensure that service standards are consistently met.	_____
16. **Theme or event meals**	The food and beverage department plans and provides at least two theme meals and one food and beverage event per month. The dining room manager and staff work closely with the chef to provide a style of service geared to the theme or event, in addition to decorations, displays, costumes, and music.	_____
17. **Continental breakfast**	The continental breakfast selection is always appealing, abundant, fresh, and neat. Refills are offered on coffee. Tables are cleared and reset immediately, and trays of dirty dishes are quickly removed to the kitchen.	_____
18. **Resident survey**	The dining room staff scored well on the resident opinion survey. There is a written plan of corrective action for any negative responses.	_____
19. **Food and beverage meetings**	The executive director, chef, and dining room manager meet weekly. Minutes of these meetings are kept on file.	_____
20. **Reports**	Food checks, check-control sheets, meal count summary, payroll summary, banquet and any other function billings, and food and equipment pars and requisitions are completed daily.	_____
21. **Motivation**	The supervisor motivates the staff through incentives to achieve better service, less absenteeism, and lower breakage and loss rates.	_____
22. **Marketing**	All dining room staff members are fully informed and rehearsed in their roles in marketing the community.	_____

Departmental score _____ **Percent** _____ **Rating** _____

▰▰▰▰ HOUSEKEEPING AND LAUNDRY

Category	Standard	Score
1. **Goals and objectives**	All departmental prior-period goals and objectives are met.	_____
2. **Budget**	The department consistently meets its budgetary guidelines.	_____
3. **Ancillary revenue**	Ancillary revenue is at or above budget. All staff members are fully aware of what work is included in the service fee and what may be charged to residents. Every effort is made to maximize this source of revenue.	_____
4. **Job description and orientation**	Each housekeeping staff member has a current job description and employee handbook. Each has been thoroughly oriented to the job expectations, infection control and resident relations.	_____
5. **Training**	A training program is in place to provide employees with professional development and growth within their position.	_____
6. **Staff meetings**	Monthly staff meetings are held to discuss issues pertaining to the department and to solicit input from all department members. Daily briefing sessions are held with all members before beginning the day's schedule.	_____
7. **Master plan**	A current written master plan is consistently followed for cleaning the entire property.	_____
8. **Tasking plan**	All staff members consistently follow task lists for apartment cleaning and can communicate the limits of their services to residents when asked.	_____
9. **Work schedules**	The staff schedule is planned and posted at least one week in advance. Work schedules are approved by the executive director and strictly comply with the labor budget. Any overtime is approved in writing.	_____
10. **Cleaning schedules**	Schedules and responsibilities for cleaning all apartments and common areas are maintained and posted.	_____
11. **Nonresident apartments**	All nonresident apartments, including vacant, guest, and model and marketing units, are scheduled for regular cleaning. The executive director receives a monthly status report on all vacant apartments, whether leased or not.	_____
12. **Furnishings**	Cleaning schedules are maintained for all furnishings, fixtures, and equipment in common areas and back-of-the-house areas.	_____
13. **Cleaning log**	All housekeeping services chargeable to residents are documented (by resident, apartment, date, and time) by end of each shift.	_____
14. **Equipment manuals**	Operating and service manuals and all warranty information for equipment are on file and accessible.	_____
15. **Service contracts**	All current service contracts are on file and accessible. Each service contract has at least two competitive bids on file and is reviewed annually.	_____
16. **Vendor accounts**	A current ledger is kept of all vendor accounts, outside contractors, and technicians, by service area and contact person.	_____
17. **Safety**	OSHA regulations are kept on file and posted. A record of continuing education on chemical use is kept for each employee.	_____
18. **Deliveries and inventory**	Written procedures are followed for the check-in and security of all deliveries. All supplies are inventoried quarterly and stored in a secure area.	_____
19. **Uniforms**	All staff members wear uniforms that are clean and complete.	_____
20. **Key control**	Keys are checked out to housekeepers only for the specific units for which they have responsibility. Master keys do not leave the building. Keys are duplicated only with the approval of the executive director.	_____
21. **Tools and equipment**	All facility tools and movable equipment are marked with facility identification and inventoried.	_____
22. **Storage of chemicals**	All chemicals are properly inventoried, stored, and labeled. Staff members are fully trained in safely refilling self-dispensing chemicals. An inventory of and emergency procedures for each chemical are kept on file and accessible.	_____

Category	Standard	Score
23. **Hazardous waste**	All staff members are fully informed regarding infection control and the disposal of hazardous waste.	_____
24. **Separation of laundry**	Clean linen and dirty linen areas are kept separate and maintained to ensure adequate supplies of linens in good condition.	_____
25. **Laundry training**	Staff members are trained in the correct and safe use of all laundry equipment. Training includes the proper amounts of detergents and chemicals to be used and the checking of water temperature on a daily basis to ensure compliance with all regulations.	_____
26. **Laundry inventory**	A written inventory is used and followed to ensure adequate supplies of linens that are in good condition.	_____
27. **Laundry contract**	Laundry sent to an outside laundry service is counted or weighed before being sent out and again on delivery to confirm proper billing and control.	_____
28. **Identification of laundry**	All linens are clearly marked with identification, whether the items are processed internally or externally.	_____
29. **Marketing**	All housekeeping staff members are fully informed and rehearsed in their role in marketing the community.	_____
30. **Resident relations**	All housekeeping staff members understand the importance of alerting the management to changes in a resident's health or any resident dissatisfaction. Housekeepers understand their role in promoting a positive environment within the community and are solution-oriented.	_____
31. **Resident survey**	The department scored well on the resident opinion survey. There is a written plan of corrective action for any negative responses.	_____

Departmental score _____   **Percent** _____   **Rating** _____

ENGINEERING/MAINTENANCE

Category	Standard	Score
1. **Goals and objectives**	All departmental prior-period goals and objectives are met.	_____
2. **Budget**	The department consistently meets its budgetary guidelines.	_____
3. **Job description and orientation**	Each maintenance staff member has a current job description and employee handbook. All current staff members and new hires have passed the maintenance skills test. Each staff member has been thoroughly oriented to the job expectations and resident relations.	_____
4. **Training**	A training program is in place to provide career development for employees.	_____
5. **Work orders**	Work-order procedures are followed. Receipt and timing of work are confirmed with each resident within twenty-four hours of the order.	_____
6. **Ancillary charges**	Ancillary revenue is at or above budget. All work orders are coded as included or billable to the resident. All billable work is confirmed with the resident beforehand. Every effort is made to maximize this source of revenue.	_____
7. **Equipment manuals**	Operating and service manuals for all major and minor equipment are kept on file and accessible. All warranty information, sales receipts, and registration cards are properly filed or mailed to the manufacturer, and copies are accessible.	_____
8. **Service contracts**	Copies of all current service contracts are kept on file and accessible. All service contracts have at least two competitive bids on file and are reviewed annually. Certificates of insurance are updated as they expire. A current ledger is maintained to list all service contracts with a summary of service, pricing including off-peak hour premiums, expiry date, and contact person.	_____

Category	Standard	Score
9. **Vendor contracts**	A current ledger is kept of all vendor accounts, outside contractors, and technicians, by service area and contact person.	_____
10. **Preventive maintenance**	A current, written preventive maintenance plan is developed and implemented according to company policy, insurance company, and manufacturer instructions. (See exhibit 13.1.)	_____
11. **Service log**	Service logs are kept for all maintenance work, by location, date, time, materials, and apartment or service area. Service logs are updated at the end of each shift.	_____
12. **Safety**	OSHA regulations are kept on file and posted. A record of drills and safety training is kept for all employees.	_____
13. **Risk management**	The facility is in full compliance with life safety, fire marshal, elevator, and health department surveys, or a plan of corrective action exists. The facility is in compliance with safety and liability consultant reports, or a plan of corrective action exists.	_____
14. **Emergency procedures**	All staff are fully aware of their role in the event of an emergency. The emergency generator is tested monthly. A fire incident log is maintained. Periodic fire drills are held and logged.	_____
15. **Deliveries and inventory**	Written procedures are followed for the check-in and security of all deliveries. All supplies are inventoried quarterly and stored in a secure area.	_____
16. **Uniforms**	All staff members wear uniforms that are clean and complete.	_____
17. **Key control**	A written key-control policy is in place and followed. Master keys do not leave the building. Residents' families do not hold duplicate keys.	_____
18. **Tools and equipment**	All facility tools and movable equipment are marked with facility identification and inventoried.	_____
19. **Resident survey**	The department scored well on the resident opinion survey. There is a written plan of corrective action for any negative responses.	_____
20. **Organization**	Engineering files and blueprints or drawings are properly maintained.	_____
21. **Conservation**	An energy management and conservation plan is in use for facility mechanical operations.	_____
22. **Marketing**	All maintenance staff members are fully informed and rehearsed in their role in marketing the community.	_____

Departmental score _____ Percent _____ Rating _____

■ SALES AND MARKETING

Category	Standard	Score
1. **Budget**	The department consistently meets its budgetary guidelines, including rental allowances (if any).	_____
2. **Occupancy**	The department meets occupancy and move-in projections.	_____
3. **Marketing plan**	The department has and follows a current sales and marketing plan.	_____
4. **Job description**	Each marketing staff member has a current job description and an employee handbook.	_____
5. **Training**	The sales and marketing director has conducted a training needs assessment with input from the sales staff. A training plan is in place, and organized training events are held at least monthly.	_____
6. **Reports**	All sales and marketing reports are timely, accurate, and complete.	_____
7. **Collateral**	The department has an inventory of all collateral material and supplies.	_____
8. **Revenue**	Monthly fee increases on turnover units are managed to maximize revenue.	_____

Category	Standard	Score
9. **Communication**	Weekly departmental hot-lead meetings are conducted with the executive director present. Weekly hot-lead meetings are conducted with individual sales representatives.	_____
10. **Sales**	The sales director shadows each sales representative monthly to determine whether he or she uses relationship selling techniques effectively.	_____
11. **Advertising**	A current clipping file of competitors' ads and weblinks is kept. The lead-tracking system is current and complete. Each lead is assigned a specific response category.	_____
12. **Referrals**	The sales staff works with current residents and families to solicit referrals.	_____
13. **Follow-up of leads**	A lead-tickler system is used to schedule follow-up of leads. All active leads are contacted at least monthly.	_____
14. **Outreach**	The community outreach plan is implemented by all members of the marketing department.	_____
15. **Publicity**	Publicity opportunities are proactively identified and pursued. Press releases featuring newsworthy events at the facility are submitted to local newspapers at least quarterly.	_____
16. **Competition**	The department has a current (six months or less) comparative market analysis of the competition. The competition has been mystery-shopped within the last six months.	_____
17. **Wait list**	The department consistently meets goals for wait-list deposits.	_____
18. **Event leads**	Leads are followed up during and after all events.	_____
19. **Phone-outs**	The department consistently meets phone-out goals, including call-to-appointment conversion ratios and phone-out targets by lead classification.	_____
20. **Appointments**	The department consistently meets appointment goals, including appointment-to-sale conversion ratios and appointments-kept goals.	_____
21. **Operations**	The operations staff is fully informed about the role they play in marketing and incorporated into the tour process.	_____
22. **Move-ins**	New leases are passed to the move-in coordinator to minimize cancellations. "Not ready yet" cancellations are minimized. The average move-in time is less than sixty days.	_____
23. **Resident survey**	The marketing staff scored well on the resident opinion survey. There is a written plan of corrective action for any negative responses.	_____

Departmental score _____ **Percent** _____ **Rating** _____

▩▩▩ MOVE-IN COORDINATOR

Category	Standard	Score
1. **Initial contact**	The move-in coordinator works closely with the marketing department to develop relationships with prospects. Each prospect is contacted within one week of signing the residency agreement.	_____
2. **Ongoing contact**	Consistent (weekly) contact is maintained with future residents. Effective communication exists, with approval of family and friends.	_____
3. **Communication**	The move-in coordinator communicates the special needs and concerns of future residents with department heads well in advance of move-in dates.	_____
4. **Accelerating move-in**	The move-in coordinator is successful at maneuvering residents to move into the community sooner than anticipated (within sixty days).	_____
5. **Welcome package**	Correspondence (welcome kit, etc.) is distributed before move-in. Information is current and accurate. The move-in checklist is complete and on file for each new resident before move-in.	_____
6. **Transition**	The move-in coordinator provides support to new residents through a formal orientation program.	_____

Category	Standard	Score
7. **Resources**	The move-in coordinator maintains a file on moving companies, house-sale services, realtors, antique appraisers, decorating services, and other resources useful in expediting move-ins.	_____
8. **Move-in manual**	The move-in coordinator follows the move-in manual and networks with other move-in coordinators within the company.	_____

Departmental score _____ **Percent** _____ **Rating** _____

▰▰▰▰ PERSONAL CARE

Category	Standard	Score
1. **Budget**	The department consistently meets its budgetary guidelines.	_____
2. **Regulations**	State regulations are kept on file. All staff members understand their role and follow these regulations.	_____
3. **License**	The facility's license is posted and current. All staff members are properly licensed and have a supporting documentation in their personnel files.	_____
4. **State surveys**	Copies of state licensure inspections are kept on file and posted where required.	_____
5. **Policy and procedures**	The department has a current policy and procedures manual on hand.	_____
6. **Resident survey**	The assisted living department scored well on the resident opinion survey. There is a written plan of corrective action for any negative responses.	_____
7. **Job description and orientation**	Each staff member has a current job description and an employee handbook. Each has been fully oriented to the job expectations and resident relations.	_____
8. **Training and education**	All staff members are appropriately trained for their jobs using a monthly training plan developed by the personal care director based on the results of a needs assessment and regulatory requirements. In-service training documentation is maintained for each employee.	_____
9. **Work schedules**	Staff schedules are planned and posted in advance. Work schedules are approved by the executive director and strictly comply with the labor budget.	_____
10. **CPR**	All staff members have current and valid CPR certification and understand the company's resuscitation policy and emergency procedures. A current copy of each certification is kept on file.	_____
11. **Staff medical testing**	All staff members have documentation of a current tuberculosis test on file. The community offers the option of a hepatitis B series.	_____
12. **Residents' files**	All residents' files are organized, confidential, and up to date.	_____
13. **Records**	Records and logs for events and incidents are current and complete and can be passed from shift to shift. Any serious incidents are reported to the insurance carrier.	_____
14. **Incident reports**	All incident reports are investigated thoroughly, and any suspected neglect or abuse is reported to the executive director.	_____
15. **Supervision**	The management routinely visits all residents to ensure that the personal care plan is consistently implemented. Nurse management visits at-risk residents daily and follows up on any need to reassess resident service plans.	_____
16. **Utilization review**	The staff meets to discuss each resident's needs and problems. These needs are properly documented and, where appropriate, discussed with the resident's family.	_____
17. **Family conferences**	Staff members hold quarterly conferences with family members to update them on the residents' condition.	_____
18. **Reception**	All visitors and guests in the assisted living unit are greeted immediately and welcomed. A log is kept of all traffic in and out of the unit.	_____

Category	Standard	Score
19. **Cleanliness**	The assisted living common areas and apartments are clean and odor free.	_____
20. **Uniforms**	All staff members wear uniforms that are clean and complete.	_____
21. **Equipment and supplies**	The department has all necessary equipment and supplies. These are properly marked with the community identification and inventoried.	_____
22. **Meals**	All meals are served promptly, and the dining area is kept immaculate.	_____
23. **Special diets**	Special diet orders appropriate for the resident's needs are accommodated.	_____
24. **Medications**	All medications taken by residents are documented in the resident's file according to prescribing physician, medication, dosage, and expiration date (where appropriate). Prescription medications and treatments are administered strictly according to physician's orders.	_____
25. **Wellness program**	Ongoing wellness programs and health checks are provided to residents in assisted living and independent apartments.	_____
26. **Quality improvement plan**	A formal written quality improvement plan is in place and based upon resident outcomes to monitor performance to ensure excellence and detect areas of deficiency.	_____
27. **Marketing**	All personal care staff members are fully informed and rehearsed in their role in marketing the community.	_____
28. **Outside vendors**	Agreements with home health, private duty, and hospice organizations are current and include a copy of the vendor's certificate of insurance for each. Vendor reports and schedules are maintained for the consultant pharmacist, registered dietician, nurse consultant, etc.	_____
29. **Privacy**	HIPAA regulations are followed to protect residents' privacy. HIPAA agreements are current for each appropriate professional associate.	_____

Departmental score _____   **Percent** _____   **Rating** _____

SUMMARY AND TOTAL

Department	Score	Percent	Rating	Plan of correction
Executive director	_____/240	_____	_____	_____
Property accounting	_____/180	_____	_____	_____
Human resources	_____/250	_____	_____	_____
Concierge	_____/110	_____	_____	_____
Resident relations	_____/150	_____	_____	_____
Transportation	_____/100	_____	_____	_____
Activities and enrichment	_____/140	_____	_____	_____
Food and beverage	_____/210	_____	_____	_____
Dining room	_____/220	_____	_____	_____
Housekeeping and laundry	_____/310	_____	_____	_____
Engineering and maintenance	_____/220	_____	_____	_____
Sales and marketing	_____/230	_____	_____	_____
Move-in coordinator	_____/ 80	_____	_____	_____
Personal care	_____/290	_____	_____	_____
Total property	_____**/2,730**	_____	_____	_____

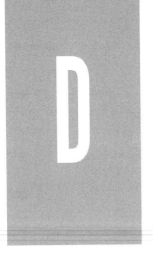

Executive Director Responsibilities

DAILY

- Arrive on site and police parking lot and grounds for trash.
- Check in with concierge and review log of all visitors overnight and enforce prescreening procedures daily.
- Visit kitchen to ensure appropriate staffing and meal prep for breakfast and lunch.
- Visit nursing station and read logbook from overnight. Review and sign any incident reports, review residents on alert charting.
- Ensure appropriate staff is on site and discuss any call-offs or shortages. Review direct care staffing schedule. Review all behavioral and fall prevention issues are addressed.
- Visit with residents at breakfast and sit and have coffee with them. Assist with meal service as needed and refresh beverages.
- Perform rounds throughout the building and extend morning greetings to all staff, residents, and visitors after breakfast.
- Prepare or fill out flash (daily status) report for daily stand-up.
- Visit units to be moved into today to verify ready status.
- Follow up on issues raised during stand-up that affect today's operations.
- Review any maintenance issues that arose overnight and respond.
- Review marketing activity and assign today's goals for follow-ups.
- Review activities for the day for planning, materials, participation.
- Review and respond to any emails pertaining to care delivery and daily operations.
- Collect messages and prioritize according to importance.
- Set up appointments as needed.
- Review and approve invoices as they are coded and verified by Business Office Manager.
- Visit kitchen to verify meal preparations for lunch and dinner.
- Perform rounds throughout the building and touch base with all staff, residents, and visitors after lunch.
- Visit nursing station at shift change to verify adequate staffing and personally approve all overtime hours in advance.
- Review reporting requirements and schedule time for completion.
- Work on "To Do" items from SWOT (see appendix A) that achieve community objectives.
- Work on any crisis issues that will impact priority list.

- Return all phone calls and emails.
- Make an appearance during all marketing tours, verify that the building presents well.
- Perform rounds throughout the building and touch base with all staff, residents, and visitors after dinner.
- Call in each day on weekends to check on operations and manager on duty.

WEEKLY

- Meet with all department heads as a group. Prepare and distribute the agenda a day prior.
- Meet with department heads individually. Each department head should bring their own agenda.
- Meet with family members. Seek out families as they come in each time and tell them something good about their loved one.
- Research invoices in question and discuss issues with vendors.
- Interview employment applicants after they have been screened. Place ads for recruitment.
- Review staff terminations and exit interview statements. Download turnover report from payroll provider.
- Review accounts receivable and take next steps for collections.
- Review weekly marketing reports for accuracy and set performance goals for marketing director.
- Review new hires to comply with budget and HR process in the hire.
- Review event planning schedule and progress to date.
- Review and assist with reportable resident incidents. Create and follow up on all Plans of Correction, implement preventive interventions.
- Review infection control plan and related reporting and follow up with county and state agencies.
- Attend any resident memorial services.
- Send handwritten thank-you notes for any referrals.
- Check Google reviews and encourage residents and staff to post positive reviews.
- Review all hot leads and propose closing strategies. Approve any discounts or waived fees.
- Review all storage areas and stairwells to remove any hazardous items.
- Check all mechanical rooms for leaks, storage of combustibles and hazardous materials.
- Stock treats in employee refrigerator/lounge area.
- Evaluate fall frequency and prevention plan for all vulnerable residents.
- Review payroll summary and OT prior to sending for processing.

MONTHLY

- Review monthly draft Profit and Loss Statement (P&L) and produce variance report.
- Review balance sheet and ensure that bank account balances are sufficient for at least two payroll cycles.
- Review marketing results and metrics.
- Review Accounts Receivable (A/R) report and summarize collection efforts to date on each. Meet with families regarding shortage of funds and collections.
- Review Accounts Payable (A/P) reports to determine if any invoices are accumulating unpaid.
- Review all major accounts to ensure the billings have been received and approved no later than the 10th of each month.
- Review utility bills for any anomalies—water usage will show leaks or open lines.
- Review SWOT to ensure objectives are being advanced and people held accountable (see Appendix A).
- Review training logs to ensure that all employees are receiving mandatory and monthly training.
- Review payroll journals and labor analysis each pay period.
- Review critical building systems—HVAC, fire, water, trash, kitchen equipment, hood condition, landscaping, winter protection.
- Conduct safety committee meeting with agenda and keep notes.
- Conduct family fireside chat with agenda and keep notes for follow-up.
- Formal system of communication is repeated (weekly department heads, monthly all staff, monthly families).

- Review level of care residents receive and revise billing to families.
- Review training plan has been achieved each month.
- Attend monthly networking meeting to maintain visibility within marketplace.
- Review monthly proposed move-outs to verify nothing can be done to accommodate resident remaining in the community.
- Inspect all kitchen coolers and freezers to ensure compliance with storage and labeling.
- Inspect all fire extinguishers to have current inspection date.
- Review narcotic logs.
- Review and recruit volunteers for activities and sitters.
- Attend monthly care plan meetings and ensure collaborative care report is kept current.
- Inspect all storage closets to control security of inventoried supplies, to include kitchen cold and dry storage.
- Review status on all rent-ready apartments. Goal is 90% or better rent-ready status on every vacant unit.
- Review monthly activity calendar to ensure standards are met to include: Cognitive, reminiscence, physical, long-term memory (LTM), short-term memory (STM), spiritual, and crafts.
- Participate in and lead one resident activity each month.
- Review residents due for rent increases and issue letters to families.

QUARTERLY

- Perform resident family survey and analyze results. Create and manage plan of correction with action steps.
- Perform employee survey and analyze results.
- Meet with family members.
- Review status on mock survey for each department head.
- Prepare and review Occupational Safety and Health Administration (OSHA) logs.
- Review status on all workers' compensation injuries and reserves. Personally contact preferred physician's office to discuss point of care issues.
- Review van checklist to ensure safety and operational integrity. Verify each licensed driver's background and status.
- Review all signage, interior and exterior, to ensure their appropriate and fresh appearance.
- Remove and replace all dead landscaping materials from property.
- Winterize all vulnerable outdoor water sources, then recharge in spring, checking for leaks.
- Review pharmacy reports and medication cart audits. Enforce destruction of discontinued medications according to policies and procedures.
- Review the price on every vacant unit to ensure maximum rent attainable on turned-over units and vacant in inventory. Ensure at least one rent-ready unit of each type is available for tours.
- Call to invite referral sources—paid and unpaid—to tour the community.
- Send EMS treats or donations to the ambulance corps.
- Reach out to ombudsman to keep them in the loop for behaviorally challenged residents and family issues.
- Ensure all staff are properly licensed with appropriate renewals. Dietary staff should all be safe-serve certified.
- Conduct resident food preference survey.
- Review status on preventive maintenance tracker.
- Review infection control practices, infection tracker, and training status of all caregiver staff.

ANNUALLY

- Review draft budget with each department head.
- Review capital expense needs with each department.
- Conduct competitor pricing evaluation.
- Conduct benefit and competitor hiring analysis.
- Conduct an annual employee file audit—I-9, TB, backgrounds, orientation, training.

- Conduct performance evaluations for all department heads, create individualized success plan. Calculate merit-based salary increases based upon goals achieved and market rates.
- Review all vendor contracts and renegotiate against competitive bids, remove all evergreen clauses for automatic renewal.
- Collect all insurance certificate from contract vendors with community named as additional insured.
- Renew operating license.
- Renew administrator/executive director license.
- Review all insurance applications for accuracy at each renewal.
- Respond to state survey issues within response deadlines with detailed plan of correction.
- Review facility emergency plan and contact book to ensure all information is current and accurate.
- Review all operations policy and procedures and educate all staff with any revisions.
- Review employee handbook and educate all staff with any revisions.
- Review rent roll and create system for rent increases each resident anniversary. Prepare notice of increase in base rents 60 days prior to responsible party.
- Invite the local fire chief to conduct a mock building evacuation to test response time and equipment placement.
- Review all cycle menus with dietician or dietary consultant for cost, caloric content, variety, product availability.
- Create vacation tracker for each department.
- Review preventive maintenance plan and revise as needed.
- Conduct departmental Operations audit (see Appendix C). Follow-up on any standards that may be out of compliance.
- Review and revise SWOT analysis to identify operational objectives for the next year.

Critical-Path Tasks
for Preopening

Task no.	Weeks before opening	Area	Task
1	48	Development	Review market feasibility and penetration
2	48	Development	Conduct competitive market analysis
3	48	Development	Develop product pricing and market positioning
4	48	Development	Review plans and evaluate operational efficiency
5	48	Development	Specify phone and emergency call system, and number, types, and locations of phones
6	48	Development	Review interior design plan and make recommendations
7	48	Development	Review unit mix and floor plans
8	48	Development	Review and evaluate administrative office plan
9	48	Development	Design and specify central kitchen equipment and layout
10	48	Development	Participate in design development
11	48	Development	Review construction drawings with architect
12	48	Development	Set up preopening accounting procedures
13	48	Development	Create financial projections: pro forma, development budget, 10-year projections, investment returns
14	48	Marketing	Write marketing plan
15	48	Marketing	Develop preopening marketing budget
16	48	Marketing	Hold concept meetings for logo, business papers, brochure
17	36	Development	Create resident lease agreement, application, and financial, medical, and other documents
18	36	Development	Develop preopening budget
19	36	Marketing	Gather media information for market area, create website and fact sheet information flyer
20	36	Marketing	Purchase business papers and #10 brochure
21	36	Marketing	Order and install computerized lead management system
22	24	Administration	Set up medical insurance carriers; collect information on each provider for distribution to employees

Task no.	Weeks before opening	Area	Task
23	24	Administration	Set up personnel files, to include application, job description, references, copies of licenses, orientation, I-9 form
24	24	Marketing	Order display boards for marketing office (floor plans and unit designs)
25	24	Marketing	Create social media campaign with Google Ads and other online resources
26	24	Marketing	Recruit marketing director
27	24	Operations	Recruit executive director
28	24	Operations	Develop resident handbook
29	24	Operations	Set up employee benefit plans
30	24	Operations	Develop employee manual, verify employment practices in current state
31	18	Administration	Develop hiring packages and benefits brochure
32	18	Administration	Set up payroll
33	18	Designer	Specify, receive, and set up model furniture
34	18	Development	Evaluate signage needs, create temporary information sign on construction site
35	18	Marketing	Prepare direct mail campaign
36	18	Marketing	Create concepts for online pay per click (PPC) advertising
37	18	Marketing	Finalize marketing budget and online advertising schedule
38	18	Marketing	Develop and implement community outreach plan
39	18	Marketing	Begin advertising
40	18	Marketing	Develop move-in coordination and resident orientation procedures
41	18	Marketing	Set up temporary sales office
42	18	Marketing	Drop first direct mail pieces
43	18	Operations	Obtain bids for vehicle leasing or purchase
44	16	Operations/marketing	Set up marketing reporting system
45	14	Marketing	Prepare press kit for information center opening
46	14	Operations/marketing	Review start-up budget and progress to date; evaluate and prioritize further needs
47	12	Food and beverage	Acquire permits and licenses
48	12	Marketing	Hold information center opening event
49	12	Operations	Review certificate of occupancy requirements
50	12	Operations	Set up operating accounting procedures; forward copies of management agreements to accounting offices
51	10	Marketing	Set up information session at an appropriate nearby location
52	10	Marketing	Recruit marketing representative
53	8	Accounting	Establish purchase order system
54	8	Accounting	Set up labor reports
55	8	Administration	Set up housekeeping and laundry operations
56	8	Administration	Recruit bookkeeper or business office manager (prequalify with skills exam)
57	8	Administration	Establish all service contracts; send notices to all providers, collect certificates of insurance
58	8	Administration	Recruit director of maintenance (prequalify with skills exam)
59	8	Administration	Recruit director of activities
60	8	Administration	Recruit housekeeping director

Task no.	Weeks before opening	Area	Task
61	8	Administration	Train all managers on interviewing and hiring practices; conduct training and develop manual
62	8	Administration	Hold department head meetings to discuss communications procedures
63	8	Administration	Orient maintenance director on all building systems; obtain all manuals and manufacturer recommendations
64	8	Administration	Develop job descriptions for all positions
65	8	Administration	Recruit supervisor of assisted living
66	8	Administration	Review health codes
67	8	Food and beverage	Order linen, china, silverware, and glassware
68	8	Food and beverage	Establish purchasing practices; set up vendors and pricing; negotiate group discounts
69	8	Food and beverage	Order menu board (framed and glass covered, writable) with easel
70	8	Food and beverage	Develop dining room controls, meal accounting, sanitation procedures, and side-work sheets
71	8	Food and beverage	Order smallware package; arrange delivery date after burnoff of kitchen (see below)
72	8	Food and beverage	Review wine and beer licensing (if needed)
73	8	Food and beverage	Create staffing schedules
74	8	Food and beverage	Select uniforms for kitchen and housekeeping staff
75	8	Food and beverage	Establish all work schedules for dining room and kitchen; evaluate job descriptions; review ratios
76	8	Food and beverage	Recruit director of food service (prequalify with skills exam)
77	8	Food and beverage	Create menus (menus, cycles, and presentations must correspond to budgeted amounts)
78	8	Housekeeping	Establish cleaning schedules and master housekeeping plan
79	8	Maintenance	Develop contact list for local contractors
80	8	Maintenance	Establish key-control procedures; distribute policy and review with department heads
81	8	Maintenance	Draw up construction punch list for apartments and common areas; review with architect
82	8	Maintenance	Collect all vendor information and set up accounts; summarize contract terms and conditions
83	8	Maintenance	Set up maintenance office; order tools and supplies; inventory and mark all equipment
84	8	Maintenance	Arrange utility contracts; investigate deposit requirements
85	8	Maintenance	Recruit housekeeper to clean models; maintenance director to supervise housekeeping
86	8	Marketing	Begin resident assessments, sign leases, collect deposits
87	8	Marketing	Prepare move-in packet
88	8	Operations	Establish EEOC procedures
89	8	Operations	Order property, liability, and general insurance
90	7	Administration	Lease pagers
91	6	Accounting	Set up budget and declining-balance ledgers for each department head (budget should reflect count of actual residents with signed leases)
92	6	Accounting	Set up accounting, ordering, receiving, inventory, production, and reporting systems
93	6	Administration	Create delivery, inventory, and security systems for supplies; inspect supply storage areas and review procedures
94	6	Food and beverage	Recruit kitchen personnel

Task no.	Weeks before opening	Area	Task
95	6	Food and beverage	Research local purveyors
96	6	Food and beverage	Assemble training material and food and beverage manual
97	6	Food and beverage	Set up employee lounge
98	6	Maintenance	Arrange for manufacturer training on equipment; record training on video
99	6	Maintenance	Purchase preopening maintenance and housekeeping equipment and inventory
100	6	Maintenance	Receive as-built drawings and manuals from architect
101	6	Maintenance	Review maintenance work-order procedures; review maintenance log and procedures
102	6	Maintenance	Arrange preopening security if needed
103	6	Maintenance	Accept attic stock of excess materials from general contractor
104	6	Maintenance	Establish preventive maintenance schedules according to manufacturer recommendations
105	5	Accounting	Confirm local tax laws
106	5	Accounting	Set up resident ancillary billing system
107	5	Activities	Confirm vehicle licensing and insurance; collect driver documents
108	5	Activities	Set up transportation procedures and log
109	5	Administration	Contract with local beautician; obtain beauty shop permit
110	5	Administration	Create emergency plan from master; create "red book" for emergency procedures and contacts
111	5	Administration	Allocate community storage areas; price resident storage if appropriate
112	5	Food and beverage	Organize storerooms
113	5	Food and beverage	Confirm receivable and storage plans
114	5	Food and beverage	Set up sanitation program; assign responsibility for same
115	4	Accounting	Develop monthly reports and variance summaries; train executive director on format and function
116	4	Accounting	Acquire accounting forms from regional accounting office
117	4	Accounting	Set up computer system
118	4	Accounting	Set up accounts payable
119	4	Accounting	Set up file system for contracts
120	4	Accounting	Set up local bank account
121	4	Accounting	Set up petty cash account
122	4	Accounting	Acquire tax identification number and business license
123	4	Accounting	Set up time clock
124	4	Accounting	Create credit information sheet
125	4	Activities	Develop activity calendar of events
126	4	Activities	Order, set up, check out, and inventory activities and craft supplies
127	4	Activities	Develop transportation plan, schedule, and staffing; set up Uber and Lyft procedures
128	4	Activities	Review activity and recreation manual
129	4	Activities	Develop leisure interest surveys
130	4	Administration	Perform operations audit (see appendix C); meet with department heads to discuss purpose and implementation
131	4	Administration	Recruit personal care aides (consider a job fair for rapid recruitment)
132	4	Administration	Conduct orientation for all employees (six-hour orientation and video training)

Task no.	Weeks before opening	Area	Task
133	4	Administration	Recruit receptionist (provide orientation to marketing materials and procedures)
134	4	Assisted living	Perform prep survey to assure regulatory compliance prior to licensing survey
135	4	Assisted living	Set up quality assurance program; create quality assurance and safety committee
136	4	Assisted living	Hold training program for certified nurses' aides and formal training for aides
137	4	Food and beverage	Acquire food service manual; set up systems and procedures
138	4	Food and beverage	Receive dry and frozen goods
139	4	Food and beverage	Order supplies and paper goods
140	4	Food and beverage	Review order of service; set up side-work sheets for all dining rooms and assign ongoing responsibility for them
141	4	Food and beverage	Recruit dining room staff (consider a job fair for rapid recruitment)
142	4	Food and beverage	Set up sanitation control
143	4	Food and beverage	Place initial dry goods order
144	4	Food and beverage	Recruit and train lead server
145	4	Human resources	Train local human resources person on employee orientation; train all staff on emergency evacuation policies and procedures
146	4	Human resources	Train concierge and implement lobby control procedures; set up training for all shifts and part-timers
147	4	Human resources	Review OSHA requirements with regional human resources office
148	4	Human resources	Acquire risk management manual and train staff
149	4	Maintenance	Develop computer software system for work orders
150	4	Maintenance	Test emergency call system
151	4	Maintenance	Test sprinkler and fire alarm systems; establish monitoring or testing contracts if appropriate
152	4	Maintenance	Confirm chemical setup and training; post material safety data sheets; install eyewash stations
153	4	Maintenance	Stock maintenance supplies; create master inventory for all supplies
154	4	Maintenance	Recruit housekeeping staff
155	4	Marketing	Prepare press kit for grand opening
156	4	Marketing	Send out invitations to preview opening ("sneak peek")
157	3	Food and beverage	Organize all coolers
158	3	Food and beverage	Turn over kitchen equipment; video equipment orientation training from kitchen supplier
159	3	Food and beverage	Burn off kitchen (operate all appliances to remove protective grease coating)
160	3	Food and beverage	Set up cooking line
161	3	Food and beverage	Place first perishables order
162	3	Food and beverage	Train dining room staff with manual, video, and skill practice sessions
163	3	Food and beverage	Start cook and utility training
164	3	Food and beverage	Break out smallwares and utility equipment
165	3	Food and beverage	Receive dining room uniforms; develop cost, inventory, and control systems; install purchasing manual
166	3	Maintenance	Supervise final cleaning
167	3	Maintenance	Review emergency call system condition and installation

Task no.	Weeks before opening	Area	Task
168	2	Activities	Develop newsletter
169	2	Administration	Establish resident advisory committee
170	2	Administration	Establish relationship for in-house banking services
171	2	Food and beverage	Deep-clean kitchen
172	2	Human resources	Post required personnel posters
173	2	Human resources	Create all employee rosters and organization charts, including rate of pay, hire date, and date of next review
174	2	Maintenance	Review landscaping issues with builder
175	2	Marketing	Counsel initial move-ins; schedule elevator use
176	1	All	Preview opening event for prospects
177	1	All	Preview event for referral sources
178	1	Marketing	Coordinate grand opening
179	1	Maintenance	Complete punch list with general contractor and architect; videotape all equipment orientation, especially preventive maintenance, critical parts and reorder numbers, and normal operating settings
180	0	All	Enjoy your success!

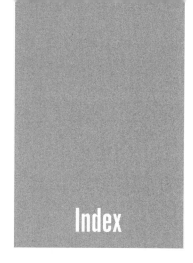

Index

Where an entry refers to a subject discussed on several pages, only the number of the page on which the discussion begins may be listed in this index.